The Dynamic Brain

The Dynamic Brain
An Exploration of Neuronal Variability and Its Functional Significance

Edited by

MINGZHOU DING, PhD
The J. Crayton Pruitt Family
Department of Biomedical Engineering
University of Florida
Gainesville, FL

DENNIS L. GLANZMAN, PhD
Theoretical and Computational Neuroscience Program
National Institute of Mental Health
Bethesda, MD

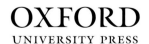

OXFORD
UNIVERSITY PRESS

2011

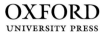

OXFORD
UNIVERSITY PRESS

Oxford University Press, Inc., publishes works that further
Oxford University's objective of excellence
in research, scholarship, and education.

Oxford   New York
Auckland   Cape Town   Dar es Salaam   Hong Kong   Karachi
Kuala Lumpur   Madrid   Melbourne   Mexico City   Nairobi
New Delhi   Shanghai   Taipei   Toronto

With offices in
Argentina   Austria   Brazil   Chile   Czech Republic   France   Greece
Guatemala   Hungary   Italy   Japan   Poland   Portugal   Singapore
South Korea   Switzerland   Thailand   Turkey   Ukraine   Vietnam

Copyright © 2011 by Oxford University Press, Inc.

Published by Oxford University Press, Inc.
198 Madison Avenue, New York, New York 10016
www.oup.com

Library of Congress Cataloging-in-Publication Data
The dynamic brain : an exploration of neuronal variability and its functional significance /
edited by Mingzhou Ding, Dennis L. Glanzman.
      p.; cm.
  Includes bibliographical references and index.
  ISBN 978-0-19-539379-8
  1. Neural circuitry. 2. Neural networks (Neurobiology) 3. Evoked potentials (Electrophysiology)
4. Variability (Psychometrics) I. Ding, Mingzhou. II. Glanzman, Dennis.
[DNLM: 1. Neurons—physiology. 2. Brain—physiology. 3. Models, Neurological. 4. Nerve Net—physiology.
WL 102.5 D9966 2011]
  QP363.3.D955 2011
  612.8′2–dc22

                                                                          2010011278

ISBN-13 9780195393798

9 8 7 6 5 4 3 2 1

Printed in China
on acid-free paper

To our families

Preface

Neuronal responses to identical stimuli vary significantly from trial to trial. This variability has been conventionally attributed to noise at various levels from single signaling proteins to overt behavior, and was often dealt with simply by using signal averaging techniques. Recent work is changing our perspective on this issue. For example, attempts to measure the information content of single neuron spike trains have revealed that a surprising amount of information can be coded in spike trains, even in the presence of trial-to-trial variability. In learning, trial-to-trial variability appears to be exploited by the brain as it provides a larger range of input–output options (generalizability). In the absence of stimulation, spontaneous synaptic activity can in many cases be shown to be well-organized both in time and in space, and can have a significant impact on stimulus processing. Clinically, disruptions of normal variability may play a role in neurological and neuropsychiatric disorders. For example, the greater variability seen in clinically weaker muscles may account for differences in patients with bulbar palsy and classical amyotrophic lateral sclerosis. Functional connectivity analysis with fMRI examines interregional correlations in neuronal variability, and disruptions in these correlations have been demonstrated in patients with schizophrenia. To bring together various disciplines where the issue of neuronal variability plays an important role, a conference entitled "Dynamical Neuroscience XVI: Neuronal Variability and Noise" was held in November 2008 in Washington, DC. This book, which had its origin in that meeting, is organized along four broadly defined themes: (1) characterizing neuronal variability, (2) dynamics of neuronal ensembles, (3) neuronal variability and cognition, and (4) neuronal variability and brain disorders.

Characterizing Neuronal Variability

A recurring theme throughout this volume is that spontaneous neuronal activity is stochastic and stimulus-evoked neuronal responses are extremely variable. Development of methods to characterize such variability is thus an important pursuit in neuroscience. Three chapters are devoted to this topic. Coleman et al., propose to evaluate the dynamics of learning by applying state space models to analyze neuronal spike trains. The model was tested on a simulation example and on simultaneously recorded neuronal spiking data and behavioral data from a monkey performing a sensorimotor association task. The significance of the new insights revealed by the approach is highlighted. Miller and Katz note that traditional approaches such as averaging at once remove variability as well as the potential information contained in it. After a critical review of such commonly used methods of spike train analysis as the PSTH, they propose a hidden Markov model to analyze the state transitions in multiple single neuron recordings. Two computational systems are used to test the method: (1) taste processing and (2) decision making. Stein and Everaert consider sensory representation from several perspectives, including information theory, rate coding and temporal coding. Using examples from sensory physiology, they show that neuronal variability may play an essential role in increasing a neuron's sensitivity to different profiles of temporal input; and for precise timing inference, both temporal code and rate code are employed by sensory neurons. A brief historic review of Shannon information theory and its adoption in neuroscience is included.

Dynamics of Neuronal Ensembles

A neuronal ensemble may refer to a group of interconnected cells or a population of cells embedded in a large network. Its dynamics can be studied both experimentally and from a computational point of view. Abbott et al. examine how intrinsic ongoing network dynamics impacts stimulus processing. Computational models are used to simulate both chaotic and non-chaotic spontaneous activities. They find that the spatiotemporal patterns of ongoing activity can help explain stimulus selectivity as well as trial-to-trial variability. They further point out that the methods used for analyzing model data should be equally applicable to the analysis of experimental data. Hung et al. recorded from pairs of single neurons in the visual cortex of the cat during baseline and during stimulus processing. Synchronous activity was revealed by a cross correlation analysis and shown to be different between the two conditions. A possible gain modulation mechanism during the baseline period is suggested. Achuthan et al. studied oscillatory activity and synchronization in the nervous system. Both model circuits and hybrid circuits consisting of model neurons and biological neurons are considered. In particular, these authors showed that a mathematical technique called the phase resetting curve can be applied to predict phase locking between different neuronal oscillators and assess its robustness to random noise perturbation. Prinz et al. note the tremendous animal-to-animal variability in cellular properties. They then proceed to pose the following question: Why, despite several-fold ranges of animal-to-animal variability in many biological parameters, does the level and temporal patterning of electrical activity in neuronal networks stay remarkably consistent? Both experimental and modeling perspectives are employed to address this question. Abarbanel et al. write that biophysically-realistic computational models contain multiple tunable parameters, and how to choose the values of these parameters for a given neural system remains a challenging problem. These authors address the problem by proposing a new method, called dynamical parameter estimation (DPE), to estimate model parameter values from observed membrane voltage data. It was proven effective when tested on two network models of neurons.

Neuronal Variability and Cognition

The origins of neuronal variability and behavioral variability and how these two are related to each other are not well understood. Four chapters are devoted to this topic in the context of cognitive operations in humans and non-human primates. The chapter by Tang et al. attempts to analyze the context upon which such variability arises. These authors identify the state of the brain prior to stimulus onset as a possible physiological correlate of context and propose to use EEG as an appropriate experimental tool for quantifying such states in humans. Various techniques used for EEG analysis are introduced and applied to both lab and real world experiments. Sajda et al. directly addresses the link between neuronal and behavioral variability. After pointing out the inability of the averaging method in accomplishing this objective, they propose a framework in which advanced signal processing methods are combined with EEG and fMRI recordings to explain reaction time variability in terms of single-trial brain activity in human decision making. Turning to primate studies, Gray and Goodell note that neuronal activity in individual areas of the brain is noisy, highly variable and only weakly correlated with behavior and external events. They hypothesize that spatially distributed patterns of synchronous activity play a fundamental role in cognitive brain function. Preliminary data from a macaque monkey viewing natural images are presented to support the hypothesis. Also employing primate subjects, Lee and Seo explore the neural basis of stochastic decision making as a strategy to achieve optimal performance in competitive environments. Single neuron activities are recorded from multiple brain areas while the animal performed a computer-simulated mixed strategy game. It is found that neuronal variability exceeds that predicted by a Poisson model and some of the variability can be explained by behavioral events.

Neuronal Variability and Brain Disorders

While characterizing variability in spike trains in the normal brain helps us understand the neuronal basis of cognition, characterizing the variability associated with brain disorders may be essential to understanding disease pathophysiology and designing effective therapeutic strategies. Schiff reviews patient data on variability in treatment outcomes following severe brain injuries and recovery from unconsciousness (coma, vegetative state, etc.). A circuit theory consistent with the observed clinical manifestations is proposed in which the key role played by the central thalamus is emphasized. A case study involving an unconscious patient receiving central thalamus deep brain stimulation (DBS) is presented. Mandell et al. consider resting state MEG data from 10 patients suffering from schizophrenia and 10 controls. Applying a wide variety of analysis techniques, including spectral measures and nonlinear measures, they test the hypothesis that randomly fluctuating MEG time series during rest can be used to differentiate global states of dysfunction from that of normal operation in humans. Lane argues that it is possible to attribute observed neuronal variability to the effect of some underlying state variable and modeling the root cause of neuronal variability using the theory of latent variables can produce highly informative outcome. He proceeds to develop a Bayesian inference framework and apply it to neuroimaging data from clinical populations. While much work remains to validate the approach, the preliminary data nonetheless is promising.

Summary

The role of variability in neuronal responses is receiving increased attention at national and international meetings where neuroscientists, statisticians, engineers, physicists, mathematicians and computer scientists congregate. We now have a general appreciation of variability at all organizational levels of the nervous system. The use of computational models provides a foundation for further enhancing our ability to understand how the brain continues to function dependably, despite the lack of consistent performance in the very elements from which it is composed. Chapters in this book serve as a starting point for an exploration of this emerging research direction.

–M.D. and D.L.G.

Contents

Contributors

Henry D.I. Abarbanel, PhD
Department of Physics; and
Marine Physical Laboratory
  (Scripps Institution of
  Oceanography)
University of California,
San Diego
La Jolla, CA

Larry F. Abbott, PhD
Departments of Neuroscience
  and Physiology and Cellular
  Biophysics
Columbia University College
  of Physicians and Surgeons
New York, NY

Srisairam Achuthan, PhD
Neuroscience Center of
  Excellence
LSU Health Sciences Center
School of Medicine
New Orleans, LA

Emery N. Brown, MD, PhD
Department of Brain &
  Cognitive Sciences
Massachusetts Institute of
  Technology
Cambridge, MA

Paul H. Bryant, PhD
Institute for Nonlinear
  Science
University of California,
San Diego
La Jolla, CA

Carmen C. Canavier, PhD
Departments of
  Ophthalmology and
  Neuroscience
Neuroscience Center of
  Excellence
LSU Health Sciences Center
School of Medicine
New Orleans, LA

Todd P. Coleman, PhD
Department of Electrical and
  Computer Engineering
University of Illinois at
  Urbana-Champaign
Urbana, IL

Richard Coppola, DSc
NIMH Core MEG Laboratory
Bethesda, MD

Dirk G. Everaert, PhD
Department of Physiology
Centre for Neuroscience
University of Alberta
Edmonton, AB
Canada

Philip E. Gill, PhD
Department of Mathematics
University of California
San Diego
La Jolla, CA

Baldwin Goodell, MSEE
Department of Cell Biology
  and Neuroscience
Center for Computational
  Biology
Montana State University
Bozeman, MT

Charles M. Gray, PhD
Department of Cell Biology and
  Neuroscience
Center for Computational
  Biology
Montana State University
Bozeman, MT

Hauke Heekeren, MD, PhD
Max Planck Institute for
  Human Development
Berlin, Germany

Tom Holroyd, PhD
NIMH Core MEG Laboratory
Bethesda, MD

Amber E. Hudson, BS
Department of Biomedical
  Engineering,
Emory University and Georgia
  Institute of Technology,
Atlanta, GA

Chou P. Hung, PhD
Institute of Neuroscience
  and Brain Research Center
National Yang Ming University
Taipei, Taiwan

Donald B. Katz, PhD
Department of Psychology and Volen
  Center for Complex Systems
Brandeis University
Waltham, MA

Mark Kostuk, PhD
Department of Physics; and
  Institute for Nonlinear Science
University of California
San Diego
La Jolla, CA

Terran Lane, PhD
Department of Computer Science
University of New Mexico
Albuquerque, NM

Daeyeol Lee, PhD
Department of Neurobiology
Yale University School of Medicine
New Haven, CT

Arnold J. Mandell, MD
Cielo Institute, Inc.
Asheville, NC

Paul Miller, PhD
Department of Biology and Volen
  Center for Complex Systems
Brandeis University
Waltham, MA

Marios G. Philiastides, PhD
Max Planck Institute for
  Human Development
Berlin, Germany

Astrid A. Prinz, PhD
Department of Biology
Emory University
Atlanta, GA

Kanaka Rajan, PhD
Lewis-Sigler Institute for Integrative
  Genomics, Carl Icahn Laboratories
Princeton University
Princeton, NJ

Benjamin M. Ramsden, PhD
Department of Neurobiology
  and Anatomy
West Virginia University School
  of Medicine
Morgantown, WV

Roger Ratcliff, PhD
Department of Psychology
Ohio State University
Columbus, OH

Anna Wang Roe, PhD
Department of Psychology
Vanderbilt University
Nashville, TN

Justin Rofeh
Department of Physics
University of California
La Jolla, CA

Lindsay Rutter, BS
Undergraduate Fellow
NIMH Core MEG Laboratory
Bethesda, MD

Paul Sajda, PhD
Department of Biomedical
  Engineering
Columbia University
New York, NY

Nicholas D. Schiff, MD
Laboratory of Cognitive
  Neuromodulation
Department of Neurology and
  Neuroscience
Weill Cornell Medical College
New York, NY

Karen A. Selz, PhD
Cielo Institute, Inc.
Asheville, NC

Hyojung Seo, PhD
Department of Neurobiology
Yale University School of Medicine
New Haven, CT

Fred H. Sieling, PhD
Department of Biology
Emory University; and
 The Georgia Institute
 of Technology
Atlanta, GA

Zakary Singer
Department of Bioengineering
University of California
La Jolla, CA

Tomasz G. Smolinski, PhD
Department of Computer and
 Information Sciences,
Delaware State University,
Dover, DE

Haim Sompolinsky, PhD
Racah Institute of Physics
Interdisciplinary Center for
 Neural Computation
Hebrew University
Jerusalem, Israel

Richard B. Stein, DPhil
Department of Physiology
Centre for Neuroscience
University of Alberta
Edmonton, AB
Canada

Matthew T. Sutherland, PhD
Neuroimaging Research Branch
National Institute on Drug Abuse–
 Intramural Research Program
NIH/DHHS
Baltimore, MD

Wendy A. Suzuki, PhD
Center for Neural Science
New York University
New York, NY

Akaysha C. Tang, PhD
Department of Psychology
University of New Mexico
Albuquerque, NM

Bryan Toth
Department of Physics
University of California
La Jolla, CA

Elizabeth Wong
Department of Mathematics
University of California
La Jolla, CA

Zhen Yang
Department of Psychology
University of New Mexico
Albuquerque, NM

Marianna Yanike, PhD
Department of Neuroscience
Columbia University
New York, NY

Part I: Characterizing Neuronal Variability

I

A Mixed-Filter Algorithm for Dynamically Tracking Learning from Multiple Behavioral and Neurophysiological Measures

Todd P. Coleman, Marianna Yanike,
Wendy A. Suzuki, and Emery N. Brown

Introduction

Learning is a dynamic process generally defined as a change in behavior as a result of experience (Barnes et al., 2004, Jog et al., 1999; Wirth et al., 2003; Gallistel, 2008; Siegel and Castellano, 1988; Smith et al. 2004; Smith et al., 2010).Understanding how processes at the molecular and neuronal levels integrate so that an organism can learn is a central question in neuroscience. Most learning experiments consist of a sequence of trials. During each trial, a subject is given a fixed amount of time to execute a task and the resulting performance is recorded. During each trial, performance can be measured with a continuous variable (i.e. reaction time) as well as a binary one (whether or not the subject executes task correctly). The spiking behavior of certain neurons can also be used to characterize learning (Wirth et al., 2003; Yanike et al., 2009; Chiu et al., 2009).Learning is usually illustrated by using the behavioral variables to show that the subject has successfully performed the previously unfamiliar task with greater reliability than would be predicted by chance. When neural activity is recorded at the same time as the behavioral measures, an important question is the extent to what neural correlates can be associated with the changes in behavior.

We have developed a state–space model to analyze binary behavioral data (Wirth et al., 2003; Smith et al., 2004; Smith et al., 2010; Smith and Brown, 2003). The model has been successfully applied in a number of learning studies (Wirth et al, 2003; Law et al., 2005; Williams and Eskander, 2006; Karlsson and Frank, 2008; Smith et al, 2005). Recently, we have extended this model to analyze simultaneously recorded continuous and binary measures of behavior (Precau et al., 2008; Precau et al., 2009). An open problem is the analysis in a state–space framework of simultaneously recorded continuous and binary performance measures along with neural spiking activity modeled as a point process.

To develop a dynamic approach to analyzing data from learning experiments in which continuous and binary and responses are simultaneously recorded along with neural spiking activity, we extend our previously developed state–space model of learning to include a lognormal probability model for the continuous measurements, a Bernoulli probability model for the binary measurements and a point process model for the neural spiking activity. We estimate the model using an approximate EM algorithm (Smith and Brown, 2003; Smith et al., 2004; Rrecau et al., 2009) to conduct the model fitting. We illustrate our approach in the analysis of a simulated learning experiment, and an actual learning experiment, in which a monkey rapidly learns new associations within a single session.

A State–Space Model of Learning

We assume that learning is a dynamic process that can be analyzed with the well-known state–space framework used in engineering, statistics and computer science . The state–space model is comprised of two equations: the state equation and the observation equation. The state equation defines the temporal evolution of an unobservable process. State models with unobscrvable processes are also referred to as latent process or hidden Markov models (Durbin and Koopman, 2001; Doucet et al., 2001; Fahrmeir et al, 2001; Kitagawa and Gersch, 1996; Mendel, 1995; Smith and Brown, 2003). The subject's understanding of the task. We track the evolution of this cognitive state across the trials in the experiment. We formulate our model so that as learning occurs, the state increases, and when learning does not occur, it decreases. The observation equation relates the observed data to the cognitive state process. The data we observe in the learning experiment are the neural spiking activity and the continuous and binary responses. Our objective is to characterize learning by estimating the cognitive state process using simultaneously all three types of data.

To develop our model we extend the work in (Precau et al, 2008; Precau et al., 2009) and consider a learning experiment consisting of K trials in which on each trial, a continuous reaction time, neural spiking activity, and a binary response measurement of performance are recorded. Let Z_k and M_k be respectively the values of the continuous and binary measurements on trial k for $k = 1...., K$. We assume that the cognitive state model is the first-order autoregressive process:

$$X_k = \gamma + \rho X_{k-1} + V_k \tag{1}$$

where $\rho \in (0,1)$ represents a forgetting factor, γ is a learning rate, and the V_k's are independent, zero mean, Gaussian random variables with variance. $\sigma^2 v$. Let $X = [X_1,...,X_K]$ be the unobserved cognitive state process for the entire experiment.

For the purpose of exposition, we assume that the continuous measurements are reaction times and that the observation model for the reaction times is given by

$$Z_k = \alpha + hX_k + W_k \tag{2}$$

where Z_k is the logarithm of the reaction time on the Kth trial, and the W_k's are independent zero mean Gaussian random variables with variance $\sigma^2 w$. We assume that $h < 0$ to insure that on average, as the cognitive state X_k increases with learning, then the reaction time decreases. We let $Z = [Z_1,...,Z_K]$ be the reaction times on all K trials.

We assume that the observation model for the binary responses, the M_k's obey a Bernoulli probability model

$$P(M_k = m \mid X_k = x_k) = p_k^m (1 - p_k)^{1-m} \tag{3}$$

where $m = 1$ if the response is correct and 0 if the response is incorrect. We take p_k to be the probability of a correct response on trial k, defined in terms of the unobserved cognitive state process x_k as

$$p_k = \frac{\exp(\mu + \eta x_k)}{1 + \exp(\mu + \eta x_k)} \tag{4}$$

Formulation of p_k as a logistic function of the cognitive state process (4) ensures that the probability of a correct response on each trial is constrained to lie between 0 and 1, and that as the cognitive state increases, the probability of a correct responses approaches 1.

Assume that each of the K trials lasts T seconds. Divide each trial into $J = \dfrac{T}{\Delta}$ bins of width Δ so that there is at most one spike per bin. Let $N_{k,j} = 1$ if there is a spike on trial k in bin j and 0 otherwise for $j = 1, \ldots, T$ and $k = 1, \ldots, K$. Let $N_k = [N_{k,1}, \ldots, N_{k,J}]$ be the spikes recorded on trial k, and $N^k = [N_1, \ldots, N_k]$ be the spikes observed from trial 1 to k. We assume that the probability of a spike on trial k in bin j may be expressed as

$$P(N_{k,j} = n_{k,j} \mid X^k = x^k, N^{k-1} = n^{k-1}, N_{k,1} = n_{k,1}, \ldots, N_{k,j-1} = n_{k,j-1})$$

$$= (\lambda_{k,j}\Delta)^{n_{k,j}} e^{-\lambda_{k,j}\Delta} \tag{5}$$

and thus the joint probability mass function of N_k on trial k is

$$P(N_k = n_k \mid X^k = x^k) = \exp\left(\sum_{j=1}^{J} \log(\lambda_{k,j}) n_{k,j} - \lambda_{k,j}\Delta \right) \tag{6}$$

where (6) follows from the likelihood of a point process (Brown et al., 2002). We define the conditional intensity function $\lambda_{k,j}$ as

$$\log \lambda_{k,j} = \psi + g x_k + \sum_{s=1}^{S} \beta_s n_{k,j-s}. \tag{7}$$

The state model (1) provides a stochastic continuity constraint (Kitagawa and Gersch, 1998) so that the current cognitive state, reaction time (2), probability of a correct response (4), and the conditional intensity function (7) all depend on the prior cognitive state. In this way, the state–space model provides a simple, plausible framework for relating performance on successive trials of the experiment.

We denote all of our observations at trial k as $Y_k = (M_k, N_k, Z_k)$. Because X is unobservable, and because $\theta = (\gamma, \rho, \sigma_v^2, \alpha, h, \sigma_w^2, \mu, \eta, g, \psi)$ is a set of unknown parameters, we use the Expectation-Maximization (EM) algorithm to estimate them by maximum likelihood (Smith et al., 2004; Smith et al., 2005; Smith and Brown, 2003; Fahrmeir et al., 2001; Percau et al., 2009). The EM algorithm is a well-known procedure for performing maximum likelihood estimation when there is an unobservable process or missing observations. The EM algorithm has been used to estimate state–space models from point process and binary observations with linear Gaussian state processes (Dempster et al., 1977). The current EM algorithm combines features of the ones in

(Shumway and Stoffer, 1982; Smith et al., 2004; Smith et al., 2005).The key technical point that allows implementation of this algorithm is the combined filter algorithm in (8)-(12). Its derivation is given in Appendix A.

Discrete-Time Recursive Estimation Algorithms

In this section, we develop a recursive, causal estimation algorithm to estimate the state at trial k, X_k, given the observations up to and including time k, $Y^k = y^k$. Define

$$x_{k|k'} \triangleq E[X_k \mid Y^{k'} = y^{k'}]$$

$$\sigma^2_{k|k'} \triangleq \mathrm{var}\left[X_k \mid Y^{k'} = y^{k'} \right]$$

as well as $p_{k|k}$ and $\lambda_{k,j|k,j}$ by (4) and (7), respectively, with with x_k replaced by $x_{k|k}$.

In order to derive closed form expressions, we develop a Gaussian approximation to the posterior, and as such, assume that the posterior distribution on X at time k given $Y^k = y^k$ is the Gaussian density with mean $x_{k|k}$ and variance $\sigma^2_{k|k}$. Using the Chapman-Kolmogorov equations (25) with the Gaussian approximation to the posterior density, i.e. X_k given y^k, we obtain the following recursive filter algorithm:

One – Step Prediction

$$x_{k|k-1} = \gamma + \rho x_{k-1|k-1} \tag{8}$$

One – Step Prediction Variance

$$\sigma^2_{k|k-1} = \rho^2 \sigma^2_{k-1|k-1} + \sigma^2_V \tag{9}$$

Gain Coefficient

$$C_k = \frac{\sigma^2_{k|k-1}}{h^2 \sigma^2_{k|k-1} + \sigma^2_W} \tag{10}$$

Posterior Mode

$$x_{k|k} = x_{k|k-1} + C_k \left[h\left(z_k - \alpha - h x_{k|k-1} \right) + \eta \sigma^2_W (m_k - p_{k|k}) \right]$$
$$+ \sum_{j=1}^{J} C_k \sigma^2_W \left[g(n_{k,j} - \lambda_{k,j|k,j}\Delta) \right] \tag{11}$$

Posterior Variance

$$\sigma_{k|k}^2 = \left[\frac{1}{\sigma_{k|k-1}^2} + \frac{h^2}{\sigma_W^2} + \eta^2 p_{k|k}(1-p_{k|k}) + \sum_{j=1}^{J} g^2 \lambda_{k,j|k,j} \Delta \right]^{-1}$$

(12)

Details can be found in Appendix A. Because there are three observation processes, (11) has a continuous-valued innovation term, $(z_k - \alpha - hx_{k|k-1})$, a binary innovation term, $(m_k - p_{k|k})$, and a point-process innovation term, $(n_{k,j} - \lambda_{k,j|k,j}\Delta)$. As is true in the Kalman filter, the continuous-valued innovation compares the observation z_k with its one-step prediction. The binary innovation compares the binary observation m_k with $p_{k|k}$, the probability of a correct response at trial k. Finally, the point process innovation compares the $n_{k,j}$, whether or not a spike occurred in bin j on trial k, with the expected number of occurrences, $\lambda_{k,j|k,j}\Delta$. As in the Kalman filter, C_k in (10), is a time-dependent gain coefficient. At trial k, the amount by which the continuous-valued innovation term affects the update is determined by $C_k h$, the amount by which the binary innovation affects the update is determined by $C_k \eta \sigma_W^2$, and the amount by which the point process innovation for neuron j affects the update is determined by the sum of $C_k \sigma_W^2 g$. Unlike in the Kalman filter algorithm, the left and right hand sides of the posterior mode (11) and the posterior variance (12) depend on the state estimate $x_{k|k}$. That is, because $p_{k|k}$ and $\lambda_{k,j|k,j}$ depend on $x_{k|k}$ through (4) and (7). Therefore, at each step k of the algorithm, we use Newton's methods (developed in Appendix A) to compute $x_{k|k}$ in (11).

An Expectation-Maximization Algorithm for Efficient Maximum Likelihood Estimation

We next define an EM algorithm (Dempster et al., 1977) to compute jointly the state and model parameter estimates. To do so, we combine the recursive filter given in the previous section with the fixed interval smoothing algorithm and the covariance smoothing algorithms to efficiently evaluate the E-step.

E-Step

The E-step of the EM algorithm only requires the calculation of the posterior $f_{X_k|Y}(x_k \mid y)$. As mentioned in Section 3, we use a Gaussian approximation to the posterior. Although in general this is a multi-dimensional Gaussian, we need only compute the mean and certain components of the covariance of this distribution.

E-STEP I: NONLINEAR RECURSIVE FILTER

The nonlinear recursive filter is given in (8) through (12).

E-STEP II: FIXED INTERVAL SMOOTHING (FIS) ALGORITHM

Given the sequence of posterior mode estimates $x_{k|k}$ and the variance $\sigma^2_{k|k}$, we use the fixed interval smoothing algorithm [20, 3] to compute $x_{k|K}$ and $\sigma^2_{k|K}$

$$A_k \triangleq \rho \frac{\sigma^2_{k|k}}{\sigma^2_{k+1|k}} \tag{13}$$

$$x_{k|K} = x_{k|k} + A_k \left(x_{k+1|K} - x_{k+1|k} \right) \tag{14}$$

$$\sigma^2_{k|K} = \sigma^2_{k|k} + A_k^2 \left(\sigma^2_{k+1|K} - \sigma^2_{k+1|k} \right) \tag{15}$$

for $k = K-1,\dots,1$ with initial conditions $x_{K|K}$ and $\sigma^2_{K|K}$ computed from the last step in (8) through (12).

E-STEP III: STATE–SPACE COVARIANCE ALGORITHM

The conditional covariance, $\sigma_{k,k'|K}$, can be computed from the state–space covariance algorithm and is given for $1 \le k \le k' \le K$ by

$$\sigma_{k,k'|K} = A_k \sigma_{k+1,k'|K} \tag{16}$$

Thus the covariance terms required for the E-step are

$$\tilde{W}_{k,k+1} = \sigma_{k,k+1|K} + x_{k|K} x_{k+1|K} \tag{17}$$

$$\tilde{W}_k = \sigma^2_{k|K} + x^2_{k|K} \tag{18}$$

M-Step

The M-step requires maximization of the expected log likelihood given the observed data. Appendix B gives the computations that lead to the following approximate update equations:

$$\begin{bmatrix} \gamma \\ \rho \end{bmatrix} = \begin{bmatrix} K & \sum_{k=1}^{K} x_{k-1|K} \\ \sum_{k=1}^{K} X_{k-1|K} & \sum_{k=1}^{K} \tilde{W}_{k-1} \end{bmatrix} \begin{bmatrix} \sum_{k=1}^{K} x_{k|K} \\ \sum_{k=1}^{K} \tilde{W}_{k-1,k} \end{bmatrix} \tag{19}$$

$$
\begin{bmatrix} \alpha \\ h \end{bmatrix} = \begin{bmatrix} K & \sum_{k=1}^{K} x_{k|K} \\ \sum_{k=1}^{K} xk \mid K & \sum_{k=1}^{K} \tilde{W}_k \end{bmatrix}^{-1} \begin{bmatrix} \sum_{k=1}^{K} z_k \\ \sum_{k=1}^{K} Z_{z_k x_{k|K}} \end{bmatrix} \tag{20}
$$

$$
\sigma_W^2 = \frac{1}{K} \left[\sum_{k=1}^{K} (z_k - \alpha)^2 - 2(z_k - \alpha) h x_{k|K} + h^2 \tilde{W}_k \right] \tag{21}
$$

$$
\psi = \log \left(\frac{\sum_{k=1}^{K} \sum_{j=1}^{J} n_{k,j.}}{\sum_{k=1}^{K} \sum_{j=1}^{J} \Delta \exp\left(gx_{k|K} + \frac{1}{2} \sigma_{k|K}^2 g^2 + \sum_{s=1}^{S} \beta_s n_{k,j-s} \right)} \right) \tag{22}
$$

To solve for $\mu, \eta, \psi, g, \{\beta_s\}$, we use Newton's method techniques, described in Appendix C.

Algorithm Performance and Simulation

Application of the Methods to Simulated Data

To illustrate our analysis paradigm, we apply it first to simulated data. We simulated neural spiking activity, reaction times and binary responses for a twenty-five trial learning experiment during which each trial lasted five seconds. We discretized time into 5000 one-millisecond bins. To simulate the state process, we used the parameter values $\gamma = 0.1, \rho = 0.99$, and $\sigma_V^2 = 0.03$. For the continuous-valued reaction time process, we used the parameters $\alpha = 3.69, h = -0.38$, and $\sigma_W^2 = 0.75$. For binary-valued data, we used the parameter values $\mu = -1.4170$ and $\eta = 1.75$. For the point process parameters we chose $\psi = -3.5$, $g = 2.0$, and $\beta = (-20, -5, 1, 3)$. The simulated data are shown in Figure 1. 1.

The state estimates are in close agreement with the true state for all trials (Figure 1.2A). The Kolmogorov-Smirnov plot (Brown et al., 2002) confirms that the model describes well the point process component of the model (Figure 1.2B). These results demonstrate that the mixed analysis is capable of recovering the unobserved states and the components the three observation models from simulated data.

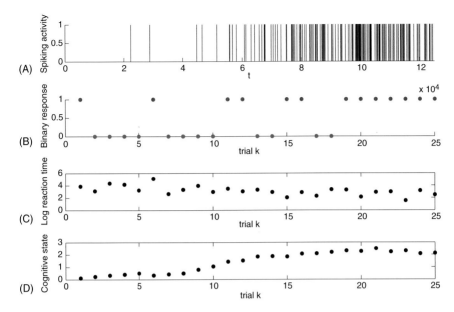

FIGURE I.I Visualization of the simulated data. Panel A shows the simulated spiking activity. Panel B shows the binary responses, with blue (red) corresponding to correct (incorrect) responses. Panel C shows the log reaction times. Panel D shows the cognitive state.

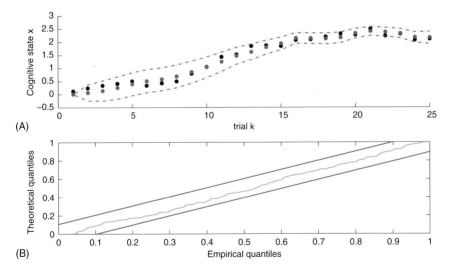

FIGURE I.2 (A): performance of the recursive estimation procedure. The true cognitive state is given in black, while estimates are given in red. 95% Confidence intervals are given with the red dashed lines. (B): Kolmogorov-Smirnov plot confirms that the model describes well the point process component of the model.

Application of the Methods to Experimental Data

In this section we apply the analysis paradigm to an actual learning experiment in which neural spiking activity was recorded along with binary and continuous performance measures as a rhesus monkey executed a location-scene association task described in detail in (Wirth et al., 2003). The experiment consists of forty-five trials with each trial lasting 3,300 msec. In this task, each trial started with a baseline period (0 to 400 msec) during which the monkey fixated on a cue presented on a computer screen. The animal was then presented with three identical targets (north, east, and west) superimposed on a novel visual scene (401 to 900 msec). The scene disappeared and the targets remained on the screen during a delay period (901 to 1600 msec). At the end of the delay period, the fixation point disappeared cueing the animal to make an eye-movement to one of the three targets (1,600 to 3,300 msec). For each scene, only one target was rewarded and three novel scenes were typically learned simultaneously. Trials of novel scenes were interspersed with trials in which three well-learned scenes were presented. The probability of a correct response occurring by chance was 0.33 because there were three locations the monkey could choose as a response. To characterize learning we reported for all trials the reaction times (time from the go-cue to the response), the correct and incorrect responses, and neural spiking activity recorded in the perirhinal cortex.

The correct and incorrect responses and neural spiking activity are shown in Figure 1.3A for one scene. The spiking activity on a trial is red if the behavioral response was incorrect on that trial and blue if the response was correct. The response times are shown in Figure 1.3B. The animal clearly showed a change in responses from all incorrect to correct around trial 23 or 24. The response time decreased from trial 1 to 45. The spiking rate of the neural firing increased with learning. To analyze the spiking activity we used one milliseconds time bins and chose the order of the autoregressive for the spiking activity equal to 10 milliseconds.

The cognitive state estimates in Figure 1.4A are consistent with the animal learning the task. The KS plot in Figure 1.4B suggests that the point process component of the model describes the neural spiking activity well. The learning curve plot of the probability of correct response, overlayed with the binary responses, is given by techniques in (Precau, 2009) and shown in Figure 1.5A. This information, as well as the decrease in the reaction time of Figure 1.5B, is consistent with learning. The estimated value of the parameter $\hat{g} = 0.0232$ is consistent with increasing spiking activity as the animal learned whereas the estimated coefficients

$$\hat{\beta} = (-3.0278, -2.3581, -0.4836, -0.9458, -0.1914, -0.3884,$$
$$-0.7690, 0.1783, -0.4119, 0.1066)$$

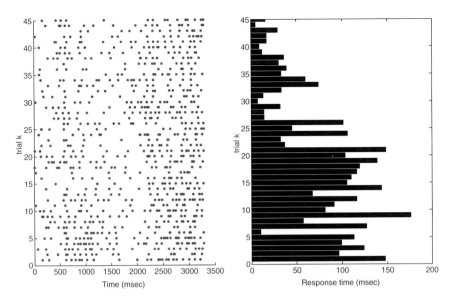

FIGURE I.3 A: correct/incorrect responses in blue/red rows; a spike in bin *j* of trial *k* is present if a dot appears in the associated (*k*, *j*) row and column. A change in responses from correct to incorrect is clear around trial 23 or 24. B: The response times in milliseconds on each trial. The response times on average decreased from trial 1 to 45.

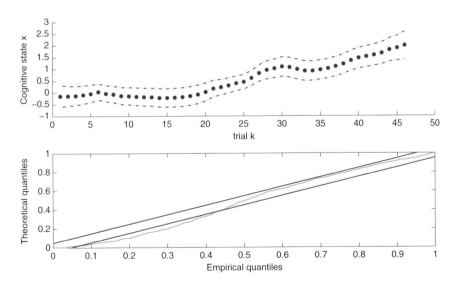

FIGURE I.4 Mixed modality recursive filtering results. A: the estimate and confidence interval of the cognitive state process. B: a Kolmogorov-Smirnov plot of the time-rescaled interspike intervals from the learned parameters.

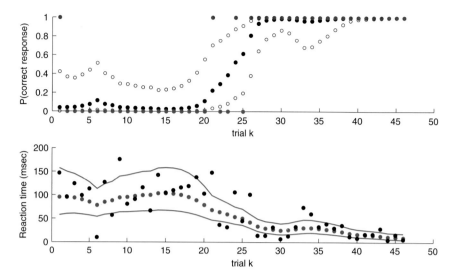

FIGURE 1.5 A: plot of the estimated probability of correct response (black filled circles), along with 95% confidence intervals (black hollow circles), as well as the correct (blue) and incorrect (red) behavioral responses. B: plot of the estimated reaction times, along with 95% confidence intervals (red), as well as the true reaction times (black).

are consistent with a refractory period and a relative refractory period for the neuron. The results establish the feasibility of conducting simultaneous analysis of continuous and binary behavioral data along with neural spiking activity using the mixed model.

Discussion and Conclusion

Continuous observations, such as reaction times and run times, neural spiking activity,and binary observations, such as correct/incorrect responses, are frequently recorded simultaneously in behavioral learning experiments, however, The two types of performance measures and neurophysiological recordings, however, are not analyzed simultaneously to study learning. We have introduced a state–space model in which the observation model makes use of simultaneously recorded continuous and binary measures of performance, as well as neural spiking activity to characterize learning. Using maximum likelihood implemented in the form of an EM algorithm we estimated the model from these simultaneously recorded performance measures and neural spiking activity.

We illustrated the new model and algorithm in the analysis of simulated data and data from an actual learning experiment.

The computational innovation that enabled our combined model analysis is the recursive filter algorithm for mixed observation processes, i.e. continuous, point process and binary observations, the fixed-interval smoothing algorithm, and an approximate EM algorithm for combined cognitive state and model parameter estimation. Our mixed recursive filter algorithm (Smith et al., 2004) combines the well-known Kalman filter with a recently developed binary filter (Precau et al., 2008) and the point process filter (Brown et al., 1998; Barbieri et al., 2004; Eden et al., 2004). In this way, the mixed filter makes possible simultaneous dynamic analysis of behavioral performance data and neural spiking activity.

Several extensions of the current work are possible to more complex models of performance and neural spiking data. These model extensions could be fit by constructing the appropriate extensions of our EM algorithm. An alternative approach would be to formulate the model parameter estimation as a Bayesian question and take advantage of readily available Bayesian analysis software packages such as BUGS to conduct the model fitting (Smith et al., 2007).

The question we have studied here of simultaneously analyzing performance data and neural spiking activity offers a solution to the now ubiquitous problem of combining information dynamically from different measurement types. Possible extensions of this paradigm in neuroscience include combining information from local field potentials and ensemble neural spiking activity to devise algorithms for neural prosthetic control. Another extension of this approach is to functional neural imaging studies in which combinations of functional magnetic resonance imaging, electroencephalographic and magnetoencephalographic recordings are made simultaneously or in sequence. Again, the state–space modeling framework provides an optimal strategy for combining the information from the various sources. We will investigate these theoretical and applied problems in future investigations.

Acknowledgments

Support was provided by National Institutes of Health Grants DA-015644 to E. N. Brown and W. Suzuki; DPI0D003646, MH-59733, and MH-071847 to E. N. Brown; and by the AFOSR Complex Networks Program via Award No. FA9550-08-1-0079 to T. P. Coleman.

REFERENCES

Barbieri, R., Frank, L.M., Nguyen, D.P., Quirk, M.C., Solo, V., Wilson, M. A. and
 Brown, E.N. (2004). Dynamic analyses of information encoding by neural
 ensembles. *Neural Computation, 16, 2*: 277–308.

Barnes, T.D., Kubota, Y., Hu, D., Jin, D.Z., and Graybiel, A.M. (2005). Activity of
 striatal neurons reflects dynamic encoding and recoding of procedural memories.
 Nature, 437 (7062), 1158–1161.

Brown, E.N., Frank, L.M., Tang, L.M., Quirk, M.C. and Wilson, M. (1998). A statistical
 paradigm for neural spike train decoding applied to position prediction from
 ensemble firing patterns of rat hippocampal place cells. *J of Neuroscience, 18,*
 7411–7425.

Brown, E.N., Barbieri, R., Kass, R.E., and Frank, L.M. (2002) The time-rescaling
 theorem and its application to neural spike train data analysis. *Neural
 Computation, 14, 2*, 325–346.

Chiu, C.C., Varun, S., Smith, A.C., Brown, E.N., Suzuki, W.A., Wirth, S. and Avsar, E.
 (2009). Trial outcome and associative learning signals in the monkey
 hippocampus. *Neuron, 61, 6*, 930–940.

Dempster, A.P., Laird, N.M., Rubin, D.B. (1977). Maximum likelihood from
 incomplete data via the EM algorithm. *J of the Royal Statistical Society. Series B
 (Methodological), 39, 1*, 1–38.

Doucet, A., De Freitas, N., and Gordon, N. (2001). *Sequential Monte Carlo methods in
 practice*. New York, NY: Springer Verlag.

Durbin, J. and Koopman, S.J. (2001). *Time series analysis by state space methods*.
 Oxford, UK: Oxford University Press.

Eden, U.T., Frank, L.M., Barbieri, R., Solo, V. and Brown, E.N. (2004). Dynamic
 analyses of neural encoding by point process adaptive filtering. *Neural
 Computation, 16, 5*, 971–998.

Fahrmeir, L., Tutz, G., and Hennevogl, W. (2001). *Multivariate statistical modeling based
 on generalized linear models*. New York, NY: Springer Verlag.

Gallistel, C.R. (2008). Learning and representation. *Learning and memory: A
 comprehensive reference*. Maryland Heights, MO: Elsevier, 2008.

Jog, M.S., Kubota, Y., Connolly, C.I., Hillegaart, V. and Graybiel, V. (1999). Building
 neural representations of habits. *Science, 286, 5445*, 1745–1749.

Karlsson, M.P. and Frank, L.M. Network dynamics underlying the formation
 of sparse, informative representations in the hippocampus. *J of Neuroscience,
 28, 52*, 14271.

Kitagawa, G. and Gersch, W. (1996). *Smoothness priors analysis of time series*. New York,
 NY: Springer Verlag.

Law, J.R., Flanery, M.A., Wirth, S., Yanike, M., Smith, A.C., Frank, L.M., Suzuki, W.A.,
 Brown, E.N. and Stark, C.E.L. (2005). Functional magnetic resonance imaging

activity during the gradual acquisition and expression of paired-associate memory. *J of Neuroscience, 25, 24,* 5720–5729.

Mendel, J.M. (1995). Lessons in estimation theory for signal processing, communications, and control. Englewood Cliffs, N.J.: Prentice Hall.

Prerau, M.J., Smith, A.C., Eden U.T., Kubota, Y., Yanike, M., Suzuki, W., Graybiel, A.M., and Brown, E.N. (2009). Characterizing learning by simultaneous analysis of continuous and binary measures of performance. *J of Neurophysiology,* 3060–3072.

Prerau, M.J., Smith, A.C., Eden, U.T., Yanike, M., Suzuki, W.A. and Brown, E.N. (2008). A mixed filter algorithm for cognitive state estimation from simultaneously recorded continuous and binary measures of performance. *Biological Cybernetics, 99,* 1, 1–14.

Shumway, R.H. and Stoffer, D.S. (1982). An approach to time series smoothing and forecasting using the EM algorithm. *J of Time Series Analysis, 3, 4,* 253–264.

Siegel, S. and Castellan, N. J. (1988). *Nonparametric statistics for the behavioral sciences.* New York: McGraw-Hill.

Smith, A.C. and Brown, E.N. (2003). Estimating a state–space model from point process observations. *Neural Computation, 15,* 965–991.

Smith, A.C., Frank, L. M., Wirth, S., Yanike, M., Hu, D., Kubota, Y., Graybiel, A. M., Suzuki, W. and Brown, E. N. (2004). Dynamic analysis of learning in behavioral experiments. *J of Neuroscience, 24, 2,* 447–461, 2004. E.N.

Smith, A.C., Scalon, J. D., Wirth, S., Yanike, M., Suzuki, W. A. and Brown, E. N. (2010). State–space algorithms for estimating spike rate functions. *Computational Intelligence and Neuroscienc, vol.* 2010, article ID 426539, 14 pages. doi:10.1155/2010/426539.

Smith, A.C., Stefani, M. R., Moghaddam, B., and Brown, E. N. (2005). Analysis and design of behavioral experiments to characterize population learning. *J of Neurophysiology, 93,* 1776–1792.

Smith, A.C., Wirth, S., Suzuki, W.A. and Brown, E.N. (2007). Bayesian analysis of interleaved learning and response bias in behavioral experiments. *J of Neurophysiology, 97, 3,* 2516–2524.

Williams, Z.M., and Eskandar, E.N. (2006). Selective enhancement of associative learning by microstimulation of the anterior caudate. *Nature Neuroscience, 9, 4,* 562–568.

Wirth,S., Yanike, M., Frank, L.M., Smith, A.C., Brown, E.N. and Suzuki, W.A. Single neurons in the monkey hippocampus and learning of new associations. *Science, 300, 5625,* 1578–1581.

Yanike, M., Wirth, S., Smith, A.C., Brown, E.N. and Suzuki, W.A. (2009). Comparison of associative learning-related signals in the macaque perirhinal cortex and hippocampus. *Cerebral Cortex, 19, 5,* 1064–1078.

APPENDIX

A. Details of the Recursive Filter

In this section, we provide details of the derivation of equations (8)-(12). Our objective is to construct a recursive filter to estimate the state X_k at trial k from $Y^k = \{Z^k, M^k, N^k\}$. The standard approach to deriving such a filter is to express recursively the probability density of the state given the observations. For events $\{A, B, C\}$, we have from Bayes' rule that

$$P(A \mid B,C) = \frac{P(A,B \mid C)}{P(B \mid C)} = \frac{P(A \mid C)P(B \mid A,C)}{P(B \mid C)} \tag{23}$$

Denote A according to $\{X_k = x_k\}$, B according to $\{Y_k = y_k\}$, and C according to $\{Y^{k-1} = y^{k-1}\}$. Then we have

$$f_{X_k \mid Y^k}\left(x_k \mid y^k\right) = \frac{f_{X_k \mid Y^{k-1}}\left(x_k \mid y^{k-1}\right) f_{Y_k \mid X_k}\left(y_k \mid x_k\right)}{f_{Y_k \mid Y^{k-1}}\left(y_k \mid y^{k-1}\right)}$$

$$= \frac{f_{X_k \mid Y^{k-1}}\left(x_k \mid y^{k-1}\right) P_{M_k \mid X_k}\left(m_k \mid x_k\right) P_{N_k \mid X_k}\left(n_k \mid x_k\right) f_{Z_k \mid X_k}\left(z_k \mid x_k\right)}{f_{Y_k \mid Y^{k-1}}\left(y_k \mid y^{k-1}\right)}$$

$$\propto f_{X_k \mid Y^{k-1}}\left(x_k \mid y^{k-1}\right) P_{M_k \mid X_k}\left(m_k \mid x_k\right) P_{N_k \mid X_k}\left(n_k \mid x_k\right) f_{Z_k \mid X_k}\left(z_k \mid x_k\right) \tag{24}$$

and the associated one-step prediction probability density or Chapman-Kolmogorov equation is

$$f_{X_k \mid Y^{k-1}}\left(x_k \mid y^{k-1}\right) = \int\!\!\int f_{X_{k-1} \mid Y^{k-1}}\left(x_{k-1} \mid y^{k-1}\right) f_{X_k \mid X_{k-1}}\left(x_k \mid x_{k-1}\right) dx_{k-1} \tag{25}$$

Together (24) and (25) define a recursion that can be used to compute the probability of the state given the observations.

We derive the mixed filter algorithm by computing a Gaussian approximation to the posterior density $f_{X_k \mid Y^k}(x_k \mid y^k)$ in (24). At time k, we assume the one-step prediction density (25) is the Gaussian density

$$f_{X_k \mid Y^{k-1}}\left(x_k \mid y^{k-1}\right) \sim \mathcal{N}\left(x_{k \mid k-1}, \sigma^2_{k \mid k-1}\right). \tag{26}$$

To evaluate $x_{k|k-1}$ and $\sigma^2_{k|k-1}$, we note that they follow in a straightforward manner:

$$x_{k|k-1} = \mathbb{E}\left[X_k \mid Y^{k-1} = y^{k-1}\right] = \gamma + \rho x_{k-1|k-1} \qquad (27)$$

$$\sigma^2_{k|k-1} = var\left(X_k \mid Y^{k-1} = y^{k-1}\right) \qquad (28)$$

$$= var\left(\gamma + \rho X_{k-1} + V_k \mid Y^{k-1} = y^{k-1}\right) \qquad (29)$$

$$= \rho^2 \sigma^2_{k-1|k-1} + \sigma^2_V \qquad (30)$$

Substituting all these equations together, then we have that the posterior density can be expressed as

$$f_{X_k|Y^k}\left(x_k \mid y^k\right) \propto \exp\{-\frac{(x_k - x_{k|k-1})^2}{2\sigma^2_{k|k-1}} + m_k \log[p_k(1-p_k)^{-1}] + \log(1-p_k)$$

$$-\frac{(z_k - \alpha - hx_k)^2}{2\sigma^2_W} + \sum_{j=1}^{J} n_{k,j} \log\left(\lambda_{k,j}\right) - \lambda_{k,j}\Delta\}$$

$$\Rightarrow \log f_{X_k|Y^k}\left(x_k \mid y^k\right)$$

$$= C(y^k) - \frac{(x_k - x_{k|k-1})^2}{2\sigma^2_{k|k-1}} + m_k \log[p_k(1-p_k)^{-1}] + \log(1-p_k) \qquad (31)$$

$$-\frac{(z_k - \alpha - hx_k)^2}{2\sigma^2_W} + \sum_{j=1}^{J} n_{k,j} \log\left(\lambda_{k,j}\right) - \lambda_{k,j}\Delta \qquad (32)$$

Now we can compute the maximum-a-posteriori estimate of x_k and its associated variance estimate. To do this, we compute the first and second derivatives of the log posterior density with respect to x_k, which are respectively

$$0 = \frac{\partial \log f_{X_k|Y^k}\left(x_k \mid y^k\right)}{\partial x_k} = -\frac{(x_k - x_{k|k-1})}{\sigma^2_{k|k-1}} + \frac{h(z_k - \alpha - hx_k)}{\sigma^2_W} + \eta(m_k - p_k)$$

$$+ \sum_{j=1}^{J} g(n_{k,j} - \lambda_{k,j}\Delta)$$

$$\frac{\partial^2 \log f_{X_k|Y^k}\left(x_k\,|\,y^k\right)}{\partial x_k^2} = -\frac{1}{\sigma_{k|k-1}^2} - \frac{h^2}{\sigma_W^2} - \eta^2 p_k(1-p_k) - \sum_{j=1}^{J} g^2 \lambda_{k,j} \Delta$$

where we have exploited the fact that from (4) and (7), the following properties hold:

$$\frac{\partial p_k}{\partial x_k} = \eta p_k(1-p_k) \Rightarrow \begin{cases} \dfrac{\partial \log(1-p_k)}{\partial x_k} = -\eta p_k, \\[2mm] \dfrac{\partial \log p_k}{\partial x_k} = \eta(1-p_k) \end{cases} \tag{33}$$

$$\frac{\partial \lambda_{k,j}}{\partial x_k} = g\lambda_{k,j} \tag{34}$$

$$\frac{\partial \log \lambda_{k,j}}{\partial x_k} = g \tag{35}$$

Combining all this together, using the Gaussian approximation, we arrive at (8)-(12).

B. Details of the M Step Update Equations

In this section, we derive details of the update equations provided in the previous section, "M Step." Note that the joint distribution on all (observed and latent) variables is given by

$$\log f_{X^K|Y^K}\left(x^K\,|\,y^K;\theta\right) = C(y^K) + \sum_{k=1}^{K} -\frac{1}{2\sigma_V^2}(x_k - \gamma - \rho x_{k-1})^2$$

$$-\frac{1}{2\sigma_W^2}(z_k - \alpha - hx_k)^2$$

$$+\sum_{k=1}^{K} m_k\left(\mu + \eta x_k\right) - \log\left(1 + \exp(\mu + \eta x_k)\right)$$

$$+\sum_{k=1}^{K}\sum_{j=1}^{J} n_{k,j}\left[\psi + gx_k + \sum_{s=1}^{S}\beta_s n_{k,j-s}\right]$$

$$-\Delta \exp\left(\psi + gx_k + \sum_{s=1}^{S}\beta_s n_{k,j-s}\right)$$

Note that the expected log-likelihood $Q(\theta) \triangleq \mathbb{E}\left\{\log f_{X^K|Y^K}\left(x^K \mid Y^K; \theta\right) \mid Y^K = y^K\right\}$ has linear terms in $E[X_k \mid Y^k = y^k]$ along with quadratic terms involving $\tilde{W}_{k,j} \triangleq \mathbb{E}\left\{X_k X_j \mid Y^K = y^K\right\}$, except for a couple of terms, including $E[e^{gx_k} \mid Y^k = y^k]$. We note that if $\tilde{X} \sim \mathcal{N}\left(\mu, \sigma^2\right)$ then its moment generating function $M(t) \triangleq E[e^{\tilde{x}t}]$ is given by

$$M(t) = e^{ut + \frac{1}{2}\sigma^2 t^2}. \tag{36}$$

With this, we have

$$Q(\theta) \simeq C(y^K) - \sum_{k=1}^{K} \frac{1}{2\sigma_V^2} \mathbb{E}\left[(X_k - \gamma - \rho X_{k-1})^2 \mid Y^K = y^K\right]$$

$$- \frac{1}{2\sigma_W^2} \mathbb{E}\left[(Z_k - \alpha - hX_k)^2 \mid Y^k = y^k\right]$$

$$+ \sum_{k=1}^{K} m_k \left(\mu + \eta x_{k|K}\right) - \mathbb{E}\left[\log\left(1 + \exp(\mu + \eta X_k)\right) \mid Y^k = y^k\right] \tag{37}$$

$$+ \sum_{k=1}^{K} n_{k,j} \left(\psi + g x_{k|K} + \sum_{s=1}^{S} \beta_s n_{k,j-s}\right)$$

$$- \mathbb{E}\left[\exp\left(\psi + gX_k + \sum_{s=1}^{S} \beta_s n_{k,j-s}\right) \Delta \mid Y^K = y^K\right] \tag{38}$$

$$= C(y^K) - \frac{1}{2\sigma_V^2}\left[\sum_{k=1}^{K} \tilde{W}_k - 2\gamma x_{k|K} - 2\rho \tilde{W}_{k-1,k} + \gamma^2 + 2\gamma\rho x_{k-1|K} + \rho^2 \tilde{W}_{k-1}\right]$$

$$- \frac{1}{2\sigma_W^2}\left[\sum_{k=1}^{K} (z_k - \alpha)^2 - 2(z_k - \alpha)h x_{k|K} + h^2 \tilde{W}_k\right]$$

$$+ \sum_{k=1}^{K} m_k \left(\mu + \eta x_{k|K}\right) - \mathbb{E}\left[\log\left(1 + \exp(\mu + \eta x_k)\right) \mid Y^K = y^K\right] \tag{39}$$

$$+ \sum_{k=1}^{K} n_{k,j} \left(\psi + g x_{k|K} + \sum_{s=1}^{S} \beta_s n_{k,j-s}\right)$$

$$- \Delta \exp\left(\psi + g x_{k|K} + \frac{1}{2}\sigma_{k|K}^2 g^2 + \sum_{s=1}^{S} \beta_s n_{k,j-s}\right) \tag{40}$$

where in going from (38) to (40), we have used the (36).

We now rely upon the Taylor series approximation around $x_{k|K}$

$$E[\rho(X_k) | Y^K = y^K] \simeq \rho(x_{k|K}) + \frac{1}{2} \sigma^2_{k|K} \rho''(x_{k|K})$$

Let us now consider the conditional expectation term involves

$$\log(1 + \exp(\mu + \eta x_k))$$

$$\rho_1(x_k) \triangleq \frac{\partial \log(1 + \exp(\mu + \eta x_k))}{\partial \mu} = \frac{\exp(\mu + \eta x_k)}{1 + \exp(\mu + \eta x_k)} = p_k, \qquad (41)$$

$$\rho_2(x_k) \triangleq \frac{\partial \log(1 + \exp(\mu + \eta x_k))}{\partial \eta} = \frac{x_k \exp(\mu + \eta x_k)}{1 + \exp(\mu + \eta x_k)} = x_k p_k \qquad (42)$$

Note from before that

$$\rho_1'(x_k) = \eta p_k (1 - p_k) = \eta(p_k - p_k^2)$$

$$\Rightarrow \rho_1''(x_k) = \eta[\eta p_k (1 - p_k) - 2 p_k \eta p_k (1 - p_k)]$$

$$= \eta^2 p_k (1 - p_k)(1 - 2 p_k)$$

Thus we have that

$$f_1(\mu, \eta) = \frac{\partial}{\partial \mu} \left\{ \sum_{k=1}^{K} m_k \left(\mu + \eta x_{k|K} \right) - \mathbb{E}\left[\log(1 + \exp(\mu + \eta X_k)) | Y^K = y^K \right] \right\} \quad (43)$$

$$= \sum_{k=1}^{K} m_k - \mathbb{E}[\rho_1(X_k) | Y^K = y^K] \qquad (44)$$

$$\simeq \sum_{k=1}^{K} m_k - p_{k|K} - \frac{1}{2} \sigma^2_{k|K} \eta^2 p_{k|K} (1 - p_{k|K})(1 - 2 p_{k|K}) \qquad (45)$$

Let us now consider $\rho_2(x_k) = x_k p_k$. Note from (42) that

$$\rho_2'(x_k) = [x_k \rho_1(x_k)]'$$

$$= x_k \rho_1'(x_k) + \rho_1(x_k)$$

$$\Rightarrow \rho_2''(x_k) = \rho_1'(x_k) + \rho_1'(x_k) + x_k \rho_1''(x_k)$$

$$= 2\rho_1'(x_k) + x_k \rho_1''(x_k)$$

$$= 2\eta p_k(1-p_k) + x_k \eta^2 p_k(1-p_k)(1-2p_k)$$

$$= \eta p_k(1-p_k)\left[2 + x_k \eta(1-2p_k)\right]$$

Thus we have that

$$f_2(\mu,\eta) = \frac{\partial}{\partial \eta}\left\{ \sum_{k=1}^{K} m_k\left(\mu + \eta x_{k|K}\right) - \mathbb{E}\left[\log\left(1+\exp(\mu+\eta x_k)\right) \mid Y^K = y^K\right]\right\} \quad (46)$$

$$= \sum_{k=1}^{K} m_k x_{k|K} - \mathbb{E}\left[\rho_2(X_k) \mid Y^K = y^K\right] \quad (47)$$

$$\simeq \sum_{k=1}^{K} m_k x_{k|K} - x_{k|K} p_{k|K} - \frac{1}{2}\sigma_{k|K}^2 \eta p_{k|K}(1-p_{k|K})\left[2 + x_{k|K}\eta(1-2p_{k|K})\right] \quad (48)$$

Thus we differentiate to find a local minimum

$$0 = \frac{\partial Q}{\partial \gamma} = -\frac{1}{\sigma_V^2}\left[\sum_{k=1}^{K} -x_{k|K} + \gamma + \rho x_{k-1|K}\right]$$

$$0 = \frac{\partial Q}{\partial \rho} = -\frac{1}{\sigma_V^2}\left[\sum_{k=1}^{K} -\tilde{W}_{k-1,k} + \gamma x_{k-1|K} + \rho \tilde{W}_{k-1}\right]$$

$$0 = \frac{\partial Q}{\partial \alpha} = -\frac{1}{\sigma_W^2}\left[\sum_{k=1}^{K} \alpha - z_k + h x_{k|K}\right]$$

$$0 = \frac{\partial Q}{\partial h} = -\frac{1}{\sigma_W^2}\left[\sum_{k=1}^{K} -(z_k - \alpha)x_{k|K} + h\tilde{W}_k\right]$$

$$0 = \frac{\partial Q}{\partial \sigma_W^2} = \frac{1}{2[\sigma_W^2]^2}\left[-K\sigma_W^2 + \sum_{k=1}^{K}(z_k-\alpha)^2 - 2(z_k-\alpha)h x_{k|K} + h^2\tilde{W}_k\right]$$

$$0 = \frac{\partial Q}{\partial \mu} = \sum_{k=1}^{K} m_k - p_{k|K} - \frac{1}{2}\sigma_{k|K}^2 \eta^2 p_{k|K}(1-p_{k|K})(1-2p_{k|K}) \quad (49)$$

$$0 = \frac{\partial Q}{\partial \eta} = \sum_{k=1}^{K} m_k x_{k|K} - x_{k|K} p_{k|K} - \frac{1}{2} \sigma_{k|K}^2 \eta p_{k|K} (1 - p_{k|K}) \left[2 + x_{k|K} \eta (1 - 2 p_{k|K}) \right] \quad (50)$$

$$0 = \frac{\partial Q}{\partial \psi} = \sum_{k=1}^{K} \sum_{j=1}^{J} n_{k,j} - \Delta \exp \left(\psi + g x_{k|K} + \frac{1}{2} \sigma_{k|K}^2 g^2 + \sum_{s=1}^{S} \beta_s n_{k,j-s} \right) \quad (51)$$

$$0 = \frac{\partial Q}{\partial g} = \sum_{k=1}^{K} \sum_{j=1}^{J} n_{k,j} x_{k|K}$$
$$- \Delta (x_{k|K} + g \sigma_{k|K}^2) \exp \left(\psi + g x_{k|K} + \frac{1}{2} \sigma_{k|K}^2 g^2 + \sum_{s=1}^{S} \beta_s n_{k,j-s} \right) \quad (52)$$

$$0 = \frac{\partial Q}{\partial \beta_s} = \sum_{k=1}^{K} \sum_{j=1}^{J} n_{k,j} n_{k,j-s}$$
$$- \Delta n_{k,j-s} \exp \left(\psi + g x_{k|K} + \frac{1}{2} \sigma_{k|K}^2 g^2 + \sum_{s=1}^{S} \beta_s n_{k,j-s} \right) \quad (53)$$

Simplifying, we get

$$\begin{bmatrix} \gamma \\ \rho \end{bmatrix} = \begin{bmatrix} K & \sum_{k=1}^{K} x_{k-1} \mid K \\ \sum_{k=1}^{K} X_{k-1|K} & \sum_{k=1}^{K} W_{k-1} \end{bmatrix}^{-1} \begin{bmatrix} \sum_{k=1}^{K} x_{k|K} \\ \sum_{k=1}^{K} W_{k-1,k} \end{bmatrix} \quad (54)$$

$$\begin{bmatrix} \alpha \\ h \end{bmatrix} = \begin{bmatrix} K & \sum_{k=1}^{K} x_{k|K} \\ \sum_{k=1}^{K} x_{k \backslash K} & \sum_{k=1}^{K} \tilde{W}_k \end{bmatrix}^{-1} \begin{bmatrix} \sum_{k=1}^{K} z_k \\ \sum_{k=1}^{K} z_k x_{k \backslash K} \end{bmatrix} \quad (55)$$

$$\sigma_W^2 = \frac{1}{K} \left[\sum_{k=1}^{K} (z_k - \alpha)^2 - 2(z_k - \alpha) h x_{k|K} + h^2 \tilde{W}_k \right] \quad (56)$$

$$\psi = \log \left(\frac{\sum_{k=1}^{K} \sum_{j=1}^{J} n_{k,j}}{\sum_{k=1}^{K} \sum_{j=1}^{J} \Delta \exp \left(g x_{k|K} + \frac{1}{2} \sigma_{k|K}^2 g^2 + \sum_{s=1}^{S} \beta_s n_{k,j-s} \right)} \right) \quad (57)$$

Details for solving for the remaining parameters $\mu, \eta, g, \{\beta_s\}$ using Newton-like methods are given in Appendix 9.

C. Newton Algorithms to Solve Fixed Point Equations

Newton Algorithm for the Posterior Update

We note that $x_{k|k}$ as defined in (11) is the root of the function ρ:

$$\rho(x_{k|k}) = -x_{k|k} + x_{k|k-1} + C_k \left[h\left(z_k - \alpha - h x_{k|k-1} \right) + \eta \sigma_W^2 \left(m_k - p_{k|k} \right) \right]$$

$$+ \sum_{j=1}^{J} C_k \sigma_W^2 \left[g(n_{k,j} - \lambda_{k,j|k,j} \Delta) \right]$$

$$\Rightarrow \rho'(x_{k|k}) = -1 - C_k \sigma_W^2 \left[\eta^2 p_{k|k} (1 - p_{k|k}) + \sum_{j=1}^{J} g^2 \lambda_{k,j|k,j} \Delta \right]$$

Either the previous state estimate, $x_{k-1|k-1}$, or the one-step prediction estimate, $x_{k|k-1}$, can provide a reliable starting guess.

Binary Parameters

In this section we develop derivatives of the functions f_3 and f_4 for the purpose of enabling a Newton-like algorithm to find the fixed point pertaining to (49)–(50). Define:

$$f_3 = \sum_{k=1}^{K} m_k - p_k - \frac{1}{2} \sigma_{k|K}^2 \eta^2 p_k (1 - p_k)(1 - 2p_k)$$

$$f_4 = \sum_{k=1}^{K} m_k x_{k|K} - x_{k|K} p_k - \frac{1}{2} \sigma_{k|K}^2 \eta p_k (1 - p_k) \left[2 + x_{k|K} \eta (1 - 2p_k) \right]$$

We arrive at the Jacobian:

$$\frac{\partial}{\partial \mu} \{f_3\} = -\sum_{k=1}^{K} p_k (1 - p_k) \left[1 + \frac{1}{2} \sigma_{k|K}^2 \eta^2 \left[(1 - 2p_k)^2 - 2p_k (1 - p_k) \right] \right]$$

$$\frac{\partial}{\partial \eta} \{f_3\} = -\sum_{k=1}^{K} p_k (1 - p_k)$$

$$\left[x_{k|K} + \frac{1}{2} \sigma_{k|K}^2 \eta^2 (1 - 2p_k)^2 x_{k|K} + \sigma_{k|K}^2 \eta [1 - 2p_k - \eta x_{k|K} p_k (1 - p_k)] \right]$$

$$\frac{\partial}{\partial \mu}\{f_4\} = -\sum_{k=1}^{K} p_k (1 - p_k)$$

$$\left[x_{k|K} + \sigma_{k|K}^2 (1 - 2p_k) + \frac{1}{2}\sigma_{k|K}^2 \eta^2 \left[(1 - 2p_k)^2 - 2p_k (1 - p_k) \right] \right]$$

$$\frac{\partial}{\partial \eta}\{f_4\} = -\sum_{k=1}^{K} p_k (1 - p_k)[x_{k|K}^2 + \sigma_{k|K}^2 \left[\eta x_{k|K} (1 - 2p_k) + 1 \right]$$

$$+ \frac{1}{2}\sigma_{k|K}^2 x_{k|K} \left[2\eta \left(1 - 2p_k - \eta x_{k|K} p_k (1 - p_k) \right) + \eta^2 (1 - 2p_k)^2 x_{k|K} \right]$$

Spiking Parameters

Finding g

In this section we develop derivatives of the functions f_5 and f_6 for the purpose of enabling a Newton-like algorithm to find the fixed point pertaining to (52). From (57), note that

$$\psi = \log \left(\frac{\sum_{k=1}^{K}\sum_{j=1}^{J} n_{k,j}}{\sum_{k=1}^{K}\sum_{j=1}^{J} \Delta \exp \left(g x_{k|K} + \frac{1}{2}\sigma_{k|K}^2 g^2 + \sum_{s=1}^{S} \beta_s n_{k,j-s} \right)} \right)$$

$$\text{or } \Delta \exp(\psi) = \frac{\sum_{k=1}^{K}\sum_{j=1}^{J} n_{k,j}}{\sum_{k=1}^{K}\sum_{j=1}^{J} \exp \left(g x_{k|K} + \frac{1}{2}\sigma_{k|K}^2 g^2 + \sum_{s=1}^{S} \beta_s n_{k,j-s} \right)} \qquad (58)$$

Define:

$$f_5 = \frac{\partial Q}{\partial g} = \sum_{k=1}^{K}\sum_{j=1}^{J} n_{k,j} x_{k|K}$$

$$- \Delta(x_{k|K} + \sigma_{k|K}^2 g) \exp \left(\psi + g x_{k|K} + \frac{1}{2}\sigma_{k|K}^2 g^2 + \sum_{s=1}^{S} \beta_s n_{k,j-s} \right)$$

$$= \left(\sum_{k=1}^{K}\sum_{j=1}^{J} n_{k,j} x_{k|K} \right)$$

$$-\sum_{k=1}^{K}\sum_{j=1}^{J}\frac{\left(\sum_{k=1}^{K}\sum_{j=1}^{J}n_{k,j}\right)(x_{k|K}+\sigma_{k|K}^2 g)\exp\left(gx_{k|K}+\frac{1}{2}\sigma_{k|K}^2 g^2+\sum_{s=1}^{S}\beta_s n_{k,j-s}\right)}{\sum_{k=1}^{K}\sum_{j=1}^{J}\exp\left(gx_{k|K}+\frac{1}{2}\sigma_{k|K}^2 g^2+\sum_{s=1}^{S}\beta_s n_{k,j-s}\right)}$$

$$=\left(\sum_{k=1}^{K}n_{k,j}x_{k|K}\right)-\left(\sum_{k=1}^{K}n_{k,j}\right)\left(\frac{a(g)}{b(g)}\right)$$

$$\Rightarrow f_5'(g)=-\left(\sum_{k=1}^{K}\sum_{j=1}^{J}n_{k,j}\right)\frac{\partial}{\partial g}\left\{\frac{a(g)}{b(g)}\right\}=-\left(\sum_{k=1}^{K}\sum_{j=1}^{J}n_{k,j}\right)\frac{b(g)a'(g)-a(g)b'(g)}{b(g)^2}$$

$$a(g)\triangleq\sum_{k=1}^{K}\sum_{j=1}^{J}(x_{k|K}+\sigma_{k|K}^2 g)\exp\left(gx_{k|K}+\frac{1}{2}\sigma_{k|K}^2 g^2+\sum_{s=1}^{S}\beta_s n_{k,j-s}\right)$$

$$b(g)\triangleq\sum_{k=1}^{K}\sum_{j=1}^{J}\exp\left(gx_{k|K}+\frac{1}{2}\sigma_{k|K}^2 g^2+\sum_{s=1}^{S}\beta_s n_{k,j-s}\right)$$

$$a'(g)=\sum_{k=1}^{K}\left[\left(x_{k|K}+\sigma_{k|K}^2 g\right)^2+\sigma_{k|K}^2\right]\exp\left(gx_{k|K}+\frac{1}{2}\sigma_{k|K}^2 g^2+\sum_{s=1}^{S}\beta_s n_{k,j-s}\right)$$

$$b'(g)=\sum_{k=1}^{K}\left(x_{k|K}+\sigma_{k|K}^2 g\right)\exp\left(gx_{k|K}+\frac{1}{2}\sigma_{k|K}^2 g^2+\sum_{s=1}^{S}\beta_s n_{k,j-s}\right)=a(g)$$

$$\Rightarrow\frac{f_5(g)}{f_5'(g)}=\frac{\left(\sum_{k=1}^{K}n_{k,j}x_{k|K}\right)b(g)^2-\left(\sum_{k=1}^{K}\sum_{j=1}^{J}n_{k,j}\right)a(g)b(g)}{\left(\sum_{k=1}^{K}\sum_{j=1}^{J}n_{k,j}\right)\left(a(g)^2-b(g)a'(g)\right)}$$

Finding β_s

In this section we develop the derivative of the functions f_6 to find the fixed point pertaining to (53). Note that the equation for $\frac{\partial Q}{\partial\beta_s}=0$ in (53) can be expressed as

$$f_6(\beta_s)=\tilde{f}_5(\phi(\beta_s))$$

$$=a_0-a_1\phi(\beta_s),$$

$$\phi(\beta_s) = \exp(\beta_s),$$

$$\Rightarrow f_6'(\beta_s) = -a_1 \phi'(\beta_s) = -a_1 \exp(\beta_s)$$

where

$$a_0 = \sum_{k=1}^{K} \sum_{j=1}^{J} n_{k,j} n_{k,j-s},$$

$$a_1 = \sum_{k,j:n_{k,j-s}=1} \Delta \exp\left(\psi + g x_{k|K} + \frac{1}{2}\sigma_{k|K}^2 g^2 + \sum_{s'\neq s}\beta_{s'} n_{k,j-s'}\right)$$

Note that since each $a_0 \geq 0$, $a_1 > 0$, and $\phi > 0$, it follows that $f_6'(\beta_s) < 0$ and thus f is monotonically decreasing. Moreover, since $f_6(0) \geq 0$, it follows that f has a unique zero x^* and thus a unique fixed point β_s^*, when considering all other parameters $\beta_{s'}$ fixed.

2

Stochastic Transitions between States of Neural Activity

Paul Miller and Donald B. Katz

Introduction

Measurements of neural spike trains, particularly *in vivo* measurements, reveal strong variability across successive trials that persist despite scientists' best efforts to hold all external variables fixed (Arieli et al., 1996; Holt et al., 1996; Shadlen and Newsome, 1998; Kisley and Gerstein, 1999). Such trial-to-trial variability in the brain of a living creature may not be surprising from an ecological or evolutionary perspective: our brains evolved in nonstationary environments, predictability puts one at a competitive disadvantage, and a lack of variability can prevent one from discovering better responses. Such variability, however, renders nontrivial the analysis of neural responses to environmental stimuli. In the face of point processes with Poisson-like variability, the traditional solution is to assume the brain produces an identical underlying response to each stimulus presentation—the response code—such that by averaging across trials one removes only undesirable variability within individual spike trains. Such trial averaging into peri-stimulus time histograms (PSTHs) for individual cells has been at the heart of neural analysis, because traditionally it has been essential to combine information across trials to obtain sufficient statistical power.

Nowadays, of course, multiple electrode recordings are more commonplace, so such trial averaging is not necessary. This has allowed for the recent development of state–space generalized linear models (Truccolo et al., 2005; Czanner et al., 2008), which prove to be particularly useful for real-time decoding of spike trains (Lawhern et al., 2010). Analysis via PSTHs remains the norm, however, so the typical method for analyzing data from multiple cells is to first average cell responses individually across trials (which are assumed identical) before carrying out a more sophisticated analysis such as Principle Components Analysis (PCA). In the absence of a clearly superior alternative or strong evidence that any important information is lost by such trial averaging, the use of PSTHs as the basis for neural data analysis remains *de rigueur*.

In this chapter we describe a method for analysis of data from multiple simultaneously recorded neurons that does not assume identical behavior across trials, but, indeed, uses the trial-to-trial variability to extract correlations and produce states of network activity. This method, Hidden Markov modeling (HMM), produces a description of neural taste responses in gustatory cortex that performs significantly better than other techniques, such as PSTH and PCA. We begin by recapitulating some of these results in the next section.

HMM assumes that network activity proceeds through distinct states, with relatively sharp transitions between them. It is important to note that while states are fixed, the transitions between them can vary across trials. If the data match these assumptions—if transitions are inherently sharp but not set in their timing from trial to trial—then the HMM solution will differ from PSTH-based analyses in important ways: HMM will detect these sharp transitions, whereas standard analyses will interpret the data as containing gradually changing and ramping activity. We demonstrate these properties in a model attractor-based network, which reproduces the key features of cortical activity during taste processing: simulated taste input causes activity to progress through a reliable, taste-specific sequence of states of distributed cortical activity, with high trial-to-trial variability in the timing of transitions between the states (Miller and Katz, 2010).

In the final sections of the chapter, we consider a role for stochastic transitions between neural states (Deco et al., 2009) in decision-making (Deco and Romo, 2008; Sakai et al., 2006) and in timing (Okamoto and Fukai, 2001). We show that stochastic transitions can, using an appropriate measure of reliability of decision making, perform better than standard models of decision making based on integration of inputs. In a similar network designed to reproduce timing behavior, we show that stochastic transitions between discrete states naturally lead to a standard deviation proportional to the mean time to reach a particular state of the system. Such proportionality between standard deviation and mean is well known as Weber's law of timing, which formalizes the high trial-to-trial variability in timing of mental responses (Gibbon, 1977). In fact, the conceptual beauty of models based on stochastic transitions between discrete states arises because the one process that produces the system's dynamics also accounts for its variability. Thus the between-trial variability of perception can be explained without the need for adding any "extra" unbeneficial noise.

Hidden Markov Modeling (HMM)

HMM is a statistical method most commonly used in speech recognition software in engineering and for analysis of DNA sequences in biology. Use of HMM in neuroscience has been infrequent to date, particularly with regard to the purpose described here (Abeles et al., 1995; Seidemann et al., 1996; Jones et al., 2007).

HMM assumes the presence of two Markov processes, each of which, by definition, depends only on the current state of the system and is independent of the history of prior states. When applied to neural spike trains, one of the Markov processes is the emission of spikes by a neuron at any point in time. The Markov assumption for spike emission assumes that spike trains follow a Poisson process at a fixed mean rate, given a particular state of the system. The state of the system is defined by the mean rates of each neuron within the state (see Figure 2.1). The second Markov assumption pertains to the state of the system itself and assumes that when the system is in a specific state, its probability of transition to another state is both independent of prior states and constant in time.

It is important to note that this procedure is at best a first approximation to the possible coherent population process—in fact, the Markov assumptions contained within the statistical model do not match the neural data, as neither state durations nor inter-spike-intervals within a state are distributed exponentially, as they would be for Poisson processes which perfectly obey the Markov assumptions. The non-Poissonian nature of real data arises from biological processes with real time constants. In principle, these extra time constants could be incorporated into an HMM analysis, but doing so would render it non-Markovian and would add hand-picked parameters, perhaps making it less simple and unbiased than the standard historyless Markovian method. We find that the standard HMM method is of sufficient benefit to be used even without including specific temporal aspects of the real data. In fact, we suggest

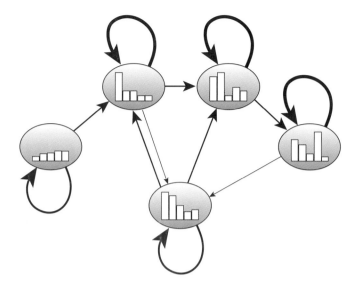

FIGURE 2.1 A Hidden Markov model of spike trains from multiple cells produces a set of states (ovals), in which each state is defined by the mean firing rate of cells within that state (histograms within ovals). The system is doubly stochastic, as the emission of spikes within a state is assumed to be Poisson (and therefore a Markov process) with the given rate for each cell, while transitions between states (thick arrows) are also a stochastic Markov process. In order for the states to be meaningful in neural terms, the state durations should be significantly longer than the times between spike emissions, so in practice, from one time bin to the next, it is much more likely for the system to remain in the same state (thickest recurrent arrows) than to transition to another (smaller directed arrows).

that one use of the HMM analysis could be to uncover some of the biological processes that it does not include within itself.

Method for Analyzing Neural Data via HMM

Statistical software for running a HMM analysis is available in Matlab and "R." We used Matlab for the calculations and results described below. The algorithms require that time be binned, and that each time bin contains a single event—either no spike or the label of a cell that spikes. Currently, if two or more cells spike in the same time bin (an uncommon event given time bins of 1–2ms and ten or fewer simultaneously recorded cells with average rates of 10Hz or lower) we simply select one spike at random and ignore others. Thus for each trial we produce a single series of emissions labeled 0 to N, where N is the number of neural spike trains recorded. We initialize the HMM scheme with randomized emission probabilities representing random estimates of the firing rates of each state. From random initial conditions we use the Baum-Welch algorithm, which iteratively improves the Hidden Markov model, adjusting transition probabilities between states and emission probabilities within a state, to maximize the log likelihood of the set of spike trains arising from the final model. Since the Baum-Welch algorithm is guaranteed to converge to a local optimum, but not a global one, the process is repeated up to ten times with different random number seeds and the model with highest log likelihood selected. It is also possible to evaluate the set of ten solutions—both their form and their log likelihoods—for reliability.

As a result, HMM outputs a set of states, indexed by the firing rate of each cell within the state and the probability of transition from one state to another per unit time. For each trial, the probability that the actual ensemble activity is in any particular state is calculated. The evolution of such probabilities with time is represented by the solid lines in Figure 2.2, in which the solid shading indicates that at that time the probability of one particular state is greater than 0.85.

Intertrial Variability in Taste-Processing Data

In the work of Jones et al, the authors analyzed neural spike trains from gustatory cortex of rats, while delivering tastes to their tongues. The authors recorded simultaneous spike trains from multiple (typically 8–10) taste-responsive cells across up to ten trials with each of four taste stimuli. They then analyzed the data both with standard methods that implicitly assume all trials contain the same network dynamics, such that spike trains can be averaged across trials, and also with HMM, which uses the intertrial variability to extract coherent states of activity.

The two schemes of analysis could be compared in two ways. In the first comparison, each method was implemented on a subset of the data, where at least one trial was removed from each stimulus set. The authors then categorized the missing data set according to which of the four taste stimuli it had the greatest likelihood of belonging. In such a categorization task, HMM significantly outperformed Principle Components Analysis (which relies upon PSTHs) and direct comparison of the novel spike train with trial-averaged spike rates produced by each taste stimulus.

In the second comparison, the authors used all spike trains to produce two types of models of the trial-by-trial firing rate of all cells. In one model,

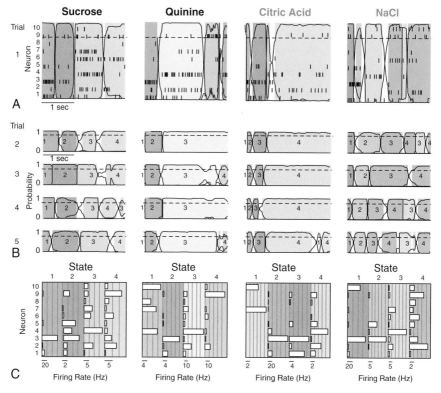

FIGURE 2.2 Sequences of state transitions in gustatory cortex* A) The response in a
single trial of a set of 10 simultaneously recorded neurons to each of the four taste
stimuli. Vertical dashes indicate the individual spikes during the trial. Color denotes a
specific Hidden Markov state whose probability (solid black line) has exceeded 85%.
B) Three more example trials for each taste, demonstrating the variability in times of
transition between states. C) Histograms of firing rate for each cell in each state, show
that the transitions correspond to correlate changes in rate across multiple cells.
*Taken with permission from (Jones et al., 2007).

produced by trial-averaging, the number of different firing rates per trial could
be large (equal to the number of time bins) but the firing rate is assumed identical on each trial. In the second model, produced by HMM, the number of
firing rates per trial is small (equal to the number of activity states), but the
transition times between states could vary from trial to trial. These two models
could be adjusted to have the same number of unconstrained parameters.
Using these two models of firing rate across trials, the authors carried out a
post-hoc analysis of the set of spike trains, to calculate the log likelihood of the
entire set of spike trains being produced by a set of cells with the underlying

firing rates given by the analyses. Again, HMM produced a significantly better fit to the data, showing at a very minimum level, trial by trial changes in activity are significantly stronger than the activity changes that occur across the majority of small time windows within a trial.

Given the advantage of HMM models over analyses based on across trial-averaging, one should take the output of HMM seriously—that is, it must be considered that state sequences are a reliable, useful, and perhaps used output of neural network activity. When applied to taste-processing data, HMM produces sequences of neural activity states, which are highly reliable in their order for each specific taste, but for which the transitions between states are highly variable from one trial to the next. In fact the variability can be so high that the time windows for the presence of a particular state may not overlap on different trials (see Figure 2.2B). That is, the variability in transition times is of the same order as the duration of activity states, which in taste processing is measured in hundreds of milliseconds. Moreover, the time between activity states, during which a transition occurs, is an order of magnitude smaller than the state duration (averaging 60ms). Indeed, analysis of surrogate data using the spiking rates of experimentally measured cells suggests that HMM analysis of cells firing in a Poisson manner in networks with instantaneous transitions between the observed sets of firing rates could not produce measured state transitions significantly shorter than the 60ms calculated from the empirical data. HMM analyses of shuffled empirical data, matching spike trains of different cells from different trials, produced state transitions significantly longer than those of the unshuffled data, however. Thus, one can conclude that abrupt state transitions, which are not aligned across trials, comprise a significant aspect of the real data.

A Stochastic Model of State Transitions in Taste Processing

To be consistent with HMM analyses of neural activity during taste processing (Jones et al., 2007), a model of the underlying circuitry should be able to produce sequences of activity states, in which firing rates are relatively constant, with short transition periods between states where firing rates change quickly and coherently across cells. Different inputs to the circuitry, corresponding to different tastes, should push the network into the initial state of a reliable sequence of states, but with high variability across trials in the timing of the transitions between states. A conceptual framework capable of producing these desired results is a network possessing discrete attractor states that transitions stochastically between the attractor wells (Durstewitz and Deco, 2008;

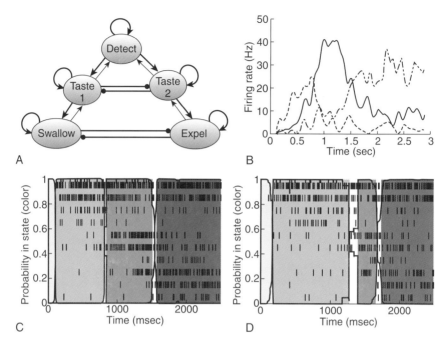

FIGURE 2.3 Model taste processing network and binary classification A) Schematic figure showing the model's architecture. Each oval represents a group of 80 excitatory and 20 inhibitory cells with similar response properties. Arrows indicate the dominant excitatory connections in the network, while solid balls denote strong cross-inhibition between groups. B) Trial-averaged firing rate of 3 example cells shows gradual ramping behavior. C),D) Two trials of the HMM output (bold solid lines) overlying spike trains for each of 10 cells (horizontal rows). The probability of being in a specific state is typically close to 1, with sharp transitions between successive states that do not align across trials.

Miller and Katz, 2010). In this section, we describe an implementation of such a conceptual framework via spiking neurons. In the next section we describe one computational advantage of such a framework.

The network structure shown in Figure 2.3 was designed to reproduce dynamic information described within gustatory cortical single neurons during taste processing (Katz et al., 2001; Di Lorenzo et al., 2003; Katz, 2005), as well as the more recently discovered population state transitions (Jones et al., 2007). In particular, three successive phases of taste processing have been characterized via the similarity of neural responses as a function of time across diverse taste stimuli. Initial activity is somatosensory, indiscriminate of the specific stimulus. In our model, we assume such activity primes the network to undergo later transitions. The second stage of neural activity, lasting on average from 200ms until 1000ms from stimulus onset, contains the most information on taste identity. The final stage, which on average starts by 1000ms after stimulus delivery, contains primarily information on palatability, which in our model we treat as a binary classification needed to produce one of two possible motor responses: "swallow" for a palatable substance and "spit" for an unpalatable substance.

We simulate our network with two different inputs, representing two different tastes, where the only difference between inputs is a 10% increase to one of the pools of cells most responsive to taste identity for one stimulus, and to the other pool for the second stimulus. Such a relatively small change in overall input (all five pools receive stimulus) is sufficient to drive the network along a different sequence of attractors. The network is designed such that in the absence of noise, even with inputs, its activity remains in a constant state. The presence of noise, however—in our simulations arising from uncorrelated Poisson synaptic inputs delivered to each cell—the activity switches abruptly from one state to another. The internal connections of the network assure that when one state is active, in the presence of a stimulus, another state is "primed" so that the stochastic transition will occur to the "primed" state in a directed manner, but at a nonspecified time.

HMM analysis of the output of our network in the presence of appropriate stimuli reveals a stimulus-specific sequence of states with duration significantly longer than the brief transition times between states (Miller and Katz, 2010). On the other hand, trial-averaging of spike trains to produce a single mean firing rate for each cell, suggests slow variations in activity, in spite of the abrupt changes present in each trial.

Thus a network containing a set of attractor states, with the network's activity switching between states in a temporally stochastic manner, but in a reliable direction determined by a bias produced by the inputs to the network, can reproduce the key features of neural activity in gustatory cortex during taste processing. One can then ask, "What is such activity good for?"

Stochastic Decision Making

One of the outcomes of taste processing that is most amenable to analysis is the resulting binary motor output based on palatability. A classification of palatability that is separate from one of identity allows a taste-processing network to be reconfigured across learning, so that previously palatable substances can become unpalatable (for example, as a result of conditioned taste aversion) or vice versa. One would like, in such a case, to be able to produce reliable, strong changes in the binary output (to spit out a substance instead of swallow it) with the minimal possible change to the internal structure of the network. Thus one can assess a binary classifier (or decision-making network) by asking how reliably it produces one particular output over another, given a small difference in its inputs. In this section, we compare a network (Wang, 2002; Wong and Wang, 2006), whose parameters can be adjusted so that when receiving inputs, its initial spontaneous state of activity can be made more or less stable (Miller and Katz, 2010).

When the spontaneous state is unstable, the network drifts to one of two distinct attractor states in a process considered by many to correlate with decision-making (Wang, 2002), in which activity of some cells "ramp" up their firing rate (Figure 2.4 A and B) (Shadlen and Newsome, 2001; Huk and Shadlen, 2005; Wong and Wang, 2006; Ratcliff and McKoon, 2008). The favoring of one

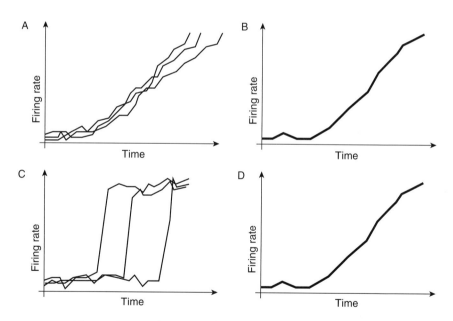

FIGURE 2.4 Two modes in a decision-making network: "ramping" or "jumping"
A) Sketch of three typical trials of the population activity of a group of ramping cells with random noise. B) The average ramping response produced from multiple trials. C) Sketch of three typical trials showing the average rate of a group of cells which makes a stochastic transition from the spontaneous state to a discrete active state. D) The average firing rate over multiple trials of such "jumping" activity can be indistinguishable from ramping activity.

attractor state over another can arise from biases in the inputs, in initial conditions, from biases in external or internal connections in the network, or a combination of the above. The drift to an attractor state would occur deterministically to one state over the other in the absence of fluctuations in the system, but fluctuations cause the non-favored attractor state to be reached on a minority of trials. We label this the "ramping" mode operation.

When the spontaneous state is more stable (or the inputs are weaker) the system remains in its initial state with no drift, until a fluctuation causes the activity to switch to one attractor state over another (Figure 2.4 C and D). This latter condition produces neural activity, which matches that observed across multiple trials during taste processing. The need for a random fluctuation to cause a state change results in large trial-to-trial variability, with a significantly large time of relatively constant activity in an attractor state in between comparatively rapid changes (or "jumps") in activity (Marti et al., 2008). Indeed, HMM analysis of spike trains from a network in this "jumping" mode of decision making produces transitions between states that last on average 20ms, whereas in the "ramping" mode, the transitions last on average over 100ms (and an extra, specious "state" is interpolated between initial and final activity states). Analysis of population activity demonstrates significantly larger trial-to-trial variability in the time from stimulus onset until activity changes significantly from baseline in the "jumping" mode compared to "ramping" mode. Averaging activity across multiple trials produces similar average behavior across both modes, however. Thus, only analysis based on multiple spike trains observed simultaneously in each trial can identify the general mode of network operation.

Comparison of the outputs of the network in the two modes of operation indicates that in the presence of typical internal noise, the "jumping" mode responds more reliably to a small bias in its inputs than does the "ramping" mode (Miller and Katz, 2010). Surprisingly, under these conditions, and when a response is required in limited time, addition of purely uninformative noise to the inputs allows the network to more reliably respond to the mean difference in inputs. The latter result corresponds to stochastic resonance, in this case where the level of noise produces a timescale for transition in the network, which is required to match the timescale of input duration for optimal performance. That is, if the total noise is too weak, the network remains in its initial state too often, without responding to the inputs in the short duration when they are present. On the other hand, with too much noise, even though transitions are rapid, they are less informative of differences in the input signal, which can be overwhelmed by noise. Thus the "jumping" mode possesses an optimal level of noise, which one sees from Figure 2.5 can be approached with

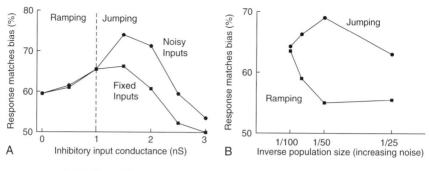

FIGURE 2.5 Reliability of "jumping" versus "ramping" modes of binary classification
A) By increasing the inhibitory conductance, one can stabilize the spontaneous state
more and more and move the network from a mode where inputs deterministically
produce an increase in activity (ramping) to a mode in which fluctuations are needed
to produce a change in activity state (jumping). Two pools of cells receive inputs, with
a small bias to one of the pools. We plot here how often the pool with the greater input
becomes the more active pool. Note that the peak reliability for the output to best
match the small bias in inputs occurs in the mode of "jumping" rather than
"ramping." Moreover, if noisy Poisson trains with the same mean replace the fixed
input currents, the peak reliability increases, since the additional fluctuations allow
the "jumping" mode to produce responses more often within the input duration of
2 seconds. B) Noise is adjusted in simulations by scaling the population size, with all
synapses scaled in inverse proportion. The "jumping" mode exhibits stochastic
resonance: a peak in performance when the time scale for noise-induced transitions
matches the 2-second duration of inputs. With too little noise, the "jumping" mode
remains in its initial state, while too much noise produces random transitions.
Conversely, the ramping mode can always do better by reducing noise, since it does
not rely on fluctuations to produce a response. Note that due to correlations, typical
levels of noise in the brain correspond to that produced by 50–100 independent
neurons (Zohary et al., 1994).

the addition of input noise. On the other hand, the ramping mode, relying
upon deterministic integration is always hampered by noise and is optimal in
the absence of noise, since its integration time is to first order unaffected by
noise. Experimentally, if one could add small fluctuations to inputs and observe
an improved ability of a subject to discriminate differences in the mean of those
inputs, then the "jumping" mode of classification would be confirmed. Since
environmental inputs are typically fluctuating and networks of cells in the brain
are bombarded by fluctuating inputs, it is not unreasonable to expect that the
brain uses such fluctuations in order to produce responses, rather than relies
upon a mode of operation that becomes optimal as fluctuations are reduced.

Timing by Stochastic Integration

Our ability to estimate time intervals is really quite poor, described by the Weber-Fechner Law of timing (Weber, 1851; Fechner, 1912; Gibbon, 1977; Gibbon and Church, 1990), which yields a constant ratio of approximately 0.3 for the standard deviation to the mean of repeated estimations (the Weber fraction). As with errors in other types of measurement, the general Weber's Law form of the distribution of estimates of time intervals are suggestive of an underlying logarithmic representation with constant errors. In general, the formalism of stochastic transitions between attractor states provides such a logarithmic representation via the barriers between states, since the time between transitions depends exponentially on barrier height (Miller and Wang, 2006). Biologically, the barrier height can be adjusted by constant background inputs to the system, which would vary logarithmically with the time interval to be estimated.

Okamoto and Fukai (2001; Kitano et al., 2003; Okamoto et al., 2007) have specifically studied how timing could emerge through a series of discrete stochastic transitions among a group of bistable units or neurons, demonstrating the Weber-Fechner Law over a timescale of seconds, while Miller and Wang (2006) produced a similar result that could generate timescales of minutes, using a model with populations of 100s of simulated cortical cells (Figure 2.6).

The models are similar in that they require more than a single transition in a bistable system; this is because, while the standard deviation is proportional to the mean time for a single transition, the ratio between the two (the Weber fraction) is approximately one. The coupling together of multiple transitions of this nature, either linearly in series, or in parallel, or nonlinearly, can produce a lower Weber fraction that reaches that measured empirically. Specifically, if a behavioral response relies on a series of N successive transitions, each Poisson, so with an exponential distribution of times, of identical mean, τ, the mean response time is $N\tau$, with variance $N\tau^2$, and thus a Weber fraction of $1/\sqrt{N}$, which becomes as low as 0.3 for $N=10$. In a parallel system, if one assumes that the behavioral response requires a subset, K, out of N independent bistable switches each with the same mean transition time and standard deviation, τ, then the mean response time is given by $\langle T \rangle = \tau \left(\dfrac{1}{N} + \dfrac{1}{N-1} + \cdots + \dfrac{1}{N-K+1} \right)$

while the variance is given by $\mathrm{var}(T) = \tau^2 \left(\dfrac{1}{N^2} + \dfrac{1}{(N-1)^2} + \cdots + \dfrac{1}{(N-K+1)^2} \right)$. The

resulting Weber fraction can fall as low as 0.3 for $N > 16$, with appropriate K, as shown in Figure 2.7.

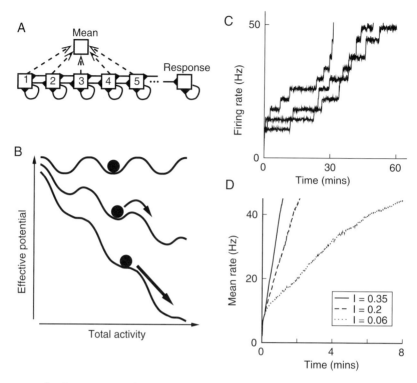

FIGURE 2.6 Slow timing and Weber's Law via a discrete stochastic integrator*
A) Schematic figure of groups of cells with recurrent excitation to produce bistable
units that are coupled together in series. Each group only becomes bistable once
primed by activity in the preceding group. Behavioral response could depend on
activity of the final population or by the mean activity of the network reaching some
threshold. The sequence of states is reproducible (similarly to that seen in taste
processing, Figure 2.2). B) Stochastic integration lies between a stable set of network
states in the absence of input (top) and deterministic integration (bottom) where input
is so strong to force a more continuous drift in network activity. C) Trial-to-trial
variability of mean network response is large. In this example, the network contains
400 cells per group, with twelve groups total. The input is low (0.1), generating very
slow integration. The Weber fraction is 0.3 as seen behaviorally. D) The mean rate
averaged over 100 trials for each of three applied currents. A wide range of ramping
rates is easily achieved (the weaker the applied current, the slower the ramping).
*Taken with permission from Miller and Wang, 2006.

In summary, while the use of stochastic transitions between discrete states
is not a very accurate method for timing, this is in fact a "selling point" of the
model, in that it does match the performance of animals, including humans,
which is far from "optimal" in this regard. Moreover, it is worth noting that

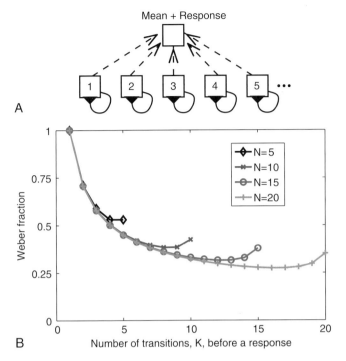

FIGURE 2.7 Weber's Law via parallel switches A) In a circuit without coupling between *N* bistable units, the mean rate depends on the number of units that have made a transition. A threshold for response would be reached when *K* of the units have transitioned to an active state. B) The Weber fraction depends on *K* and *N*. As for the serial integrator, the Weber fraction is always lower than unity and can fall to behavioral levels of 0.3. In this circuit, the sequence of states varies randomly from trial to trial, so that the trial-averaged activity of any cell resembles that of the mean population rate and slowly ramps up.

such transitions can allow behavior to arise over a range of timescales absent from the raw biological processes.

Discussion

We have reproduced evidence that cortical neurons can produce discrete states of activity, with switches between states that are reliable in content but unreliable in timing. Many groups have produced models of neural activity that can switch stochastically from one state to another (Sakai et al., 2006; Moreno-Bote et al., 2007; Okamoto et al., 2007; Marti et al., 2008; Deco and Romo, 2008;

Deco et al., 2009), but at present these models await experimental verification, specifically because it is rare to see neural data analyzed using a method, such as HMM, that allows differences between trials to be relevant.

Probably, the field of perceptual rivalry has achieved most attention using the framework of stochastic transitions between attractor states (Laing, Chow, 2002; Murata et al., 2003; Kim et al., 2006; Koene, 2006; Lankheet, 2006; Tong et al., 2006; Moreno-Bote et al., 2007; Gigante et al., 2009). Even in the absence of hard evidence for discrete transitions in neural activity, the percept of a discrete transition is strong enough to encourage modelers to use the trial-to-trial variability in timing of a discrete percept (Kim et al., 2006; Lankheet, 2006; Tong et al., 2006; O'Shea et al., 2009) as a surrogate for trial-to-trial variability in discrete states of neural activity. Recent models of perceptual rivalry (Moreno-Bote et al., 2007; Gigante et al., 2009) suggest that noise in a recurrent circuit of neurons is necessary to produce switches in percepts, while other biophysical properties such as adaptation currents may determine the precise distribution of transition times (Laing and Chow, 2002; Wilson, 2003). Ultimately, multicellular recordings are needed to validate this growing modeling effort and to distinguish competing theories. Importantly the analysis of such recordings should assume both trial-to-trial variability (Arieli et al., 1996) and correlations in the spike times of cells (Averbeck et al., 2006) in order to most effectively elucidate mechanisms of network activity. HMM is one such method, but it would be highly useful to extend this and other statistical methods (Czanner et al., 2008; Lawhem et al., 2010) in order to move the field beyond the PSTH.

REFERENCES

Abeles, M.,Bergman, H., Gat, I., Meilijson, I., Seideman, E., Tishby, N., Vaadia. E. (1995) Cortical activity flips among quasi-stationary states. *Proc. Nat. Acad. of Sci. USA 92*, 8616–8620.

Arieli, A., Sterkin, A., Grinvald, A., Aertsen, A. (1996) Dynamics of ongoing activity: Explanation of the large variability in evoked cortical responses. *Science, 273,* 1868–1871.

Averbeck, B.B., Latham, P.E., Pouget, A. (2006) Neural correlations, population coding and computation. *Nat. Rev. Neurosci., 7,* 358–366.

Czanner, G., Eden, U.T., Wirth, S., Yanike, M., Suzuki, W.A., Brown, E.N. (2008) Analysis of between-trial and within-trial neural spiking dynamics. *J. Neurophysiol., 99,* 2672–2693.

Deco, G., Romo R. (2008) The role of fluctuations in perception. *Trends Neurosci., 31,* 591–598.

Deco, G., Rolls, E.T., Romo, R. (2009) Stochastic dynamics as a principle of brain function. *Prog. Neurobiol., 88,* 1–16.

Di Lorenzo, P.M., Lemon, C.H., Reich, C.G. (2003) Dynamic coding of taste stimuli in the brainstem: Effects of brief pulses of taste stimuli on subsequent taste responses. *J. Neurosci., 23*, 8893–8902.

Durstewitz, D., Deco, G. (2008) Computational significance of transient dynamics in cortical networks. *Eur. J. Neurosci., 27*, 217–227.

Fechner, G.T. (1912) *Elemente der Psychophysik*. Ed. B. Rand. Boston: Houghton Mifflin.

Gibbon, J. (1977) Scalar expectancy theory and Weber's law in animal timing. *Psychol Rev., 84*, 279–325.

Gibbon, J., Church, R.M. (1990) Representation of time. *Cognition, 37*, 23–54.

Gigante, G., Mattia, M., Braun, J., Del Giudice, P. (2009) Bistable perception modeled as competing stochastic integrations at two levels. *PLoS Comput Biol., 5*, e1000430.

Holt, G.R., Softky, W.R., Koch, C., Douglas, R.J. (1996) Comparison of discharge variability in vitro and in vivo in cat visual cortex neurons. *J. Neurophy., 75*, 1806–1814.

Huk, A.C., Shadlen, M.N. (2005) Neural activity in macaque parietal cortex reflects temporal integration of visual motion signals during perceptual decision making. *J. Neurosci., 25*, 10420–10436.

Jones, L.M., Fontanini, A., Sadacca, B.F., Miller, P., Katz, D.B. (2007) Natural stimuli evoke dynamic sequences of states in sensory cortical ensembles. *Proc. N. Acad. of Sci. U S A 104*, 18772–18777.

Katz, D.B. (2005) The many flavors of temporal coding in gustatory cortex. *Chem Senses, 30*, Suppl 1, i80–i81.

Katz, D.B., Simon, S.A., Nicolelis, M.A.L. (2001) Dynamic and multimodal responses of gustatory cortical neurons in awake rats. *J. Neurosci., 21*, 4478–4489.

Kim, Y.J., Grabowecky, M., Suzuki, S. (2006) Stochastic resonance in binocular rivalry. *Vision Res, 46*, 392–406.

Kisley, M.A., Gerstein, G.L. (1999) Trial-to-trial variability and state-dependent modulation of auditory-evoked responses in cortex. *J of Neuroscience, 19*, 10451–10460.

Kitano, K., Okamoto, H., Fukai, T. (2003) Time representing cortical activities: Two models inspired by prefrontal persistent activity. *Biol Cybern, 88*, 387–394.

Koene, A.R. (2006) A model for perceptual averaging and stochastic bistable behavior and the role of voluntary control. *Neural Comput, 18*, 3069–3096.

Laing, C.R., Chow, C.C. (2002) A spiking neuron model for binocular rivalry. *J Comput Neurosci, 12*, 39–53.

Lankheet, M.J. (2006) Unraveling adaptation and mutual inhibition in perceptual rivalry. *J Vis, 6*, 304–310.

Lawhern, V., Wu, W., Hatsopoulos, N., Paninski, L. (2010). Population decoding of motor cortical activity using a generalized linear model with hidden states. *J. Neurosci. Methods, 189*, 267–280.

Marti, D., Deco, G., Mattia, M., Gigante, G., Del Giudice, P. (2008) A fluctuation-driven mechanism for slow decision processes in reverberant networks. *PLoS ONE 3*, e2534.

Miller, P., Wang, X.J. (2006) Stability of discrete memory states to stochastic fluctuations in neuronal systems. *Chaos, 16,* 026110.

Miller, P., Katz, D.B. (2010) Stochastic transitions between neural states in taste processing and decision-making. *J. Neurosci., 30,* 2559–2570.

Moreno-Bote, R., Rinzel, J., Rubin, N. (2007) Noise-induced alternations in an attractor network model of perceptual bistability. *J. Neurophysiol., 98,* 1125–1139.

Murata, T., Matsui, N., Miyauchi, S., Kakita, Y., Yanagida, T. (2003) Discrete stochastic process underlying perceptual rivalry. *Neuroreport, 14,* 1347–1352.

O'Shea, R.P., Parker, A., La Rooy, D., Alais, D. (2009) Monocular rivalry exhibits three hallmarks of binocular rivalry: Evidence for common processes. *Vision Res, 49,* 671–681.

Okamoto, H., Fukai, T. (2001) Neural mechanism for a cognitive timer. *Phys Rev Lett., 86,* 3919–3922.

Okamoto H, Isomura Y, Takada M, Fukai T. (2007) Temporal integration by stochastic recurrent network dynamics with bimodal neurons. *J Neurophysiol* 97: 3859–3867.

Ratcliff, R., McKoon, G. (2008) The diffusion decision model: Theory and data for two-choice decision tasks. *Neural Comput, 20,* 873–922.

Sakai, Y., Okamoto, H., Fukai, T. (2006) Computational algorithms and neuronal network models underlying decision processes. *Neural Netw., 19,* 1091–1105.

Seidemann, E., Meilijson, I., Abeles, M., Bergman, H., Vaadia, E. (1996) Simultaneously recorded single units in the frontal cortex go through sequences of discrete and stable states in monkeys performing a delayed localization task. *J of Neuroscience, 16,* 752–768.

Shadlen, M.N., Newsome, W.T. (1998) The variable discharge of cortical neurons: Implications for connectivity, computation, and information coding. *J of Neuroscience, 18,* 3870–3896.

Shadlen, M.N., Newsome, W.T. (2001) Neural basis of a perceptual decision in the parietal cortex (area LIP) of the rhesus monkey. *J of Neurophysiology, 86,* 1916–1936.

Tong, F., Meng, M., Blake, R. (2006) Neural bases of binocular rivalry. *Trends Cogn Sci., 10,* 502–511.

Wang, X.J. (2002) Probabilistic decision making by slow reverberation in cortical circuits. *Neuron, 36,* 955–968.

Weber, E.H. (1851) *Annotationes annatomicae et physiologicae.* Leipsig: CF Koehler.

Wilson, H.R. (2003) Computational evidence for a rivalry hierarchy in vision. *Proc. Nat. Acad. of Sci. USA 100,* 14499–14503.

Wong, K.F., Wang, X.J. (2006) A recurrent network mechanism of time integration in perceptual decisions. *J. Neurosci., 26,* 1314–1328.

Zohary, E., Shadlen, M.N., Newsome, W.T. (1994) Correlated neuronal discharge rate and its implications for psychophysical performance. *Nature, 370,* 140–143.

3

Neural Coding
Variability and Information

Richard B. Stein and Dirk G. Everaert

The role of neuronal variability, which is the topic of this volume, has a long history. Three men, whose pictures are included as Figure 3.1, laid the basis for our understanding of this topic more than fifty years ago, and only one would be considered primarily a neuroscientist. We were not fortunate enough to meet any of them, but they were instrumental in the entry into the field of one of us (RBS) and still influence thinking and controversies today. Claude Shannon was an electrical engineer working for Bell Labs when he published a monograph on the mathematical theory of communication (Shannon, 1948). The goal was to understand how much information could be sent down a noisy communication channel. For this purpose he measured information in terms of a binary system (using only the numbers 1 and 0), which he referred to as binary digits. The term was later shortened to *bits* of information, which is widely used today. This work had a profound influence on not only communication theory, but on many other fields, including computer science and neuroscience. A related question was raised by von Neumann (1956) about how you could make a reliable machine in terms of unreliable components. Although this question is quite general, it was motivated by the idea, already prevalent at the time, that the activity of nerve cells could be quite variable, either when studied over time under apparently constant conditions or when a constant stimulus was applied repeatedly (McCulloch and Pitts, 1943). We will return to

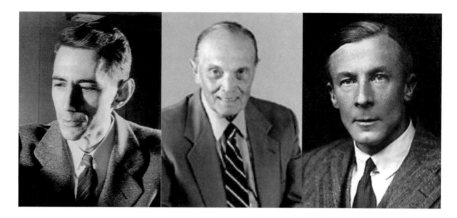

FIGURE 3.1   Three men responsible for laying the foundations for considering information in the nervous system (from left to right): Claude E. Shannon, George A. Miller, and Lord Edgar Adrian.

this point in a moment, but we first need to consider the implications of Shannon's measure of information.

Following Shannon's ideas, several papers soon appeared based on the idea that the presence or absence of an action potential in a short period of time could be considered as a 1 or a 0: namely, 1 bit of information. If the refractory period of a neuron is about 1 ms, a single neuron could be used to transmit about 1000 bits of information in a second (MacKay and McCulloch 1952; Rapoport and Horvath 1960). Since there are on the order of 10^{12} neurons in our nervous systems, this reasoning would suggest that 10^{15} bits/s of information might flow in the nervous system. In contrast to this idea, George Miller (1956), the second of the men pictured in Figure 3.1, published an article entitled "The magic number seven plus or minus two." Miller worked in the field of psychophysics, a branch of psychology that attempts to understand the relation between the physical properties of external objects and the psychological perception of these objects by our sensory systems. Miller was struck by the fact that whatever modality he studied—for example, the intensity of a sound source or the saltiness of a solution to the taste—human subjects could separate about seven different categories. Three bits of information represents eight different categories, from 000 to 111, so the conclusion can be drawn that a nervous system capable in theory of transmitting 10^{15} bits/s of information can only discriminate 3 bits of information about various sensory stimuli presented for a second. As a young graduate student, the first author of this chapter deemed this discrepancy worth investigating further, since he had worked in a physics lab for a summer building thermocouples to try to measure heat constants to another decimal place. Here was a discrepancy of $10^{15}/3 = 300$ trillion!

The initial resolution of the discrepancy raised above came from the work of Lord Edgar Adrian, the third of the men pictured in Figure 3.1. Adrian, working with a string galvanometer in Cambridge, England, was the first person to record from single sensory and motor neurons (Adrian and Zotterman, 1926; Adrian and Bronk, 1929). Each action potential produced a brief deflection of the galvanometer, and Adrian noted that increasing either the stimulus to a sensory neuron or the motor response for a motor neuron led to an increase in the rate of these action potentials. This is now referred to as a *rate* or *frequency* code. For this work, Adrian was awarded the Nobel Prize in Physiology or Medicine in 1927. How exactly does the use of a rate code resolve the discrepancy? This is illustrated in Figure 3.2, which was originally published more than forty years ago (Stein, 1967). It considers a sensory neuron that uses a frequency code as a communications channel. In the absence of a sensory input, the neuron may have a firing rate v_{min}. The presence of a sensory stimulus will determine the mean number x action potentials that will occur in a time t ($x \sim vt$), but on any given trial a number y action potentials will be produced. Thus, there are three sets of probabilities: $p(x)$, the probability that the

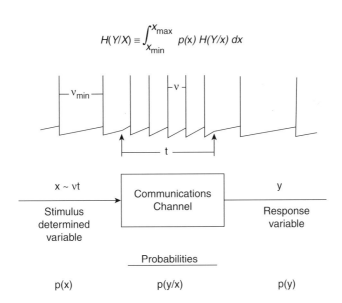

FIGURE 3.2 A nerve cell using a frequency code is considered as a communications channel and Shannon's formula is given for calculating the information transmitted (H). The other notation is explained in the text. From Stein (1967).

stimulus is x, $p(y)$ that the neuron produces y impulses, and the conditional probability $p(y/x)$ that the response is y, given that the stimulus is x. After these probabilities are measured, they can be plugged into formulae that Shannon developed to calculate the capacity of the channel. When this was done, values close to Miller's magic number 7 or 3 bits of information were obtained (Werner and Mountcastle, 1965; Matthews and Stein, 1969). This agreement is somewhat fortuitous, and a number of criticisms have been raised.

1. **Multiple pathways**. A sensory stimulus such as Miller used will activate not one neuron, but often a substantial population of neurons. With a rate code the amount of information will increase as the logarithm of the number of neurons, not linearly. A population of 10 similar neurons could generate more than twice as much information (about 6 bits) and a population of 100 neurons more than three times as much information (about 9 bits) (Stein, 1967). The information will be transmitted through several synaptic relays before reaching the level of conscious perception, however. These relays can only lose information, but whether the lost information more or less cancels the increase of information through multiple pathways is not known.

2. **Time varying inputs**. A more serious criticism is that the nervous system is not very interested in steady signals, such as the pressure of our clothing on the skin or the ambient light intensity in our surroundings. Rather, the biologically important signals are often what things are new or changing in our environment, such as the approach of a predator or the presence of prey. Information theory can be extended to time-varying signals (Stein et al., 1972), and one limiting factor is the bandwidth or range of signal frequencies that can be followed. Rapidly adapting neurons such as a Pacinian corpuscle that responds with only one or a few action potentials to a steady input can follow vibrations that are less than 1 μm in amplitude up to frequencies in the audio range (several hundred Hertz) (Sato, 1961). Thus, a Pacinian corpuscle can convey very little information about steady signals, but can provide substantial amounts of information about rapidly varying signals. The results for time-varying signals applied to a number of neurons are summarized in Table 2 in Borst and Theunissen (1999) and values tend to be in the 10's or even 100's of bits, rather than 2-3 bits.

3. **Variability and fidelity of transmission**. Another issue, which emerges from the mathematics, is that neuronal variability limits the amount

of information that can be transmitted. This applies both to steady inputs as well as to time-varying signals. The most information will be transmitted if the stimulus x in Figure 3.2 always produces the same number y impulses, yet some neurons are very regular in their firing while others are much more variable. This is seen quite dramatically in the primary and secondary muscle spindle sensory neurons that have been studied for many years. When a muscle is held at a fixed length (Figure 3.3, left) both types of neurons fire, but the secondary afferent is significantly less variable (Matthews and Stein, 1969) even when firing at a comparable frequency. Muscle spindles are unique in that they are sensory organs that contain specialized muscle fibers and these muscle fibers are innervated by specialized γ-motor neurons. The γ-motor neurons increase the firing rate of the spindles, but also increase the variability in firing markedly. The results in Figure 3.3 were obtained by studying the activity of the neurons with the ventral roots intact in a preparation with spontaneous activity of γ-motor neurons and again after cutting the ventral roots, which eliminated the activity of the γ-motor neurons.

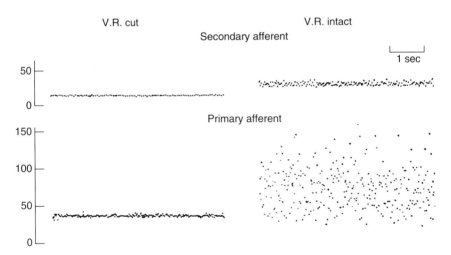

FIGURE 3.3 Instantaneous frequency in impulses/s of primary and secondary muscle spindle sensory neurons The instantaneous frequency is much more variable when the ventral roots (V.R.) are intact. This variability is due to the spontaneous activity of γ-motor neurons on the muscle spindles that is eliminated by cutting the ventral roots. However, in both situations the instantaneous frequency of the secondary afferent is less variable than that of the primary afferent. From Matthews and Stein (1969).

Why would neurons fire variably if this variability decreases information transmission? One possible answer is that neurons are operating close to physical limits of sensitivity. As we discussed in a review paper on this topic (Stein et al., 2005), the variability may be caused by the variable arrival of photons in a visual receptor or of Brownian motion affecting hair cells in the auditory system. Another possible answer was studied by using noise added as an input to a simple neural model (Figure 3.4). With low amounts of noise, the firing becomes phase-locked, i.e. one action potential is fired at the same phase of a cyclic input (cycle time =30 ms). The responses are modulated in exactly the same way when subjected to a sinusoidal stimulus as to a square wave stimulus. In other words, the nervous system would not be able to distinguish the two types of waveforms. If the firing of the neuron is more variable, then the number of action

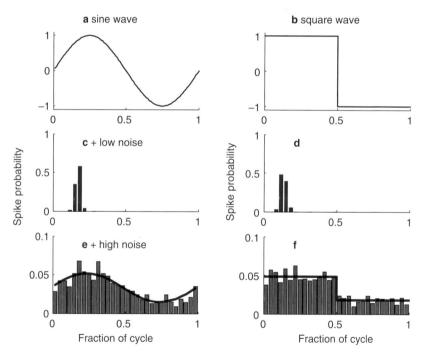

FIGURE 3.4 If a high frequency sine wave (a) or square wave (b) is applied to a neural model with low noise, the responses to the two stimuli becomes phase-locked and are indistinguishable from one another (c and d). If more noise is added to the neural model, the response is more variable but the probability of firing a spike is either modulated more sinusoidally (e) or modulated more according to the square wave (f). Modified from Stein et al. (2005).

potentials occurring at different phases of the sinusoidal stimulus
varies more sinusoidally. Similarly, the number occurring at different
phases of the square waves varies more according to this waveform.

   Although the diagram in Figure 3.4 is based on recording many
cycles of each waveform, the responses of a population of such
neurons would be similar on a cycle by cycle basis. In other words, the
fidelity of the waveform is preserved in the average response, even
though the individual responses are more variable. The primary
muscle spindle afferent responds with high gain to high frequency
signals and the variability may prevent the phase locking described in
Figure 3.4 with low noise. Auditory neurons are among the most
variable neurons in the nervous system, and this variability may help
to explain how we can distinguish the sound of two musical
instruments, such as the oboe and the violin, when both play the same
note. Other factors are probably also involved, since the notes from the
two instruments will have different harmonics, and these harmonics
will excite different places along the cochlea to different degrees.

4. **Precise timing**. Yet another issue arises when the speed of a response
   is essential. For example, if an object that is being held in the hand
   begins to slip, grip strength needs to be increased quickly; otherwise
   the object will drop. A frequency code requires at least two spikes to
   determine an "instantaneous frequency" but that may be too late to
   prevent the object from falling. Johannson and Birznieks (2004)
   studied the neural mechanisms that are involved and concluded that
   the timing of the first spikes in a population of neurons codes the
   direction of the response. The frequency of firing may signal the level
   of force that is required to hold the object. This highlights the point
   that temporal and frequency codes are not mutually exclusive and can
   be used in the same sensory neurons.

   Similar neural mechanisms may be used for maintaining balance
   in the face of perturbations. We trained cats to stand quietly on a
   platform that was suddenly tilted in each of twelve rotational
   directions. Figure 3.5 shows data from an experiment in which we
   recorded sensory neurons from the L7 dorsal root ganglion as well as
   the electrical activity of muscles (EMG), the kinematics of the
   movement and the ground reaction forces. Two opposite directions of
   perturbation are shown. In Figure 3.5A, the platform rotates upward
   against the left hind limb, causing short latency responses in both a
   skin and muscle receptor. A brief burst of EMG activity follows a short
   time later, which is the classical stretch reflex. This is an *inappropriate*

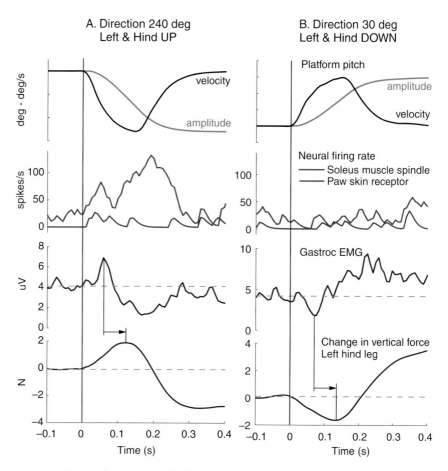

FIGURE 3.5 Postural responses of a freely standing cat on a tilting platform. If the platform is rotated in a direction of 240° (A. 8 o'clock), the left hind leg will go up. If it is rotated in a direction of 30° (B. 1 o'clock), the right front leg will go up and the left hind leg will go down. The platform movement in A flexes the leg initially, activating a muscle receptor in the soleus muscle (blue) and a skin receptor on the paw (red) of the left hind leg. A short-latency excitation is seen in the muscle (Gastrocnemius EMG) that will increase the force on the platform (bottom trace). As explained in the text, this is an inappropriate response which is reversed by a second opposite reaction, i.e. inhibition. The rotation in B in the direction of 30° initially produces an inappropriate unloading response (inhibition) that is also later reversed into excitation in order to produce the corrective forces to maintain balance. The early changes in firing rate suggest that afferents in both muscle and skin can shape the initial components of the postural response.

response, since the resultant contraction of the gastrocnemius muscle will push the cat's body even further upward and forward. The result is an initial increase in upward force in the bottom trace. There is an automatic correction that occurs slightly later, however, and it is associated with a decrease in extensor EMG. The cat's hind limb yields into flexion which, after some delay, results in a reduction of the upward force so the body is not propelled downhill and a balanced position is maintained. When the platform is moved in an opposite direction (Figure 3.5B), the left hind limb is initially unloaded. The unloading will silence the sensory receptors and lead to a decrease in extensor EMG. This decrease is again inappropriate since the body will then fall even further. An automatic correction also occurs slightly later that increases the EMG and upward force, as the limb extends to support the body in a balanced posture.

Figure 3.6 gives an overview of the firing rates of a spindle in a hind limb extensor in response to 12 different directions of perturbation for an early period (A. 20-70 ms) and a later period (B. 120-220 ms). The early period is before the start of the automatic postural response; i.e. the reversal in EMG as described above, which typically occurs at 70 to 90 ms after the onset of the perturbation (Macpherson et al., 2007). Note that these latencies in cats and the corresponding latencies in humans (Nashner, 1976) are too short to be voluntary reaction times. Figure 3.6 shows that the early and late responses were well tuned to the direction of platform rotation: the fitted sine curves accounted for more than 90% of the variance. The directional tuning was opposite for the early and late responses. A final point is that the latency of the first response (C. first spike after the perturbation) also varied with the direction of rotation, although more variably. Thus, the precise timing of the neural responses may initiate a movement in the right direction, while the firing rates over a period of time may determine the extent of the corrective movements.

A more extreme example of the same idea is used in localization of a sound source. The time of arrival of a sound at one ear relative to the other is just a fraction of one millisecond, much too short for a neuron to fire more than one spike. The earlier firing of cochlear neurons in one ear, however, can inhibit transmission in the pathway to the other ear, so that a stronger, as well as an earlier signal will be transmitted along one auditory pathway than the other. These differences can then be used to orient the head toward the sound source (Carr, 2004; Stein et al., 2005).

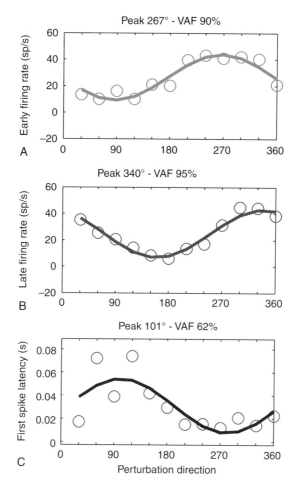

FIGURE 3.6 Responses to 12 directions of perturbation (A) in the firing rate of a spindle in an intrinsic toe plantar flexor muscle. The firing rate in spikes/s is well "tuned" to the direction of the movement, both in an early period corresponding to the reflex components (A) and the somewhat later period corresponding to the triggered postural reaction (B). The variance accounted for (VAF) by the fitted sinusoid is more than 90%. The time to the first spike is also modulated (C), although not as precisely as the firing frequency. These data suggest that first spike latency in such neurons may determine the initial direction of the response, while the firing rate may also determine the magnitude and later the reversal in EMG activity needed to maintain balance (as explained in the text).

5. **Minimum variance theory**. Section 3 above suggested that variability may have value in preserving the fidelity of the average response, but that some variability may also arise from the physical nature of the stimulus and the transmission of the signals through synaptic relays. One task of the motor system is to make movements to an end point as reliably as possible. Examples of such movements were given in the previous section to maintain balance or to orient the head. Postural stability has to be maintained despite the variability of the individual sensory and motor neurons, which again relates to von Neumann's question on how to make a reliable system out of unreliable components. This topic has been studied more recently by Wolpert and his colleagues (Harris and Wolpert, 1998; Hamilton et al., 2004). They developed a *minimum variance theory* that makes specific predictions on the assumption that the standard deviation of the motor output varies directly with the mean output. Working in Dr. Andy Schwartz' lab, we tried to test this theory. Schwartz and his colleagues train monkeys to track a variety of waveforms such as an ellipse, shown in Figure 3.7 (Schwartz, 1994; Reina and Schwartz, 2003). During the movement, the activity of cells in the motor cortex related to this movement can be recorded and the firing rate of one such cell is shown in Figure 3.7b. The firing rate of this neuron varied smoothly during the elliptical drawing task. The standard deviation of the firing rate was plotted against the mean rate, assuming this would be a reasonable measure of the motor output. In fact, the standard deviation varied as the square root of the mean rate (a slope of 0.5 on the log-log scales of Figure 3.7c) and most of the neurons recorded had a similar relationship (Figure 3.7c).

Do these experimental data disprove the minimum variance theory? May be not, since the final output is muscle force, not individual firing rates. When the standard deviation of force output is measured, it does vary linearly with the mean force output (Hamilton et al., 2004). The discrepancy arises because of the particular way in which motor neurons are recruited to fire. As first demonstrated by Henneman and his colleagues (Henneman, 1957; McPhedran et al., 1965), motor neurons tend to be recruited in order of size from small to large. The small motor neurons generate small amounts of force but the fluctuations are similarly small. Based on a model of motor units in a muscle, Figure 3.8 shows that if motor neurons were recruited randomly, then the standard deviation would vary as the square root of the mean. With Henneman's

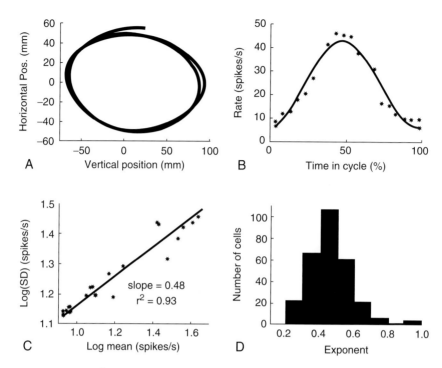

FIGURE 3.7   A monkey was trained to draw an ellipse in virtual reality (a). The mean firing rate of a cell in the motor cortex varied sinusoidally as a percentage of the average time to draw one cycle of the ellipse (b). The mean and standard deviation (SD) of the firing rate in 20 parts of the cycle were plotted on log/log coordinates. The line was fitted using linear, least mean squares techniques and had a slope near 0.5 with a high Pearson's correlation coefficient, indicative of a square root relation between these variables (c). This was typical of 286 cortical cells recorded (d). The minimum variance theory of Wolpert and his collaborators would predict a slope of 1.0, namely a linear relation between the two variables, but the discrepancy can be explained using a simulation described in Figure 3.8. Modified from Stein et al. (2005).

recruitment according to size, however, the relationship is converted to a linear one. The small motor neurons innervate muscle fibers that largely use oxidative metabolism. Therefore, they are fatigue resistant and continue to function as long as they receive oxygen through the blood system. Henneman's size principle thus serves a useful role in terms of energy utilization by the muscle, as well as minimizing the variance of the output as predicted by Wolpert.

   In conclusion, much has been learned about the processing of information in the nervous system since the pioneering work of the three men pictured in Figure 3.1. Although many neurons use the frequency coding first described by Adrian, the exact timing of a spike can also be important in localizing

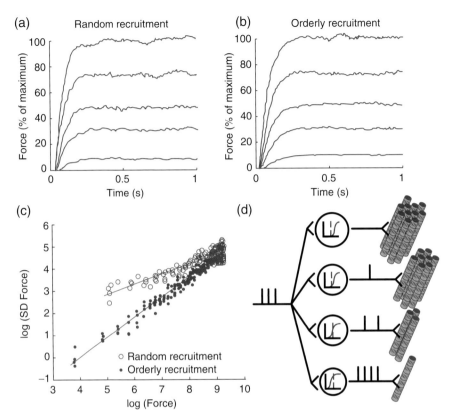

FIGURE 3.8 The variability in force was simulated using a model of a motor pool, assuming either that motor units are recruited randomly (a). Or in order of size from small to large, as first described by Henneman (b). A motor unit consists of a motor neuron and the group of muscle fibers it innervates. A motor pool is all the motor neurons innervating a given muscle. The orderly recruitment is illustrated schematically for 4 motor units of the 120 simulated in (d). Details of the simulation are given in (Jones and Bawa 1997). The orderly recruitment produces much less variability (a lower SD) at low force levels and converts the relation between the SD and the mean force from a slope near 0.5 to one near 1.0 as predicted by Wolpert's minimum variance theory. Modified from Stein et al. (2005).

a stimulus or planning a response. Neuronal variability can be unwanted noise that is minimized as described above for the motor system, but it can be also allow for more faithful transmission of a high frequency sensory signal. This flexibility in coding truly allows biological organisms to function reliably despite having somewhat unreliable neuronal elements, as first postulated by von Neumann.

REFERENCES

Adrian, E. and Bronk, D. (1929) The discharge of impulses in motor nerve fibres. Part II. The frequency of discharge in reflex and voluntary contractions. *J Physiol, 67*, 119–151.

Adrian, E and Zotterman, Y. (1926) The impulses produced by sensory nerve endings. Part 3. Impulses set up by touch and pressure. *J Physiol, 61*, 465–483.

Borst, A. and Theunissen, F.E. (1999) Information theory and neural coding. *Nat Neurosci, 2*, 947–957.

Carr, C.E. (2004) Timing is everything: organization of timing circuits in auditory and electrical sensory systems. *J Comp Neurol, 472*, 131–133.

Hamilton, A.F., Jones, K.E., Wolpert, D.M. (2004) The scaling of motor noise with muscle strength and motor unit number in humans. *Exp Brain Res, 157*, 417–430.

Harris, C.M. and Wolpert, D.M. (1998) Signal-dependent noise determines motor planning. *Nature, 394*, 780–784.

Henneman, E. (1957) Relation between size of neurons and their susceptibility to discharge. *Science, 126*, 1345–1347.

Johansson, R.S. and Birznieks, I. (2004) First spikes in ensembles of human tactile afferents code complex spatial fingertip events. *Nat Neurosci, 7*, 170–177.

Jones, K.E. and Bawa, P. (1997) Computer simulation of the responses of human motoneurons to composite 1A EPSPS: effects of background firing rate. *J. Neurophysiol., 77*, 405–420.

MacKay, D. and McCulloch, W. (1952) The limiting information capacity of a neuronal link. *Bull Math Biophys, 14*, 127–135.

Macpherson, J.M., Everaert, D.G., Stapley, P.J. and Ting, L.H. (2007) Bilateral vestibular loss in cats leads to active destabilization of balance during pitch and roll rotations of the support surface. *J. Neurophysiol., 97*, 4357–4367.

Matthews, P.B. and Stein, R.B. (1969) The regularity of primary and secondary muscle spindle afferent discharges. *J Physiol, 202*, 59–82.

McCulloch, W. and Pitts, W. (1943) A logical calculus of ideas immanent in nervous activity. *Bull Math Biophys, 5*, 115–133.

McPhedran, A.M., Wuerker, R.B., Henneman, E. (1965) Properties of motor units in a heterogeneous pale muscle (M. gastrocnemius) of the cat. *J. Neurophysiol., 28*, 85–99.

Miller, G. (1956) The magical number seven plus or minus two. Some limits on our capacity for processing information. *Psych Rev, 63*, 81–97.

Nashner, L.M. (1976) Adapting reflexes controlling the human posture. *Exp. Brain Res. 26*, 59–72.

Rapoport, A. and Horvath, W.J. (1960) The theoretical channel capacity of a single neuron as determined by various coding systems. *Information and Control, 3*, 335–350.

Reina, G.A. and Schwartz, A.B. (2003) Eye-hand coupling during closed-loop drawing: evidence of shared motor planning? *Hum Mov Sci, 22*, 137–152.

Sato. M. (1961) Response of Pacinian corpuscles to sinusoidal vibration. *J Physiol. 159*, 391–409.

Schwartz, A.B. (1994) Direct cortical representation of drawing. *Science, 265*, 540–542.

Shannon, C. (1948) A mathematical theory of communication. *Bell System Tech J, 27*, 379–423.

Stein, R.B. (1967) The information capacity of nerve cells using a frequency code. *Biophys J, 7*, 797–826.

Stein, R.B., French, A.S., Holden, A.V. (1972) The frequency response, coherence, and information capacity of two neuronal models. *Biophys J, 12*, 295–322.

Stein, R.B., Gossen, E.R., Jones, K.E. (2005) Neuronal variability: noise or part of the signal? *Nat Rev Neurosci, 6*, 389–397.

von Neumann, J. (1956) Probability logics and the synthesis of reliable organisms from unreliable components. In: Shannon, C., McCarthy, J. (Eds) *Automata Studies*. Princeton, N.J.: Princeton University Press, 43–98.

Werner, G. and Mountcastle, V.B. (1965) Neural activity in mechanoreceptive cutaneous afferents: stimulus-response relations, Weber functions, and information transmission. *J. Neurophysiol., 28*, 359–397.

Part 2: Dynamics of Neuronal Ensembles

4

Interactions between Intrinsic and Stimulus-Evoked Activity in Recurrent Neural Networks

Larry F. Abbott, Kanaka Rajan, and Haim Sompolinsky

Introduction

Trial-to-trial variability is an essential feature of neural responses, but its source is a subject of active debate. Response variability (Mast and Victor, 1991; Arieli et al., 1995, 1996; Anderson et al., 2000, 2001; Kenet et al., 2003; Petersen et al., 2003a, 2003b; Fiser et al, 2004; MacLean et al., 2005; Yuste et al., 2005; Vincent et al., 2007) is often treated as random noise, generated either by other brain areas or by stochastic processes within the circuitry being studied. We call such sources of variability "external" to stress the independence of this form of noise from activity driven by the stimulus. Variability can also be generated internally by the same network dynamics that generates responses to a stimulus. How can we distinguish between external and internal sources of response variability? Here we show that internal sources of variability inter-act nonlinearly with stimulus-induced activity, and this interaction yields a suppression of noise in the evoked state. This provides a theoretical basis and potential mechanism for the experimental observation that, in many brain areas, stimuli cause significant suppression of neuronal variability (Werner and Mountcastle, 1963; Fortier et al., 1993; Anderson et al., 2000; Friedrich and

65

Laurent, 2004; Churchland et al., 2006; Finn, Priebe and Ferster, 2007; Mitchell, Sundberg and Reynolds, 2007; Churchland et al., 2010). The combined theoretical and experimental results suggest that internally generated activity is a significant contributor to response variability in neural circuits.

We are interested in uncovering the relationship between intrinsic and stimulus-evoked activity in model networks and studying the selectivity of these networks to features of the stimuli driving them. The relationship between intrinsic and extrinsically evoked activity has been studied experimentally by comparing activity patterns across cortical maps (Arieli et al., 1995, 1996). We develop techniques for performing such comparisons in cases where there is no apparent sensory map. In addition to revealing how the temporal and spatial structure of spontaneous activity affects evoked responses, these methods can be used to infer input selectivity. Historically, selectivity was first measured by studying stimulus-driven responses (Hubel and Wiesel, 1962), and only later were similar selectivity patterns observed in spontaneous activity across the cortical surface (Arieli et al., 1995, 1996). We argue that it is possible to work in the reverse order. Having little initial knowledge of sensory maps in our networks, we show how their spontaneous activity can inform us about the selectivity of evoked responses to input features. Throughout this study, we restrict ourselves to quantities that can be measured experimentally, such as response correlations, so our analysis methods can be applied equally to theoretical models and experimental data.

We begin by describing the network model and illustrating the types of activity it produces, using computer simulations. In particular, we illustrate and discuss a transition between two types of responses: one in which intrinsic and stimulus-evoked activity coexist, and the other in which intrinsic activity is completely suppressed. Next, we explore how the spatial patterns of spontaneous and evoked responses are related. By spatial pattern, we mean the way that activity is distributed across the different neurons of the network. Spontaneous activity is a useful indicator of recurrent effects, because it is completely determined by network feedback. Therefore, we study the impact of network connectivity on the spatial pattern of input-driven responses by comparing the spatial structure of evoked and spontaneous activity. Finally, we show how the stimulus selectivity of the network can be inferred from an analysis of its spontaneous activity.

The Model

Neurons in the model we consider are described by firing-rates, they do not fire individual action potentials. Such firing-rate networks are attractive because they are easier to simulate than spiking network models and are amenable to more detailed mathematical analyses. In general, as long as there is no large-scale synchronization of action potentials, firing-rate models describe network activity adequately (Shriki et al., 2003; Wong and Wang, 2006). We consider a network of N interconnected neurons, with neuron i characterized by an activation variable x_i satisfying

$$\tau \frac{dx_i}{dt} = -x_i + g \sum_{j=1}^{N} J_{ij} r_j + I_i.$$

The time constant τ is set to 10 ms. For all of the figures, except 1.5e, $N = 1000$. The recurrent synaptic weight matrix J has element J_{ij} describing the connection from presyn aptic neuron j to postsynaptic neuron i. Excitatory connections correspond to positive matrix elements, inhibitory connections to negative elements. The input term, I_i for neuron i, takes various forms that will be described as we use them.

The firing rate of neuron i is given by $r_i = R_0 + \phi(x_i)$ with $\phi(x) = R_0 \tanh(x/R_0)$ for $x \le 0$ and $\phi(x) = (R_{max} - R_0) \tanh(x/(R_{max} - R_0))$ for $x > 0$. Here, R_0 is the background firing rate (the firing rate when $x = 0$), and R_{max} is the maximum firing rate. This function allows us to specify independently the maximum firing rate, R_{max}, and the background rate, R_0, and set them to reasonable values, while retaining the general form of the commonly used tanh function. This firing rate function is plotted in Figure 4.1 for $R_0 = 0.1 R_{max}$, the value we use. To facilitate comparison with experimental data in a variety of systems, we report all responses relative to R_{max}. Similarly, we report all input currents relative to the current $I_{1/2}$ required to drive an isolated neuron to half of its maximal firing rate (see Figure 4.1).

Although a considerable amount is known about the statistical properties of recurrent connections in cortical circuitry (Holmgren et al., 2003; Song et al., 2005), we do not have anything like the specific neuron-to-neuron wiring diagram we would need to build a truly faithful model of a cortical column or hypercolumn. Instead, we construct the connection matrix J of the model network on the basis of a statistical description of the underlying circuitry. We do this by choosing elements of the synaptic weight matrix independently and randomly from a Gaussian distribution with zero mean and variance $1/N$. We could divide the network into separate excitatory and inhibitory subpopulations, but this does not qualitatively change the network properties that we discuss (van Vreeswijk and Sompolinsky, 1996, 1998; Rajan and Abbott, 2006).

The parameter g controls the strength of the synaptic connections in the model, but because these strengths are chosen from a distribution with zero mean and nonzero variance, g actually controls the size of the standard deviation

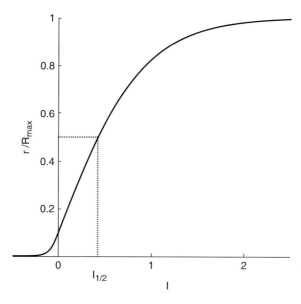

FIGURE 4.1   The firing rate function used in the network model versus the input I for $R_0 = 0.1R_{max}$ normalized by the maximum firing rate R_{max}. The parameter $I_{1/2}$ is defined by the dashed lines.

of the synaptic strengths (see discussion, page 79). Without any input ($I_i = 0$ for all i) and for large networks (large N), two spontaneous patterns of activity are seen. If $g < 1$, the network is in a trivial state in which $x_i = 0$ and $r_i = R_0$ for all neurons (all i). The case $g > 1$ is more interesting in that the spontaneous activity of the network is chaotic, meaning that it is irregular, non-repeating and highly sensitive to initial conditions (Sompolinsky et al., 1988; van Vreeswijk and Sompolinsky, 1996, 1998). We typically use a value of $g = 1.5$, meaning that our networks are in this chaotic state prior to activating any inputs.

Responses to Step Input

To begin our examination of the effects of input on chaotic spontaneous network activity, we consider the effect of a step of input (from 0 to a positive value) applied uniformly to every neuron ($I_i = I$ for all i). Before the input is turned on (Figure 4.2a and b, $t < 1000$ ms), a typical neuron of the network shows the highly irregular activity characteristic of the chaotic spontaneous state. When a sufficiently strong stimulus is applied, however, the internally generated fluctuations are completely suppressed (Figure 4.2a and b, $t > 1000$ ms). We contrast

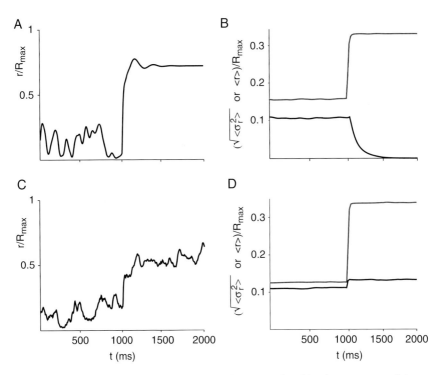

FIGURE 4.2 Firing rates and response variability normalized by the maximum firing rate, R_{max}, for a stimulus input stepping from zero to a constant, non-zero value at $t = 1000$ ms. Left column shows the firing rate of a typical neuron in a network with 1000 neurons. Right column shows the average firing rate (red traces) and the square root of the average firing-rate variance (black traces) across the network neurons. a–b) A network with chaotic spontaneous activity receiving no noise input. The response variability (b, black trace) drops to zero when the stimulus input is present. c–d) A network without spontaneous activity but receiving noise input. The response variability (d, black trace) rises slightly when the step input is turned on. The stochastic input in this example was independent white noise to each neuron, low-pass filtered with a 500 ms time constant.

this behavior to that of external noise, by turning off the recurrent dynamics and generating fluctuations with external stochastic inputs (Figure 4.2c and d). In this case, there is no reduction in the amplitude of the neuronal fluctuations when a stimulus is applied, in fact there is a small increase. Note that the increase in the mean activity is similar in both cases. These results reveal a critical distinction between internally and externally generated fluctuations – the former can be suppressed by a stimulus and therefore do not necessarily interfere with sensory processing.

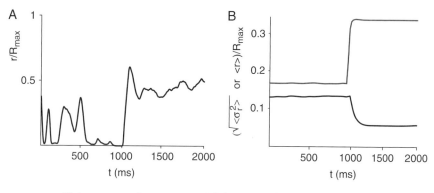

FIGURE 4.3 Firing rates and response variability normalized by the maximum firing rate, R_{max}, for the same network, stimulus and noise as in Figure 4.2, but for a network with both spontaneous activity and injected noise. a) The response of a typical neuron. b) The average firing rate (red trace) increases and the response variability (black trace) decreases when the stimulus input is present, but it does not go to zero as in Figure 4.2b.

To reveal the nature of internally generated variability, we have considered an idealized scenario in Figure 4.2, in which there was no external source of noise. In reality, we expect both external and internal sources of noise to coexist in local cortical circuits. As long as the internal noise provides a substantial component of the overall variability, our qualitative results remain valid. We can simulate this situation by adding external noise (as in Figure 4.2c and d) to a model that exhibits chaotic spontaneous activity (as in Figure 4.2a and b). The result shows a sharp drop in variance at stimulus onset, but with only partial rather than complete suppression of response variability (Figure 4.3). This result is in good agreement with experimental data (Churchland et al., 2010).

Response to Periodic Input

For Figures 4.2 and 4.3, the stimulus consisted of a step input applied identically to all neurons. To investigate the effect of more interesting and realistic stimuli on the chaotic activity of a recurrent network, we consider inputs with nonhomogeneous spatio-temporal structure. Specifically, we introduce inputs that oscillate in a sinusoidal manner with amplitude I and frequency f and examine how the suppression of fluctuations depends on their amplitude and frequency. In many cases, neurons in a local population have diverse stimulus selectivities, so a particular stimulus may induce little change in the total activity across the network. To mimic this situation, we give these oscillating inputs a different phase for each neuron (in terms of a visual stimulus, this is equivalent to presenting a drifting grating to a population of simple cells with different spatial-phase selectivities). Specifically, $I_i = I\cos(2\pi ft + \theta_i)$, where θ_i is chosen randomly from a uniform distribution between 0 and 2π. The randomly assigned phases ensure that the spatial pattern of input in our model network is not correlated with the pattern of recurrent connectivity.

In the absence of a stimulus input, the firing rates of individual neurons fluctuate irregularly, (Figure 4.4a-i) and the power spectrum across network neurons is continuous and decays exponentially as a function of frequency (Figure 4.4b-i), a characteristic features of the chaotic state of this network (Sompolinsky, Crisanti, and Sommers, 1988). When the network is driven by a weak oscillatory input, the single-neuron response is a superposition of a periodic pattern induced by the input and a chaotic background (Figure 4.4a-ii) The power spectrum shows a continuous component due to the residual chaos and peaks at the frequency of the input and its harmonics, reflecting the periodic but nonsinusoidal component of the response (Figure 4.4b-ii). For an input with a larger amplitude, the firing rates of network neurons are periodic (Figure 4.4a-iii), and the power spectrum shows only peaks at the input frequency and its harmonics, with no continuous spectrum (Figure 4.4b-iii).

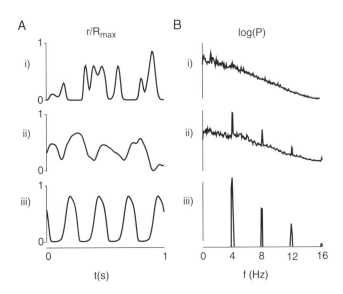

FIGURE 4.4 A chaotic network of 1000 neurons receiving sinusoidal 5 Hz input. a) Firing rates of typical network neurons (normalized by R_{max}). b) The logarithm of the power spectrum of the activity across the network . i) With no input ($I = 0$), network activity is chaotic. ii) In the presence of a weak input ($I/I_{1/2} = 0.1$), an oscillatory response is superposed on chaotic fluctuations. iii) For a stronger input ($I/I_{1/2} = 0.5$), the network response is periodic.

This indicates a complete suppression of the internally generated fluctuations as in Figure 4.2a and b.

We have used a mean-field approach similar to that developed by Sompolinsky and colleagues (1988) to analyze properties of the transition between chaotic and periodic responses to a periodic stimulus (Rajan et al., 2010). This extends previous work on the effect of input on chaotic network activity (Molgedey et al., 1992; Bertschinger and Natschläger, 2004) to continuous time models and periodic inputs. We find that there is a critical input intensity (a critical value of I) that depends on f and g, below which network activity is chaotic though driven by the input (as in Figures 4.4a-ii and b-ii) and above which it is periodic (as in Figures 4.4a-iii and b-iii.) A surprising feature of this critical amplitude is that it is a nonmonotonic function of the frequency f of the input. As a result, there is a "best" frequency at which it is easiest to entrain the network and suppress chaos. For the parameters we use, the "best" frequency is around 5 Hz, a frequency were many sensory systems tend to operate. There are some initial experimental indications that this is indeed the optimal frequency for suppressing background activity by visual stimulation (White, Abbott, Fiser, unpublished). It is interesting that a preferred input frequency for entrainment arises even though the power spectrum of the spontaneous activity does not show any resonant features (Figure 4.4b-i).

Principal Component Analysis of Spontaneous and Evoked Activity

The results of the previous two sections revealed a regime in which an input generates a nonchaotic network response, even though the network is chaotic in the absence of input. Although the chaotic intrinsic activity has been completely suppressed in this network state, its imprint can still be detected in the spatial pattern of the nonchaotic activity.

The network state at any instant can be described by a point in an N-dimensional space with coordinates equal to the firing rates of the N neurons. Over time, activity traverses a trajectory in this N-dimensional space. Principal component analysis can be used to delineate the subspace in which this trajectory predominantly lies. The analysis is done by diagonalizing the equal-time cross-correlation matrix of network firing rates, $\langle r_i(t)r_j(t)\rangle$, where the angle brackets denote an average over time. The eigenvalues of this matrix expressed as a fraction of their sum (denoted by $\tilde{\lambda}_a$), indicate the distribution of variances across different orthogonal directions in the activity trajectory. In the spontaneous state, there are a number of significant contributors to the total variance, as indicated in Figure 4.5a. For this value of g, the leading 10% of the components account for 90% of the total variance. The variance

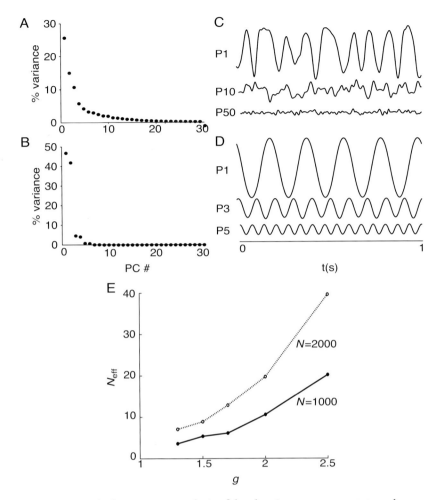

FIGURE 4.5 Principal component analysis of the chaotic spontaneous state and nonchaotic driven state. a) Percent variance accounted for by different principal components for chaotic spontaneous activity.b) Same as a, but for nonchaotic driven activity. c) Projections of the chaotic spontaneous activity onto principal component vectors 1, 10 and 50 (in decreasing order of variance). d) Projections of periodic driven activity onto principal components 1, 3, and 5. Projections onto components 2, 4, and 6 are similar except for being phase shifted by $\pi/2$. e) The effective dimension, N_{eff}, of the trajectory of chaotic spontaneous activity (defined in the text) as a function of g for networks with 1000 (solid circles) or 2000 (open circles) neurons. Parameters: $g = 1.5$ for a-d, and $f = 5$ and $I/I_{1/2} = 0.7$ for b and d.

associated with higher components falls off exponentially. It is interesting to note that the projections of the network activity onto the principal component directions fluctuate more rapidly for higher components (Figure 4.5c), revealing the interaction between the spatial and temporal structure of the chaotic fluctuations.

The nonchaotic driven state is approximately two dimensional (Figure 4.5b), with the two dimensions describing a circular oscillatory orbit. Projections of this orbit correspond to oscillations $\pi/2$ apart in phase. The residual variance in the higher dimensions reflects higher harmonics arising from network nonlinearity, as illustrated by the projections in Figure 4.5d.

To quantify the dimension of the subspace containing the chaotic trajectory in more detail, we introduce the quantity

$$N_{\text{eff}} = \left(\sum_{a=1}^{N} \tilde{\lambda}_a^2 \right)^{-1}.$$

This provides a measure of the effective number of principal components describing a trajectory. For example, if n principal components share the total variance equally, and the remaining $N - n$ principal components have zero variance, $N_{\text{eff}} = n$. For the chaotic spontaneous state in the networks we study, N_{eff} increases with g (Figure 4.5e), due to the higher amplitude and frequency content of the chaotic activity for large g. Note that N_{eff} scales approximately with N, which means that large networks have proportionally higher-dimensional chaotic activity (compare the two traces in Figure 4.5e). The fact that the number of activated modes is only 2% of the system dimensionality, even for g as high as 2.5, is another manifestation of the deterministic nature of the fluctuations. For comparison, we calculated N_{eff} for a similar network driven by external white noise, with g set below the chaotic transition at $g = 1$. In this case, N_{eff} only assumes such low values when g is within a few percent of the critical value 1. The results in Figure 4.5 illustrate another feature of the suppression of spontaneous activity by input, which is that the PCA dimension N_{eff} is reduced dramatically by the presence of the input.

Network Effects on the Spatial Pattern of Evoked Activity

In the nonchaotic regime, the temporal structure of network responses is largely determined by the input; they both oscillate at the same frequency, although the network activity includes harmonics not present in the input. The input does not, however, exert nearly as strong control on the spatial structure of the network response. The phases of the firing-rate oscillations of network neurons are only partially correlated with the phases of the inputs that drive them, and they are strongly influenced by the recurrent feedback.

We have seen that the orbit describing the activity in the nonchaotic driven state consists primarily of a circle in a two-dimensional subspace of the full N-dimensions describing neuronal activities. We now ask how this circle aligns relative to subspaces defined by different numbers of principal components that characterize the spontaneous activity. This relationship is difficult to visualize because both the chaotic subspace and the full space of network activities are high dimensional. To overcome this difficulty, we make use of the notion of "principal angles" between subspaces (Ipsen and Meyer, 1995).

The first principal angle is the angle between two unit vectors (called principal vectors), one in each subspace, that have the maximum overlap (dot product). Higher principal angles are defined recursively as the angles between pairs of unit vectors with the highest overlap that are orthogonal to the previously defined principal vectors. Specifically, for two subspaces of dimension d_1 and d_2 defined by the orthogonal unit vectors V_1^a, for $a = 1, 2, \ldots, d_1$ and V_2^b, for $b = 1, 2, \ldots, d_2$, the cosines of the principal angles are equal to the singular values of the d_1 by d_2 matrix formed from all the possible dot products of these two vectors. The resulting principal angles vary between 0 and $\pi/2$, with zero angles appearing when parts of the two subspaces overlap and $\pi/2$ corresponding to directions in which the two subspaces are completely non-overlapping. The angle between two subspaces is the largest of their principal angles. This definition is illustrated in Figure 4.6a, in which we show the irregular trajectory of the chaotic spontaneous activity, described by its two leading principal components (black curve in Figure 4.6a). The circular orbit of the periodic activity (red curve in Figure 4.6a) has been rotated by the smaller of its two principal angles. The angle between these two subspaces (the angle depicted in Figure 4.6a) is then the remaining angle through which the periodic orbit would have to be rotated to bring it into alignment with the horizontal plane containing the two-dimensional projection of the chaotic trajectory.

Figure 4.6a shows the angle between the subspaces defined by the first two principal components of the orbit of periodic driven activity and the first two principal components of the chaotic spontaneous activity. We now extend this idea to a comparison of the two-dimensional subspace of the periodic orbit and subspaces defined by the first m principal components of the chaotic spontaneous activity. This allows us to see how the orbit lies in the full N-dimensional space of neuronal activities relative to the trajectory of the chaotic spontaneous activity. The results (Figure 4.6b, red dots) show that this angle is close to $\pi/2$ for small m, equivalent to the angle between two randomly chosen subspaces. The value drops quickly for subspaces defined by progressively more of the leading principal components of the chaotic activity. Ultimately, this angle approaches zero when all N of the chaotic principal component vectors are considered, as it must, because these span the entire space of network activities.

In the periodic state, the temporal phases of the different neurons determine the orientation of the orbit in the space of neuronal activities. The rapidly falling angle between this orbit and the subspaces defined by spatial patterns

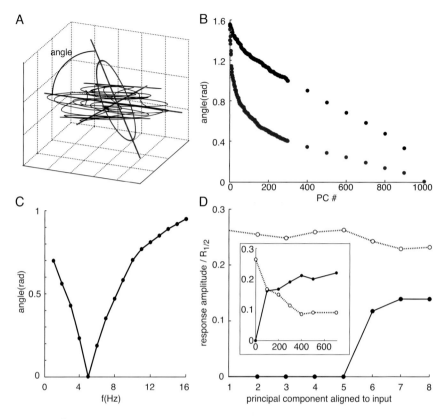

FIGURE 4.6 Spatial pattern of network responses. a) Definition of the angle between the subspace defined by the first two components of the chaotic activity (black curve) and a two-dimensional description of the periodic orbit (red curve). b) Relationship between the orientation of periodic and chaotic trajectories. Angles between the subspace defined by the two principal components of the non-chaotic driven state and subspaces formed by principal components 1 through m of the chaotic spontaneous activity, where m appears on the horizontal axis (red dots). Black dots show the analogous angles but with the two-dimensional subspace defined by random input phases replacing the subspace of the non-chaotic driven activity. c) Effect of input frequency on the orientation of the periodic orbit. The angle (vertical axis) between the subspaces defined by the two leading principal components of non-chaotic driven activity at different frequencies (horizontal axis) and these two vectors for a 5 Hz input frequency. d) Network selectivity to different spatial patterns of input. Signal (dashed curves and open circles) and noise (solid curves and filled circles) amplitudes in response to inputs aligned to the leading principal components of the spontaneous activity of the network. The inset shows a larger range on a coarser scale. Parameters: $I/I_{1/2} = 0.7$ and $f = 5$ Hz for b, $I/I_{1/2} = 1.0$ for c, and $I/I_{1/2} = 0.2$ and $f = 2$ Hz for d.

dominating the chaotic state (Figure 4.6b, red dots) indicates that these phases are strongly influenced by the recurrent connectivity that in turn determines the spatial pattern of the spontaneous activity. As an indication of the magnitude of this effect, we note that the angles between the random phase sinusoidal trajectory of the input to the network and the same chaotic subspaces are much larger than those associated with the periodic network activity (Figure 4.6b, black dots).

Temporal Frequency Modulation of Spatial Patterns

Although recurrent feedback in the network plays an important role in the spatial structure of driven network responses, the spatial pattern of the activity is not fixed but instead is shaped by a complex interaction between the driving input and the intrinsic network dynamics. It is therefore sensitive to both the amplitude and the frequency of this drive. To see this, we examine how the orientation of the approximately two-dimensional periodic orbit of driven network activity in the nonchaotic regime depends on input frequency. We use the technique of principal angles described in the previous section, to examine how the orientation of the oscillatory orbit changes when the input frequency is varied. For comparison purposes, we choose the dominant two-dimensional subspace of the network oscillatory responses to a driving input at 5 Hz as a reference. We then calculate the principal angles between this subspace and the corresponding subspaces evoked by inputs with different frequencies. The result shown in Figure 4.6c indicates that the orientation of the orbit for these driven states rotates as the input frequency changes.

The frequency dependence of the orientation of the evoked response is likely related to the effect seen in Figure 4.5b in which higher frequency activity is projected onto higher principal components of the spontaneous activity. This causes the orbit of driven activity to rotate in the direction of higher-order principal components of the spontaneous activity as the stimulus frequency increases. In addition, the larger the stimulus amplitude, the closer the response phases of the neurons will be to the random phases of their external inputs (results not shown).

Network Selectivity

We have shown that the response of a network to random-phase input is strongly affected by the spatial structure of spontaneous activity (Figure 4.6b).

We now ask if the spatial patterns that dominate the spontaneous activity in a network correspond to the spatial input patterns to which the network responds most vigorously. Rather than using random-phase inputs, we now aligned the inputs to our network along the directions defined by different principal components of its spontaneous activity. Specifically, the input to neuron i is set to IV_i^a $\cos(2\pi ft)$, where I is the amplitude factor and V_i^a is the ith component of principal component vector a of the spontaneous activity. The index a is ordered so that $a = 1$ corresponds to the principal component with largest variance and $a = N$ the least. To analyze the results of using this input, we divide the response into a signal component corresponding to the trial-averaged response, and a noise component consisting of the fluctuations around this average response. We call the amplitude of the signal component of the response the "signal amplitude" and the standard deviation of the fluctuations the "noise amplitude".

As seen in Figure 4.6d the amplitude of the signal component of the response decreases slowly as a function of which principal component is used to define the input. A more dramatic effect is seen on the noise component of the response. For the input amplitude used in Figure 4.6d, inputs aligned to the first five principal components of the spontaneous activity completely suppress the chaotic noise, resulting in periodic driven activity. For higher-order principal components, the network activity is chaotic. Thus, the "noise" shows more sensitivity to the spatial structure of the input than the signal.

Discussion

Our results suggest that experiments that study the stimulus-dependence of the typically ignored noise component of responses should be interesting and could provide insight into the nature and origin of activity fluctuations. Response variability and ongoing activity are sometimes modeled as arising from a stochastic process external to the network generating the responses. This stochastic noise is then added linearly to the signal to create the total neuronal activity in the evoked state. Our results indicate that recurrent dynamics of the cortical circuit are likely to contribute significantly to the emergence of irregular neuronal activity, and that the interaction between such deterministic "noise" and external drive is highly nonlinear. In our work (Rajan et al., 2010), we have shown that the stimulus causes a strong suppression of activity fluctuations and furthermore that the nonlinear interaction between the relatively slow chaotic fluctuations and the stimulus results in a nonmonotonic frequency dependence of the noise suppression.

An important feature of the networks we study is that the variance of the synaptic strengths across the network controls the emergence of interesting complex dynamics. This has important implications for experiments because it suggests that the most interesting and relevant modulators of networks may be substances or activity-dependent modulations that do not necessarily change properties of synapses on average, but rather change synaptic variance. Synaptic variance can be changed either by modifying the range over which synaptic strengths vary across a population of synapses, as we have done here, or by modifying the release probability and variability of quantal size at single synapses. Such modulators might be viewed as less significant because they do not change the net balance between excitation and inhibition. Network modeling suggests, however, that such modulations are of great importance in controlling the state of the neuronal circuit.

The random character of the connectivity in our network precludes a simple description of the spatial activity patterns in terms of topographically organized maps. Our analysis shows that even in cortical areas for which the underlying connectivity does not exhibit systematic topography, dissecting the spatial patterns of fluctuations in neuronal activity can reveal important insights about both intrinsic network dynamics and stimulus selectivity. Principal component analysis revealed that despite the fact that the network connectivity matrix is full rank, the effective dimensionality of the chaotic fluctuations is much smaller than the number of neurons in the network. This suppression of spatial modes is much stronger than expected from a linear network low-pass filtering a spatio-temporal white noise input. Furthermore, as in the temporal domain, active spatial patterns exhibit strong nonlinear interaction between external driving inputs and intrinsic dynamics. Surprisingly, even when the stimulus amplitude is strong enough to fully entrain the temporal pattern of network activity, spatial organization of the activity is still strongly influenced by recurrent dynamics, as shown in Figures 4.6c and 4.6d.

We have presented tools for analyzing the spatial structure of chaotic and non-chaotic population responses based on principal component analysis and angles between the resulting subspaces. Principal component analysis has been applied profitably to neuronal recordings (see, for example, Broome et al., 2006). These analyses often plot activity trajectories corresponding to different network states using the fixed principal component coordinates derived from combined activities under all conditions. Our analysis offers a complementary approach whereby principal components are derived for each stimulus condition separately, and principal angles are used to reveal not only the difference between the shapes of trajectories corresponding to different network states, but also the difference in the orientation of the low dimensional subspaces of these trajectories within the full space of neuronal activity.

Many models of selectivity in cortical circuits rely on knowledge of the spatial organization of afferent inputs as well as cortical connectivity. However, in many cortical areas, such information is not available. Our results show that experimentally accessible spatial patterns of spontaneous activity (e.g., from voltage- or calcium-sensitive optical imaging experiments) can be used to infer the stimulus selectivity induced by the network dynamics and to design spatially extended stimuli that evoke strong responses. This is particularly true when selectivity is measured in terms of the ability of a stimulus to entrain the neural dynamics, as in Figure 4.6d. In general, our results indicate that the analysis of spontaneous activity can provide valuable information about the computational implications of neuronal circuitry.

Acknowledgments

Research of Rajan and Abbott supported by National Science Foundation grant IBN-0235463 and an NIH Director's Pioneer Award, part of the NIH Roadmap for Medical Research, through grant number 5-DP1-OD114-02. Sompolinksy is partially supported by grants from the Israel Science Foundation and the McDonnell Foundation. This research was also supported by the Swartz Foundation through the Swartz Centers at Columbia and Harvard Universities.

REFERENCES

Anderson, J.S., Lampl, I., Gillespie, D.C., Ferster, D. (2000). The contribution of noise to contrast invariance of orientation tuning in cat visual cortex. *Science*, *290*, 1968–972.

Anderson, J.S., Lampl, I., Gillespie, D.C. and Ferster, D. (2001). Membrane potential and conductance changes underlying length tuning of cells in cat primary visual cortex. *J. Neurosci.*, *21*, 2104–2112.

Arieli, A., Shoham, D., Hildesheim, R. and Grinvald, A. (1995). Coherent spatiotemporal patterns of ongoing activity revealed by real-time optical imaging coupled with single-unit recording in the cat visual cortex. *J. Neurophysiol. 73*, 2072–2093.

Arieli, A., Sterkin, A., Grinvald, A. and Aertsen, A. (1996). Dynamics of ongoing activity: explanation of the large variability in evoked cortical responses. *Science*, *273*, 1868–1871.

Bertschinger, N. and Natschläger, T. (2004). Real-time computation at the edge of chaos in recurrent neural networks. *Neural Comput.*, *16*, 1413–1436.

Broome, B.M., Jayaraman, V. and Laurent, G. (2006). Encoding and decoding of overlapping odor sequences. *Neuron, 51,* 467–482.

Churchland M.M., Yu B.M., Cunningham J.P., Sugrue L.P., Cohen M.R., Corrado G.S., Newsome W.T., Clark A.M., Hosseini P., Scott B.B., Bradley D.C., Smith M.A., Kohn A., Movshon J.A., Armstrong K.M., Moore T., Chang S.W., Snyder L.H., Lisberger S.G., Priebe N.J., Finn I.M., Ferster D., Ryu S.I., Santhanam G., Sahani M., Shenoy K.V. (2010). Stimulus onset quenches neural variability: a widespread cortical phenomenon. *Nat Neurosci 13,* 369–378.

Churchland, M.M., Yu, B.M., Ryu, S.I., Santhanam, G. and Shenoy, K.V. (2006). Neural variability in premotor cortex provides a signature of motor preparation. *J. Neurosci., 26,* 3697– 3712.

Finn, I.M., Priebe, N.J. and Ferster, D. (2007). The emergence of contrast-invariant orientation tuning in simple cells of cat visual cortex. *Neuron, 54,* 137–152.

Fiser, J., Chiu, C. and Weliky, M. (2004). Small modulation of ongoing cortical dynamics by sensory input during natural vision. *Nature, 431,* 573–578.

Fortier, P.A. Smith, A.M. and Kalaska, J.F. (1993). Comparison of cerebellar and motor cortex activity during reaching: directional tuning and response variability. *J. Neurophysiol., 69,* 1136–1149.

Friedrich, R.W. and Laurent, G. (2004). Dynamics of olfactory bulb input and output activity during odor stimulation in zebrafish. *J. Neurophysiol., 91,* 2658–2669.

Holmgren, C., Harkany, T., Svennenfors, B. and Zilberter, Y. (2003). Pyramidal cell communication within local networks in layer 2/3 or rat neocortex. *J. Physiol., 551,* 139–153.

Hubel, D.H. and Wiesel, T.N. (1962). Receptive fields, binocular interaction and functional architecture in the cat's visual cortex. *J. Physiol., 160,* 106–154.

Ipsen, I.C.F. and Meyer, C.D. (1995). The angle between complementary subspaces. *Amer. Math. Monthly, 102,* 904-911.

Kenet, T., Bibitchkov, D., Tsodyks, M., Grinvald, A. and Arieli, A. (2003). Spontaneously emerging cortical representations of visual attributes. *Nature, 425,* 954–956.

MacLean, J.N., Watson, B.O., Aaron, G.B. and Yuste, R. (2005). Internal dynamics determine the cortical response to thalamic stimulation. *Neuron, 48,* 811–823.

Mast, J. and Victor, J.D. (1991). Fluctuations of steady-state VEPs: interaction of driven evoked potentials and the EEG. *Electroenceph. and Clinic. Neurophysiol., 78,* 389–401.

Mitchell, J.F., Sundberg, K.A. and Reynolds, J.J. (2007). Differential attention-dependent response modulation across cell classes in macaque visual area V4. *Neuron, 55,* 131–41.

Molgedey, L., Schuchhardt, J. and Schuster, H.G. (1992). Suppressing chaos in neural networks by noise. *Phys. Rev. Lett., 69,* 3717–3719.

Petersen, C.C., Grinvald, A. and Sakmann, B. (2003). Spatiotemporal dynamics of sensory responses in layer 2/3 of rat barrel cortex measured in vivo by voltage-sensitive dye imaging combined with whole-cell voltage recordings and neuron reconstructions. *J. Neurosci. 23,* 1298–1309.

Petersen, C.C., Hahn, T.T., Mehta, M., Grinvald, A. and Sakmann, B. (2003). Interaction of sensory responses with spontaneous depolarization in layer 2/3 barrel cortex. *Proc Natl Acad Sci USA 100*, 13638–13643.

Rajan, K. and Abbott, L.F. (2006). Eigenvalue spectra of random matrices for neural networks. *Phys. Rev. Lett.*, 97, 188104.

Rajan, K., Abbott, L.F. and Sompolinsky, H. (2010). Stimulus-dependent suppression of chaos in recurrent neural networks. *Phys Rev E 82*, 011903.

Shriki, O., Hansel, D. and Sompolinsky, H. (2003). Rate models for conductance-based cortical neuronal networks. *Neural Comput*, 15, 1809–1841.

Sompolinsky, H., Crisanti, A. and Sommers, H.J. (1988). Chaos in random neural networks. *Phys. Rev. Lett.*, 61, 259–262.

Song, S., Sjöström, P.J., Reigl, M., Nelson, S.B. and Chklovskii, D.B. (2005). Highly non-random features of synaptic connectivity in local cortical circuits. *PLoS Biol.*, 3, e68.

van Vreeswijk, C. and Sompolinsky, H. (1996). Chaos in neuronal networks with balanced excitatory and inhibitory activity. *Science*, 24, 1724–1726.

van Vreeswijk, C. and Sompolinsky, H. (1998). Chaotic balanced state in a model of cortical circuits. *Neural Comput.*, 10, 1321–1371.

Vincent, J.L., Patel, G.H., Fox, M.D., Snyder, A.Z., Baker, J.T., Van Essen, D.C., Zempel, J.M., Snyder, L.H., Corbetta, M. and Raichle, M.E. (2007). Intrinsic functional architecture in the anaesthetized monkey brain. *Nature*, 447, 83–86.

Werner, G. and Mountcastle, V.B. (1963). The variability of central neural activity in a sensory system, and its implications for the central reflection of sensory events. *J. Neurophysiol.*, 26, 958–977.

Wong, K.-F. and Wang, X.-J. (2006). A recurrent network mechanism of time integration in perceptual decisions. *J. Neurosci.*, 26, 1314–1328.

Yuste, R., MacLean, J.N., Smith, J. and Lansner, A. (2005). The cortex as a central pattern generator. *Nat. Rev. Neurosci.*, 6, 477–483.

5

Inherent Biases in Spontaneous Cortical Dynamics

Chou P. Hung, Benjamin M. Ramsden, and Anna Wang Roe

Measurements of spatial and temporal patterns of ongoing (spontaneous) activity in the "resting" (unstimulated) brain provide a valuable insight into the fundamental mechanisms underlying neural information processing. Calculations of information content and signal processing are critically dependent upon the validity of the null assumption—how we define what is "signal" and what is "noise" (Shadlen and Newsome, 1994; Gusnard and Raichle, 2001). One major issue is the level of structure present in spontaneous cortical network activity. While spontaneous neuronal activity may be thought of as "stochastic" in nature, covariations do exist between neighboring neurons and neurons with similar functional tuning (Cox, 1962; Perkel et al., 1967a, 1967b; Ts"o et al., 1986, 1988; Gray et al., 1989; Amzica and Steriade, 1995; Nowak et al., 1995; deCharms and Merzenich, 1996; Leopold et al., 2003). Furthermore, recent papers have elaborated upon this view by suggesting that noise during spontaneous activity appears as a series of random jumps between different population activity patterns that are linked to the underlying cortical structure (e.g., orientation maps in V1; Softky and Koch, 1992, 1993; Arieli et al., 1995; Tsodyks and Sejnowski, 1995; Amit and Brunel, 1997; Tsodyks et al., 1999; Kenet et al., 2003). Here, we propose that such "jumps" are not random, but that there are inherent biases (directionality) in the shift from one population activity pattern to another. We predict that such inherent biases would be seen in directional interactions between different response types during spontaneous activity.

To test this prediction, we chose to study interactions between two types of neurons in early visual cortex "oriented" and "luminance-modulated" (LM) neurons using cross-correlation methods. Orientation-selective neurons are commonly encountered in Areas 17 and 18 of the cat (the first and second visual cortical areas), and they are likely to play a role in the initial encoding of object borders and shape (e.g., Hubel and Wiesel, 1969). LM cells respond to large-field modulations of luminance without the presence of orientation cues and are hypothesized to play a role in processing surface brightness information (Rossi et al., 1996; Hung et al., 2001). That orientation-selective (e.g. Malach et al. 1993; Kisvarday et al., 1997; Kenet et al., 2003) and LM selective (Livingstone and Hubel,1984; Shoham et al., 1997; Tani et al., 2003) neurons have distinct organizations is reasonably well supported. Thus, oriented and LM cells comprise two functional cell types that are distinguishable on physiological, anatomical, and psychophysical bases. We report here that, under spontaneous conditions, a directional, non-random interaction exists between LM cells and oriented cells. Thus, in addition to spatial structure, these data suggest temporal structure in cortical baseline activity.

Methods

Surgery and confirmation of recording sites

All procedures were conducted in accordance with NIH and IACUC guidelines. The surgical, mapping, and experimental methods were previously reported (Hung et al., 2001, 2002). Recordings were obtained from areas 17 and 18 of eight cats under anesthesia (pentothal, 1–2 mg/kg/hr) and paralysis (pancuronium bromide, 100µg/kg/hr). EEG, heartrate, oxygen saturation, expired CO_2, and core temperature were monitored. The location of the 17–18 border was determined by optical imaging of spatiotemporal frequency response and visual field mapping, and by physiological mapping of changes in receptive field size and reversal of receptive field progression across the vertical meridian (Bonhoeffer et al., 1995; Hung et al., 2001). Receptive fields were located between 0 to 10 deg azimuth and 5 to -30 deg elevation.

Receptive field characterization and stimuli

All stimuli were shown in a darkened room (< 1 Cd/m^2). After isolation of single-units, receptive fields were mapped and tested for orientation tuning.

Oriented units are defined as those with a 60 deg or narrower orientation tuning width. Luminance-modulated (LM) units are defined by a significant firing rate modulation (Hung et al., 2001, 2002; bootstrap statistics) to a large sinusoidally-modulated uniform light patch (edges at least 2° outside the classical receptive field (RF), 0.5 Hz, 15% p-p contrast at mean 32 Cd/m²). Oriented cells did not respond to full-field luminance modulation. LM cells exhibited both oriented and non-oriented response. Pairs of single units, one LM and one oriented (not LM), were recorded on two separately positioned electrodes in Areas 17 and 18 (mean distance 6.9 mm, range 0.7 to 18.5 mm).

Stimuli

The stimulus was then positioned so that the receptive field of the oriented cell overlay the "border" (parallel to the contrast border) and that of the LM cell overlay the "surface" (Figure 5.1, inset bottom). In the "luminance-modulation" condition (Figure 5.1, inset top), the luminance of two brightness fields were sinusoidally counterphased at 0.5 Hz (approx. 8 frames/sec, 16 frames/cyc, 15% peak-to-peak contrast; total luminance was always 32 Cd/m²) across a stationary contrast border (reversing sign). This condition was an effective stimulus for both cells. Responses to this condition were compared to a blank "spontaneous" condition (Figure 5.1, inset middle) in which the luminance was an even gray matching the mean luminance of the luminance-modulated condition. Both conditions contained no motion content. Each stimulus condition was presented continuously (a typical ten-minute recording yielded more than 3,000 spikes for at least one neuron).

Data analysis

The synchrony between cell pairs was assessed by cross-correlation histograms ("correlograms") showing the frequency of occurrence of specific spike timing relationships between pairs of neurons recorded from separate electrodes. Specifically, we focused on the correlograms recorded from two types of cell pairs: between Area 17 oriented cells and Area 17 LM cells ('17-17') and between area 17 oriented and Area 18 LM cells ('17–18'). We recorded a total of 458 correlograms. Correlograms were analyzed for peak position only if they showed significant peak height. Significant correlation was exhibited by 98/113 17–17 and 107/116 17–18 cell pairs during luminance modulation, and by 96/113 17–17 and 99/116 17–18 cell pairs during spontaneous activity. Histograms are shown triggered by the spike of the oriented cell at time 0. Spikes were collected at 0.1 msec resolution. Correlograms consisted of 501 bins of 1.6 msec each, smoothed by a 7-bin median filter. Correlograms were normalized for

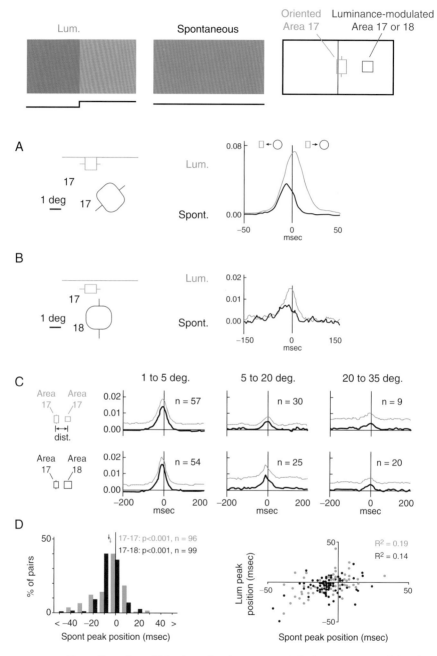

FIGURE 5.1 Recordings from LM-oriented pairs. *Inset top,* The luminance-modulated stimulus. Luminance of the two surfaces was sinusoidally modulated in antiphase across a stationary contrast border at 0.5 Hz (see Methods). Mean luminance remains constant at 32 Cd/m². *Inset middle,* Stimulus during spontaneous activity, also 32 Cd/m². *Inset bottom,* The stimulus was positioned such that one surface was centered on the

FIGURE 5.1 (Continued) LM cell's receptive field (RF shown by red box) and the border was positioned at the RF of the oriented cell (green box). (A) Example of a 17–17 pair. Schematic of RF positions is shown at left, relative to the location of the luminance-modulated contrast border (light blue line). At right are correlograms obtained during luminance-modulated (light blue) and Spontaneous (black) conditions. Negative peak position during spontaneous activity indicates a LM-to-oriented direction, and positive peak position indicates an oriented-to-LM direction. Lum: 5014 and 4453 spikes for oriented and LM cells, respectively, 2132 seconds. Spont: 815 and 3872 spikes, 2348 seconds. (B) Example of a 17–18 pair. Lum: 10490 and 3751 spikes, 984 seconds; Spont: 3491 and 1282 spikes, 622 seconds. (C) Average spontaneous correlograms for 17–17 pairs (top row, green) and 17–18 pairs (bottom row, purple) grouped according to distance between RF centers. Gray lines indicate raw correlograms, and black lines indicate correlograms after shuffle subtraction. (D) Population histograms of peak positions for 17–17 (green) and 17–18 (purple) pairs. Arrows indicate mean peak position for each population. Both populations are significantly biased (17–17: $p < 0.001$, 17–18: $p < 0.001$). (E) Peak positions during luminance-modulated versus spontaneous conditions for 17–17 and 17–18 pairs.

total spike count and peak significance was determined by bootstrap statistical methods (shuffle randomization of the two spike trains, Bonferroni corrected: individual bins at $p < 0.0001$ such that overall $p < 0.05$). For the spontaneous condition, randomization was based on an artificial 0.5 Hz cycle. All figures and calculations are based on the shuffle-subtracted correlograms, except in Figure 5.1c, where raw correlograms are also shown. Significance of peak positions in both luminance-modulation and spontaneous correlograms was determined by bootstrap analysis based on random sampling (with replacement) from the raw correlogram.

Results

INHERENT BIAS BETWEEN ORIENTED AND LM CELLS BASED ON PEAK POSITION

Figure 5.1 shows results from pairs isolated from separate electrodes in which one cell (in Area 17, green) was oriented and the other (in Area 18, red) was LM (responsive to large field luminance change). Cells were tested under two stimulus conditions (Figure 5.1 inset). In the "luminance-modulation" condition (Figure 5.1, inset top), luminance contrast was sinusoidally modulated at 0.5 Hz across a stationary contrast border. This stimulus was positioned over the receptive fields (RFs) such that the oriented cell's RF was at the contrast border and the LM cell's RF was centered on one surface (Figure 5.1, inset bottom). This condition strongly activated both cells. These responses were compared to a spontaneous condition (Figure 5.1, inset middle) in which the luminance was an even gray (no luminance modulation) matching the mean luminance of the luminance-modulation condition. Each stimulus condition was presented continuously for ten minutes, which was typically sufficient time for 3000 spikes to be collected per neuron.

Figures 5.1a and 5.1b show two examples of LM-oriented pairs, the first a 17-17 pair (both cells in Area 17) and the second a 17–18 pair (Area 17 oriented cell, Area 18 LM cell). In both cases, luminance-modulation yielded strong correlation peaks centered near zero (light blue lines). Spontaneous activity resulted in correlograms that were offset from center (black lines), however. Although the spontaneous peaks straddled the zero line, as is typical of cortical correlograms (Nowak et al., 1995; Murthy and Fetz, 1996; Roe and Ts'o, 1999), the bulk of the interactions showed the LM cell firing a few milliseconds before the oriented cell. These spontaneous peak positions are significantly offset from center ($p < 0.001$) and significantly different from the luminance-modulated peak (Figure 5.1a: luminance peak pos, 3.2 msec ± 1.11 msec; spontaneous peak position, –4.8 msec ± 0.96 msec; Figure 5.1b: luminance peak pos, –6.4 msec ± 2.39 msec; spontaneous peak position, -20.8 msec ± 5.33 msec; bootstrap tests). These shifted peaks show that spontaneous interactions may be directionally biased between oriented and LM cells.

Figures 5.1c and 5.1d show that these LM-to-oriented biases in spike timing exist across the population of 17–17 and 17–18 pairs. Figure 5.1c shows averaged spontaneous correlograms grouped according to receptive field (RF) separation distance at 1–5, 5–20, and 20–35 degrees (receptive fields were non-overlapping). Consistent with previous reports that peak height depends on RF separation, both 17–17 (top row) and 17–18 (bottom row) pairs show a decrease in peak height with RF separation. At all distances, some bias is evident in both 17–17 and 17–18 pairs (compare area left of zero msec with area right of zero msec). The bias in peak position is most evident in the peaks at the shorter RF separations (<5 deg) which are also the largest peaks. As summarized in Figure 5.1d, under spontaneous conditions peak positions for both 17–17 (green) and 17–18 (dark purple) pairs were significantly biased in the LM-to-oriented direction (17–17: mean –5.2 msec, $p < 0.001$, $n = 96$; 17–18: mean –6.2 msec, $p < 0.001$, $n = 99$; one-sample t test).

COMPARISON BETWEEN SPONTANEOUS AND EVOKED PEAK POSITIONS

Traditional correlation analyses of cortical circuitry have focused largely on correlations obtained from evoked activity, neglecting potential differences between evoked and spontaneous activity. We find, however, that evoked (luminance-modulation) and spontaneous peak positions do not necessarily coincide and can reveal different facets of the underlying circuitry. Figure 5.1e shows comparisons between evoked and spontaneous peak positions for 17–17 (green) and 17–18 (purple) pairs. For the population of 17–18 pairs, no difference was found between evoked and spontaneous peak positions (evoked: mean −5.3 msec, $p < 0.001$, $n = 107$, one-sample t test; evoked − spont: mean 0.7 msec, $p = 0.6$, $n = 95$, paired t test). For the population of 17–17 pairs, however, luminance-modulation resulted in a significant positive shift in the peak positions relative to spontaneous (evoked: mean -2.1 msec, $p > 0.05$, $n = 98$, one-sample t test; evoked − spont: mean 3.6 msec, $p = 0.01$, $n = 93$). This shift cannot be simply explained as a decrease of inherent biases and/or strengthening of common input, as we also observed shifts in the peak *away* from coincident activity, in the border-to-LM direction.

INHERENT BIAS BETWEEN ORIENTED AND LM CELLS BASED ON CORRELOGRAM SHAPE

In this section, we aim to further establish that these inherent biases are significant by examining two further measures of peak asymmetry. Whereas peak position is a convenient and simple measure of temporal relationship, it measures only one aspect of the correlogram and may at times be subject to noise in the correlogram. To further examine the strength and quality of these temporal biases, we also quantified the spontaneous correlograms with two measures that reflect correlogram shape: asymmetries of correlogram area (correlogram asymmetry, CA) and correlogram slope (peak asymmetry, PA) (Figure 5.2a) (Alonso and Martinez, 1998). These two measures indicate different aspects of temporal asymmetry; whereas CA reflects the total asynchrony, PA reflects the asymmetry around the peak, which, in ideal circumstances, can reveal the dominance of monosynaptic relationships versus asymmetric common input. For example, a CA value of 0 indicates symmetry around zero; a CA value of 0.5 (-0.5) indicates that 75% of the area is to the right (left) of zero. With respect to this data set, negative values indicate a bias in the LM-to-oriented direction, whereas positive values indicate an oriented-to-LM bias. To avoid the issue of noisy correlograms, the analysis is limited to the larger peaks (upper 50% of peak sizes).

For LM-oriented cell pairs (Figure 5.2b), CA measurements are predominantly negative, further confirming the LM-to-oriented bias revealed by peak position (Figure 5.1). Of the 17–17 pairs (green dots), 70% (31/44) have negative CA values. Of 17–18 pairs (purple dots), almost all (96%, 47/49) show negative CA, indicating virtually all of these interactions are in the LM-to-oriented 18-to-17 direction. These biases in CA cannot be simply explained by weakly luminance-modulated neurons or noisy correlograms – most of the strongest luminance-modulated neurons and strongest peak heights showed such correlogram asymmetry (Figure 5A-2).

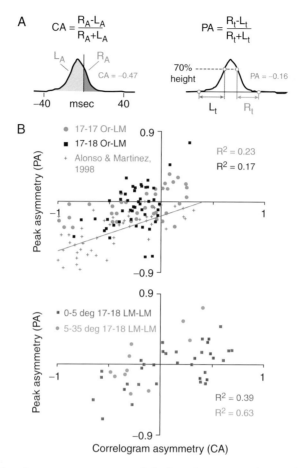

FIGURE 5.2 Correlograms were asymmetric both with respect to the zero bin (correlogram asymmetry) and with respect to the peak (peak asymmetry). Correlogram asymmetries are consistent with measurements of peak position. (A) Correlogram asymmetry (CA) is defined as $(R_A-L_A)/(R_A+L_A)$, where R_A and L_A are the areas of the shuffle-subtracted correlogram between 0 and ±40 msec. Peak asymmetry (PA) is defined as $(R_t-L_t)/(R_t+L_t)$, where R_t and L_t are the rise and decay times of the correlogram between 70% height and the shuffle-subtracted baseline. Correlogram in schematic is from example in Fig 1a. (B) Both 17-17 (green dots, N=44) and 17-18 (purple squares, N = 49) correlograms showed strongly biased CA with PA close to zero, consistent with an offset common input or network state transitions. In comparison, mono-synaptic interactions such as those seen in simple-complex pairs tend to yield more extreme PA values (gray '+' signs, Alonso and Martinez, 1998). Most 17-17 CAs and all but two 17-18 CAs were negative, consistent with measurements of peak position (Fig 1d). CA and PA values for the examples in Figure 5.1a and 5.1b are indicated by hollow dot and hollow square, respectively.

In contrast, PA values are distributed around zero, indicating that even offset peaks show a symmetric profile (symmetric slopes left and right of the peak). Indeed, 68% (17-17: 31/44, 17-18: 32/49) of the correlograms have |PA values| ≤ 0.25, and all but three (97%) have |PA| ≤ 0.5, indicating a predominance of negatively shifted symmetrical peaks. For comparison, Alonso and Martinez (1998) tended to find more extreme PA values when recording from mono-synaptic simple-complex pairs (gray "+" signs). One possible interpretation of PA symmetry coupled with CA asymmetry is that LM-oriented pairs receive offset common input (common input modified by differences in the delay to the two cell types).

Discussion

We have shown that appropriate identification of LM versus oriented responses can reveal biases in spontaneous cortical activity. Our results suggest that LM cells in Areas 17 and 18 tend to activate prior to oriented cells in area 17 (Figure 5.3a). We believe that these inherent (spontaneous) biases are likely to be related to either differential timing of common input or asymmetries in the network connections (e.g. mono- or polysynaptic connections between LM and oriented cells and/or asymmetry in common input). These are the first results to show an inherent differential timing between surface versus border networks under spontaneous conditions. We suggest that such biases need to be taken into account when evaluating neuronal interactions under stimulated versus spontaneous 'control' conditions.

How Inherent Bias Relates to Vision

These inherent biases suggest that the cortex may be actively processing information, even "at rest". Computationally, inherent biases in patterns of spontaneous activity may offer an advantage in setting the downstream neuron (e.g. the oriented cell in LM-oriented pairs) closer to an appropriate threshold, rather than at a fixed resting potential (Azouz and Gray, 1999). We speculate that the LM cells may be involved rapid dynamic normalization of response sensitivity across saccades, allowing the appropriate detection of contrast edges (which vary over a 30-fold range in reflectance) despite much wider variations in luminance (up to 10^9) within the visual field (Gilchrist et al., 1999).

Relationship of Inherent Biases to Cortical Architecture

While our data show only inherent bias between individual pairs of neurons, given what is known about cortical functional architecture, they suggest possible

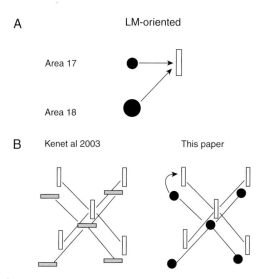

FIGURE 5.3 A) Summary of inherent biases in Areas 17 and 18. LM (black circles)-to-oriented (white rectangle) bias for both 17-17 and 17-18 cell pairs (arrows). B) *Left,* Imaging studies reveal dynamic switching of different orientation networks (white rectangles connected by lines, gray rectangles connected by lines) under spontaneous conditions (Kenet et al., 2003). *Right,* A hypothetical model based on these LM-oriented results. Dynamic switching may also occur between orientation (white rectangles connected by lines) and luminance networks (black circles connected by lines), and this switching may exhibit directionality (curved arrow).

relationships between clusters of neurons. The existence of orientation-selective networks in visual cortex is fairly well-supported (e.g. Malach et al. 1993; Kisvarday et al. 1997; Kenet et al., 2003). The presence of LM networks is also supported. As demonstrated by optical imaging, surface-responsive regions have been found in Area 18 that are distinct from orientation-selective zones (Tani et al., 2003). Area 17 contains a regular patchwork of clusters tuned to low spatial frequencies (Shoham et al., 1997), and, in monkeys it has been shown that such low spatial frequency preferring zones (blobs) form blob-selective horizontal networks (Livingstone and Hubel 1984; Ts'o and Gilbert 1988). Thus, oriented and LM cells are likely to participate in distinct horizontal networks in early visual areas that subserve border and surface information processing, respectively.

Given these distinct organizations, we view our data in the context of what has been referred to as "network state." Recent imaging evidence has shown that spontaneous cortical activity (or "network state") can be similar in structure to that of activated orientation maps, and that this network state dynamically switches from one state (one orientation map) to another (orientation map) (Figure 5.3b, left, based on Kenet et al., 2003). We speculate that dynamic switching may also occur between different types of functional networks (LM and orientation networks) and, furthermore, that this switching may be directional in nature (Figure 5.3b, right). In this scenario, the simultaneous activation of LM-dominated network activity may be quickly (~10 msec) followed by orientation-dominated activity. Thus, we suggest the hypothesis that ongoing activity is characterized not only by structured networks but also by directional interactions between surface and border networks.

Summary

The directional nature of these spontaneous interactions indicates that "at rest" there are inherent biases in cortical dynamics and suggest a more structured baseline from which to interpret cortical activity during visual perception. In the case of LM and oriented cells, we speculate that such inherent biases may indicate an underlying network for integrating edge and brightness perception. We suggest that inherent biases may also exist elsewhere in cortical circuitry, and that such inherent biases provide a view of functional circuitry "unadulterated" by the effects of sensory stimulation, attention, or working memory. Further mapping of such biases may provide a useful framework for interpreting evoked activity, both in absolute and relative terms.

Acknowledgments

The authors would like to thank Francine Healy for excellent technical assistance and Jonathan Victor and Jeff Schall for helpful comments on prevous versions of this manuscript. Supported by EY11744 and Packard Foundation.

REFERENCES

Alonso. J-M., Martinez, L.M. (1998). Functional connectivity between simple cells and complex cells in cat striate cortex. *Nature Neuroscience, 1*, 395–403.
Amit, D.J., Brunel, N. (1997). Model of global spontaneous activity and local structured activity during delay preiods in the cerebral cortex. *Cereb Cortex, 7*, 237–252.
Amzica F., Steriade M. (1995). Short- and long-range neuronal synchronization of the slow (<1 Hz) cortical oscillation. *J of Neurophysiology, 73*, 20–38.

Arieli A., Shoham D., Hildesheim R., Grinvald A. (1995). Coherent spatiotemporal patterns of ongoing activity revealed by real-time optical imaging coupled with single-unit recording in the cat visual cortex. *J Neurophysiology, 73,* 2072–2093.

Azouz. R., Gray, C.M. (1999). Cellular mechanisms contributing to response variability of cortical neurons in vivo. *J of Neuroscience, 19,* 2209–2223.

Bonhoeffer, T., Kim, D-S., Malonek, D., Shoham, D., Grinvald, A. (1995). Optical imaging of the layout of functional domains in area 17 and across the area 17/18 border in cat visual cortex. *Eur J Neurosci., 7,* 1973–1988.

Brown, H.A., Allison, J.D., Samonds, J.M.and Bonds, A.B. (2003). Nonlocal origin of response suppression from stimulation outside the classic receptive field in area 17 of the cat. *Vis Neurosci., 20,* 85–96.

DeCharms, R.C. and Merzenich, M.M. (1996). Primary cortical representation of sounds by the coordination of action-potential timing. *Nature, 381,* 610–613.

Cox, D.R. (1962). *Renewal theory.* London: Methuen.

Gilchrist, A., Kossyfidis, C., Agostini, T., Li, X., Bonato, F., Cataliotti, J., Spehar, B., Annan, V., and Economou, E. (1999). An anchoring theory of lightness perception. *Psychological Rev* 106(4): 795–834.

Gray, C.M., Konig, P., Engel, A.and Singer, W. (1989). Oscillatory responses in cat visual cortex exhibit inter-columnar synchronization which reflects global stimulus properties. *Nature, 338,* 334–337.

Gusnard, D.A. and Raichle, M.E. (2001). Searching for a baseline: functional imaging and the resting human brain. *Nature Reviews Neuroscience, 2,* 685–694.

Huang, X., MacEvoy, S.P. and Paradiso, M.A. (2002). Perception of brightness and brightness illusions in the macaque monkey. *J of Neuroscience, 22,* 9618–9625.

Hung, C.P., Ramsden, B.M. and Roe, A.W. (2002). Weakly modulated spike trains: Significance, precision, and correction for sample size. *J of Neurophysiology, 87,* 2542–2554.

Hung, C.P., Ramsden, B.M., Chen, L.M. and Roe, A.W. (2001). Building surfaces from borders in Areas 17 and 18 of the cat. *Vision Research, 41,* 1389–1407.

Kenet, T., Bibitchkov, D., Tsodyks, M., Grinvald, A.and Arieli, A. (2003). Spontaneously emerging cortical representations of visual attributes. *Nature, 425,* 954–956.

Kisvarday, Z.F., Toth, E., Rausch, M. and Eysel, U.T. (1997). Orientation-specific relationship between populations of excitatory and inhibitory lateral connections in the visual cortex of the cat. *Cereb Cortex, 7,* 7, 605–618.

Leopold, D.A., Murayama. Y. and Logothetis, N.K. (2003). Very slow fluctuations in monkey visual cortex: Implications for functional brain imaging. *Cereb Cortex, 13,* 422–433.

MacEvoy, S.P., Kim, W. and Paradiso, M.A. (1998). Integration of surface information in primary visual cortex. *Nature Neuroscience, 1,* 616–620.

Murthy, V.N. and Fetz, E.E. (1996). Synchronization of neurons during local field potential oscillations in sensorimotor cortex of awake monkeys. *J of Neurophysiology, 76,* 3968–3982.

Nowak, L.G., Munk, M.H.J., Nelson, J.I., James, A.C. and Bullier, J. (1995). Structural basis of cortical synchronization. I. Three types of interhemispheric coupling. *J of Neurophysiology, 74,* 2379–2400.

Perkel, D.H., Gerstein, G.L. and Moore, G.P. (1967a). Neuronal spike trains and stochastic point processes. I. The single spike train. *Biophys J, 7,* 391–418.

Perkel, D.H., Gerstein, G.L. and Moore, G.P. (1967b). Neuronal spike trains and stochastic point processes. II. Simultaneous spike trains. *Biophys J, 7,* 419–440.

Roe, A.W. and Ts'o, D.Y. (1999). Specificity of color connectivity between primate V1 and V2. *J of Neurophysiology, 82,* 2719–2730.

Rossi, A.F. and Paradiso, M.A. (1999). Neural correlates of brightness in the responses of neurons in the retina, LGN, and primary visual cortex. *J of Neuroscience, 19,* 6145–6156.

Rossi, A.F., Rittenhouse, C.D. and Paradiso, M.A. (1996). The representation of brightness in primary visual cortex. *Science, 273,* 1104–1107.

Shadlen, M.N., and Newsome, W.T. (1994). Noise, neural codes and cortical organization. *Current Opinion in Neurobiology,* 4, 569–579.

Shoham, D., Hubener, M., Schulze, S., Grinvald, A. and Bonhoeffer, T. (1997). Spatio-temporal frequency domains and their relation to cytochrome oxidase staining in cat visual cortex. *Nature, 385,* 529–533.

Softky, W.R. and Koch, C. (1992). Cortical cells should spike regularly but do not. *Neural Comp., 4,* 643–646.

Softky, W.R. and Koch, C. (1993). The highly irregular firing of cortical cells is inconsistent with temporal integration of random EPSPs [Review]. *J of Neuroscience, 13,* 334–350.

Tani, T., Yokoi. I., Ito, M., Tanaka, S. and Komatsu, H. (2003). Functional organization of the cat visual cortex in relation to the representation of a uniform surface. *J of Neurophysiology, 89,* 1112–1125.

Ts'o, D.Y. and Gilbert, C.D. (1988). The organization of chromatic and spatial interactions in the primate striate cortex. *J of Neuroscience, 8,* 1712–1727.

Ts'o, D.Y., Gilbert, C.D. and Wiesel, T.N. (1986). Relationships between horizontal interactions and functional architecture in cat striate cortex as revealed by cross-correlation analysis. *J of Neuroscience, 6,* 1160–1170.

Tsodyks, M.V. and Sejnowski, T. (1995). Rapid switching in balanced cortical network models. *Network, 6,* 111–124.

Tsodyks, M.V., Kenet, T., Grinvald, A. and Arieli, A. (1999). Linking spontaneous activity of single cortical neurons and the underlying functional architecture. *Science, 286,* 1943–1946.

APPENDIX

Extended Methods

Surgery

Eight cats were anesthetized (pentothal, 1-2 mg/kg/hr), paralyzed (pancuronium bromide, 100μg/kg/hr) and artificially respirated. Heart rate and EEG were continuously monitored, blood oxygenation was monitored at half-hour intervals, CO_2 was maintained at 4%, and rectal temperature maintained at 38 deg C. Eyes were refracted and fitted with contact lenses to focus upon a tangent screen. Alignment was checked before and after each recording. Proper focusing was determined by an opthalmoscope and confirmed by the physiological recording of cells with small receptive fields (less than 1 deg width in Area 17). Under aseptic conditions, a 1–2 cm² craniotomy and durotomy were made over Areas 17 and 18 (centered at Horsley-Clark coordinates A-1, L 3). All procedures were conducted in accordance with NIH and IACUC guidelines.

Confirmation of recording sites

Results of our 17/18 border mapping have been previously reported (Hung et al., 2001). Briefly, the location of the Area 17/18 border was determined by optical imaging of spatial-temporal frequency response and by visual field mapping. For mapping by optical imaging, Areas 17 and 18 were differentiated by their spatio-temporal frequency response to horizontal and vertical grating stimuli (Bonhoeffer et al., 1995; Shoham et al., 1997). High spatial frequency stimuli (0.58 cycles/deg, 4 deg/s) and low spatial frequency stimuli (0.14 cycles/ deg, 14 deg/s) were used to preferentially activate Areas 17 and 18, respectively. This optically-imaged 17/18 border was subsequently confirmed by physiological mapping, showing changes in receptive field size and reversal of receptive field progression across the vertical meridian (Tusa et al., 1978, 1979). Recorded pairs were generally separated along the rostral-caudal axis, with receptive fields located between 0 to 10 deg azimuth and 5 to −30 deg elevation.

Recording technique

All recordings were made in a darkened room (<1 Cd/m²). Because of the rarity of luminance-modulated cells (DeYoe and Bartlett, 1980), we always began recordings of oriented-LM pairs (consisting of an oriented cell in Area 17 and an LM cell in Area 17 or 18) by searching for LM units. We located potential LM units by advancing the electrode while listening to an audio monitor for multi-unit spiking response to a light flash (32 Cd/m²) 3°x3° in size from a handheld light gun. A unit was then isolated based on its waveform (Spike3, Cambridge Electronic Design, Cambridge, UK) and its autocorrelogram checked for contamination from neighboring units. Characterization of the unit as LM was based on the significance of its firing rate modulation under the luminance-modulated stimulus condition, determined by bootstrap tests of the spike train (see *Stimuli* and *Data Analysis*). For recordings from oriented-LM pairs, a second electrode was positioned in Area 17, 0.7-18.5 mm (mean 6.9 mm) away from the first electrode. We deliberately selected for pairs with nonoverlapping receptive fields in which the oriented-LM pair might encode the relationship between a surface and its border, rather than cases where both receptive fields are co-linear and likely to be directly activated by a common border. This was done by selecting for oriented units on the second electrode whose preferred orientation was orthogonal to an imaginary line between its receptive field and the receptive field of the first cell. 80% of the units were isolated from superficial layers (< 1000 μm depth), and the remainder was isolated from deep layers.

Receptive field characterization

Classical receptive fields (CRFs) were mapped with a hand-held light gun. We defined CRFs as minimal response fields whose borders were determined by flashing a small patch of light 1°x1° in size (32 Cd/m² against a black background < 1 Cd/m²). Oriented receptive fields were mapped manually using a small bar of light of the preferred orientation and optimal length. When the two mapping methods resulted in receptive fields of different sizes, we always erred on the conservative side and used the larger measured CRF. In the oriented-LM pairs we recorded, the oriented unit always had a response to the preferred orientation that was at least twice that to the non-preferred orientation, and the LM unit always exhibited a significant luminance-modulated response (see *Stimuli* and *Data Analysis*). In some cases, the oriented unit exhibited some LM response (tested with no edges in the CRF), or the LM unit exhibited some degree of orientation selectivity. Although oriented units were rarely luminance-modulated (about 10% of the units encountered were luminance-modulated), LM units often exhibited some degree of orientation selectivity (Figure 5A-1). The widths of orientation tuning encountered in LM units spanned the range from very tight (~10 deg) to non-oriented (percentages of cells described as "A"–"D", "A" sharply oriented (<20 deg width) and "D" non-oriented: 10%, 33%, 22%, and 35%).

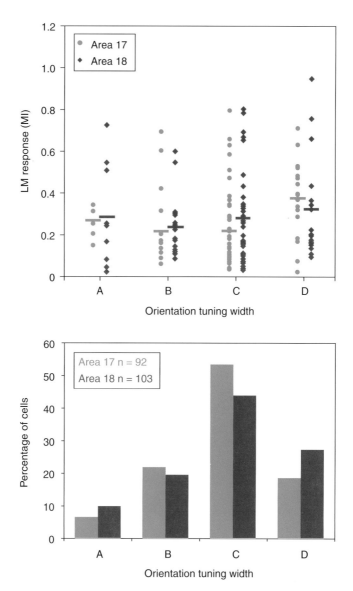

FIGURE 5A-1 Orientation tuning specificity versus LM response of LM cells.
(A) Orientation tuning specificity of Area 17 (green dots) and Area 18 (red diamonds)
LM cells are plotted versus strength of response to luminance modulation. Tuning
specificity was classified into four groups: A (less than 22.5 deg width), B (22.5 to 45 deg
width), C (45 to 67.5 deg width), and D (over 67.5 deg width). Response to luminance
modulation is given as Modulation Index, which is the contrast ratio corrected for spike
count. MIs greater than one result from sinusoidal fitting to the response histogram.
Horizontal bars indicate mean MI for each group. (B) Percentage of LM cells in each
group. Cells include those from an earlier experiment (Hung et al., 2001).

Stimuli

All stimuli were shown on a tangent screen in a darkened room (< 1 Cd/m²) under conditions identical to those previously described (Hung et al., 2001). Two stimulus conditions were tested, a "Luminance-modulation" condition and a "Spontaneous" condition (blank control; see Figure 5.1, top). Each condition was presented continuously for ten minutes. In some cases, the recording was stopped prematurely when more than 3000 spikes had been collected on each channel. Stimuli contained no motion content. In the Luminance-modulation condition, the stimulus had the appearance of a non-moving contrast border between two sinusoidally alternating brightness fields. This stimulus consisted of two adjoining rectangular surfaces (each approximately 5°x8°) whose outline was covered by a non-reflective black mask. The stimulus was positioned and oriented such that the edge between the two surfaces overlay the oriented cell"s receptive field, and one of the two surfaces was centered over the (potential) LM unit"s receptive field. The luminances of the two surfaces were counterphased (crossing sign) sinusoidally around a mean luminance of 32 Cd/m² (approx. 8 frames/sec, 16 frames/cyc, 8-15% peak-to-peak contrast; total luminance was always 32 Cd/m²). The slow sinusoidal modulation was chosen because it was well within the limits of psychophysical measures of filling-in (< 4 Hz), and the slow frame rate allowed us to distinguish phasic (< 15 msec) from tonic LM responses. Although we could clearly distinguish between tonic and phasic responses by the presence of sharp frame-locked bins in the PSTH, subsequent cross-correlation analysis revealed no difference in the results from transient versus tonic LM cells, and so their results are pooled here. In the Spontaneous condition, the cell"s spontaneous activity was recorded during continuous presentation of a static gray stimulus (also 32 Cd/m²) of the same size and location as the Luminance-modulation stimulus.

Data analysis

Characterization of a surface unit as "luminance-modulated" (LM) was based upon the significance of its response to the sinusoidal luminance modulation (determined by bootstrap statistical methods, based on shuffling the spike order of the recorded spike train while preserving the exact inter-spike interval distribution (Hung et al., 2002)). Briefly, significance of the luminance response was measured by fitting the firing-rate response with a sinusoid at the frequency of the stimulus and comparing the strength of the response modulation against those generated by 1000 bootstrap randomizations of the recorded spike train.

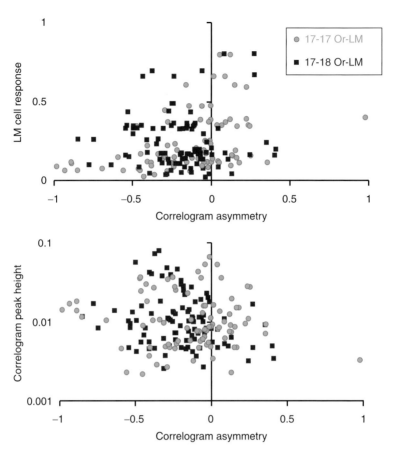

FIGURE 5A-2 Significance of Correlogram Asymmetry (A) Comparison of
Correlogram Asymmetry versus LM cell response. As suggested by a reviewer, we
have plotted the correlogram asymmetry of spontaneous correlograms against the
LM cell's luminance modulation response for 17–17 (green) and 17–18 (purple) pairs.
Asymmetry correlates poorly with LM response magnitude, as expected, because
LM cells (like oriented cells) respond best at specific stimulus contrasts. At the low
stimulus contrasts tested (15% peak-to-peak), many LM cells yielded only moderate
responses. (B) Comparison of correlogram asymmetry versus peak height for
spontaneous correlograms (shuffle-subtracted). Strong correlogram asymmetry is
seen for both 17–17 and 17–18 pairs across the entire range of peak sizes.

For each randomization, the order of the spikes was randomized while preserving the set of inter-spike intervals. We found light-modulated responses in
approximately 10% of the cells we encountered. This finding is consistent with
the results of DeYoe and Bartlett (1980), considering the stringency of their
luxotonic cell criteria compared to our LM cell criteria.

For the paired recordings, we used cross-correlation histograms ('correlo-grams') to show the frequency of occurrence of specific spike timing relation-ships between pairs of neurons. For oriented-LM pairs, the histograms are shown triggered by the spike of the oriented cell at time 0. For LM-LM pairs, histograms are triggered by the spike of the Area 17 cell. Spikes were collected at 0.1 ms resolution. Correlograms were normalized for total spike count and peak significance was determined by bootstrap statistical methods. Briefly, 10000 random correlograms were generated from randomizations of the two spike trains (Hung et al., 2002), thereby preserving the profile of the peri-stimulus time histogram (PSTH) of the two spike trains but destroying the specific timing relationships within and between the two spike trains. For ran-domization under the Spontaneous condition, an artificial cycle trigger was generated at 2-second intervals. Each correlogram consisted of 501 bins of 1.6 msec each, smoothed with a 7-bin median filter. Both raw and shuffle-subtracted correlograms are shown in Figure 5.1c. The other figures show only the shuffle-subtracted correlogram. Only peaks of significant height (Bonferroni-corrected: individual bins at $p < 0.0001$ such that overall $p < 0.05$) were consid-ered. We recorded a total of 644 correlograms. Of these, 98/113 17-17, 107/116 17-18, and 80/93 LM-LM pairs were significant during Luminance-modulation, and 96/113 17-17, 99/116 17-18, and 73/93 LM-LM pairs were significant during spontaneous activity.

Alternative explanations considered

Given that we observed inherent biases for both 17-17 and 17-18 pairs, it seemed unlikely that the LM-to-oriented bias could be simply explained as an area-to-area bias. However, because biases in inter-areal anatomical connectivity have been suggested to relate to receptive field overlap, we also analyzed pairs of simultaneously recorded LM cells, one in area 17 and the other in area 18. An area-related explanation would predict the same direction of bias (either 17-to-18 or 18-to-17) for all 17-18 interactions regardless of cell type. However, although oriented-LM pairs tended to show an 18-to-17 bias, LM-LM pairs showed no overall bias (Figure 5A-3). This also argues that differences in RF size between Areas 17 and 18 (Area 18 RFs larger than Area 17 RFs) do not account for the biases. Neither is RF separation sufficient to explain our results: although we observed clear 18-to-17 bias for LM-oriented pairs at short RF separations, LM-LM pairs showed a weakly opposite 17-to-18 bias at similar RF separations.

Finally, because stimuli were presented continuously for several minutes, we considered whether the spontaneous bias might be due to short-term

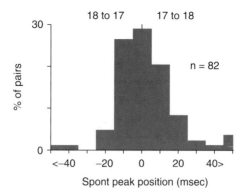

FIGURE 5A-3 Spontaneous peak positions are centered for LM-LM pairs LM-LM pairs consisting of one cell in area 17 and the other in area 18 were recorded during spontaneous activity. No systematic bias is seen in the population of peak latencies, either in the 17-to-18 direction (right side, area 17 fires first) or the 18-to-17 direction (left side) (peak position mean: 2.5 msec, std error: 3.2 msec, p > 0.05). Thus, not all interactions exhibit bias under spontaneous conditions.

experience-dependent plasticity (Fu et al., 2002) resulting from differences in response latencies of LM (surface) and oriented (border) cells during luminance-modulation. Such an explanation would predict that the magnitude of spontaneous bias should depend on whether Luminance-modulation was presented prior to the spontaneous condition, or vice versa. The order of stimulus presentation had no effect upon the spontaneous bias recorded (for all oriented-LM pairs, Luminance condition before spontaneous: peak position mean −6.1 msec, n = 167; Spontaneous condition before luminance: peak position mean −3.7 msec, n = 28; p > 0.3, unpaired t-test). Furthermore, if the spontaneous bias were due to short-term plasticity, then Luminance-modulation bias should be greater than spontaneous bias (assuming that before stimulation the interactions are synchronous, that Luminance modulation induces a short-term bias in spike timing, and that the bias seen during spontaneous conditions occurs during the adaptation decay). However, as shown by the example in Figure 5.1a, b, e the magnitude of spontaneous bias was often larger than the magnitude of Luminance-modulation bias, and in many cases the Luminancemodulation and spontaneous biases were in opposite directions. In fact, for 17–17 oriented-LM pairs, Luminance-modulation peak positions were not significantly biased whereas spontaneous peak positions were. Thus, we feel that short-term experience-dependent plasticity does not account for our findings of spontaneous bias.

APPENDIX REFERENCES

DeYoe, E.A., Bartlett, J.R. (1980). Rarity of luxotonic responses in cortical visual areas of the cat. *Exp Brain Res, 39*, 125–132.

Fu, Y.X., Djupsund, K., Gao, H., Hayden, B., Shen, K., Dan, Y. (2002). Temporal specificity in the cortical plasticity of visual space representation. *Science, 296*, 1999–2003.

Tusa, R.J., Palmer, L.A. and Rosenquist, A.C. (1978). The retinotopic organization of area 17 (striate cortex) in the cat. *J Comp Neurol, 177*, 213–235.

Tusa, R.J., Rosenquist, A.C. and Palmer, L.A. (1979). Retinotopic organization of areas 18 and 19 in the cat. *J Comp Neurol, 185*, 657–678.

6

Phase Resetting in the Presence of Noise and Heterogeneity

Srisairam Achuthan, Fred H. Sieling, Astrid A. Prinz, and Carmen C. Canavier

There has been a recent explosion of interest (Strogatz, 2003) in synchronization, i.e. the spontaneous organization of individual oscillators such as pendulum-based clocks, fireflies, or neurons, each exhibiting rhythmic activity at its own individual rate, into a coherent entity with a common frequency. The result is a phase-locked pattern in which the phasic relationships among all oscillators remain constant. Synchronization and phase-locking, the focus of this chapter, are relevant to a number of important biological problems. Transiently synchronized assemblies of neurons are believed to underlie cognitive functions (Buzsaki, 2006). For example, in humans, the presence of synchronization among distant brain regions predicts whether a word will be recalled (Fell et al., 2001) and whether an image is recognized as a face (Rodriguez et al., 1999). Exposure to rhythmic cycles of light and dark can entrain the circadian oscillators in the mammalian suprachiasmatic nucleus (de la Iglesia et al., 2004), and in photosensitive epilepsy, exposure to rhythmic bright lights can induce a paroxysm of synchronous brain activity resulting in a seizure. Absence epileptic seizures have been postulated to arise from phase-locking between thalamic and cortical sites (Perez-Velasquez et al., 2007). Pathological synchrony could also lead to tremor (Hammond et al., 2007), and there is consistent evidence for a reduction of synchronization in schizophrenia (Uhlhaas and Singer 2006). Phase-locking is also relevant to central pattern generators (CPGs), which are neural circuits that produce a repetitive pattern of motor activity (Stein et al., 1997), such as locomotion or respiration, even in the absence of sensory feedback or patterned input from higher brain centers. An influential theory (Llinas 2002; Yuste et al., 2005) suggests that cortical rhythms and circuits evolved from motor rhythms and circuits, and are therefore likely to share basic principles of organization and dynamic function. In this chapter, we show that an approach to understanding synchronization and phase-locking based on the phase resetting curve (PRC) can be extended to predict whether such lockings are robust to variability in the form of noise and heterogeneity in frequency between neural oscillators.

Neurons that spontaneously burst or spike repetitively can be considered to be limit cycle oscillators. A limit cycle oscillator can be visualized as tracing out a closed orbit (or curve) on every cycle in some appropriate state space. At any time point within the cycle, a single number from 0 to 1 is called the phase and represents the position along the limit cycle. Phase is modulo 1 and is measured from an arbitrary reference point. We define this reference point as spike or burst onset and assign it a phase of 0. Phase resetting theory (Glass and Mackey 1988; Winfree 1987) further assumes that an input instantaneously displaces the trajectory along the limit cycle, with a phase advance causing the trajectory to skip ahead on the limit cycle and a delay causing it to jump backwards. This has the effect of either shortening or lengthening the cycle in which the perturbation occurs. Phase resetting curves tabulate the effect of an input depending upon the phase at which the input is received. The response to an input is assumed to be characterized entirely by transient changes in the cycle period. The phase resetting curves of individual neural oscillators have often been used to study the oscillators' synchronization as well as phase-locking tendencies in reciprocally connected networks (Achuthan and Canavier 2009a; Netoff et al., 2005a, 2005b; Acker et al., 2003; Goel and Ermentrout, 2002; Canavier et al., 1997, 1999; Oprisan et al., 2004; Sieling et al., 2009; Canavier et al., 2009).

There are two general theoretical approaches based on the PRC, one that assumes weak coupling such that inputs add linearly, and one that simply assumes pulsatile coupling, that the effects of an input dissipate by the time the next one is received. Weak coupling implies that many cycles are required to converge to a phase-locked mode such as synchrony, and it is therefore not appropriate for the analysis of circuits in which synchronization must occur quickly, such as cortical circuits that mediate binding (Singer 1999) or CPGs that synchronize their activity quickly. Neural circuits frequently contain inputs that can produce resetting that is a substantial fraction of the cycle period.

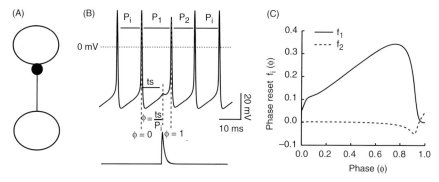

FIGURE 6.1 Phase Resetting Curve. (A) Open loop configuration. (B) The voltage waveform represents a regular spiking neuron with intrinsic period P_i. The lower trace corresponds to the postsynaptic conductance resulting from a spike in a presynaptic neuron. The normalized change in cycle period length as a result of the perturbation received at a phase $\phi=ts/P_i$ is the phase resetting. P_1 represents the period of the cycle in which the stimulus is received. The following cycle period is represented by P_2. (C) Example of first order ($f_1(\phi)$, solid line) and second order ($f_2(\phi)$, dashed line) phase resetting curves.

We therefore use the pulsatile coupling approach. This approach requires the PRC (see Figure 6.1) measured directly with the stimulus waveform that will be received by each neuron in the network (Canavier et al., 1997, 1999; Canavier, 2005; Luo et al., 2004). The PRC is measured in an open loop configuration (see Figure 6.1A) such that the neuron whose PRC is to be measured receives input from the neuron(s) that will be presynaptic to it in the closed loop network configuration, but it is isolated in that it does not affect the driving presynaptic neuron. In the example shown, this input is the synaptic conductance waveform (lower trace Figure 6.1B) that results from an action potential in the presynaptic neuron, such that the PRC is equivalent to the spike time response curve (Acker et al., 2003; Pervouchine et al., 2006). Although spiking neurons are used in this illustration, the same procedure applies to bursting neurons except that burst onset rather than spike onset is assigned a phase of 0, and the perturbation in conductance results from a presynaptic burst rather than a single action potential. Any effect on the cycle containing the start of the perturbation is tabulated as the first order resetting calculated as $(P_1-P_i)/P_i$ (solid trace Figure 6.1C)), and any effect on the next cycle is tabulated as second order resetting calculated as $(P_2-P_i)/P_i$ (dashed trace Figure 6.1C). According to this definition, delays of the event (spike or burst) following the perturbation correspond to positive values of the PRC, and advances correspond to negative values.

The assumptions required in order to use this type of PRC for network analysis are that 1) each neuron in the network can be represented as a limit cycle oscillator, 2) the trajectory of each neuron returns to its limit cycle between inputs (this is the assumption of pulsatile coupling), and 3) the input received by each neuron has the same effect in the closed loop circuit as in the open loop circuit used to generate the phase response curves. Pulsatile coupling implies that the effect of one input has died out before the next is received. In order to predict network activity using the PRCs, we must either 1) assume a firing pattern and solve for all possible sets of phases that can produce that firing pattern, or 2) pick a set of initial phases in order to iteratively identify the next firing time and update the phases accordingly. We will first illustrate here the assumed firing pattern method (Dror et al., 1999) for the simplest case of an alternating firing pattern for a two-neuron network (Figure 6.2A). For purposes of illustration, we will use a hybrid circuit, constructed using one biological bursting neuron and one bursting model neuron (Oprisan et al., 2004; Sieling et al., 2009), although the assumed firing pattern generalizes to any two network elements. The recovery interval (*tr*) is defined as the time elapsed from when a neuron receives an input until it next fires. The stimulus interval (*ts*) in a network is the time from when a neuron fires to when it receives an input. By definition, $tr_b[n] = ts_m[n]$ and $tr_m[n] = ts_b[n+1]$.

The next step is to use the assumption of pulsatile coupling in order to define the intervals in terms of the phase and the phase resetting. Although we assume that the effect of one input has dissipated by the time the next is received, we do not need to assume that the effect has dissipated by the time the next spike or burst is generated, because the total resetting is divided into two parts. The first order resetting is contained in the recovery interval $tr = P_i(1-\phi+f_1(\phi))$, whereas the second order resetting is contained in the stimulus interval $ts = P_i(\phi+f_2(\phi))$. Note that the definition of the stimulus interval is different in the closed and open loop configurations, because in contrast to the open loop, in the closed loop prior perturbations have to be considered. We next assume a steady locking point in which the neurons receive an input at the steady phases ϕ_b^* and ϕ_m^*. Since the steady values of both *tr* and *ts* depend only on phase, *tr* for each neuron can be considered a function of *ts*, $tr = g(ts)$. When phase-locking occurs, $tr_b = ts_m$ and $tr_m = ts_b$, so the intersection of the $tr_m = g(ts_m)$ and $ts_b = g^{-1}(tr_b)$ curves (Figure 6.2B) yields any fixed point(s) of the discrete map given in Figure 6.2A. The stability of the fixed point can be calculated using discrete linear systems theory if one assumes a small perturbation from the fixed point, and further assumes that the PRCs are linear in a small neighborhood about the fixed point.

The roots λ of the characteristic equation of the linearized system must all have absolute value less than 1, such that perturbations from the fixed point

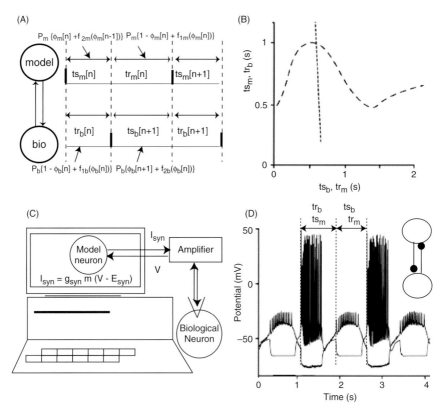

FIGURE 6.2 Prediction of Closed Loop Network Activity Using Open Loop PRCs.
A. Assumed firing pattern and definition of intervals using the PRC. B. Graphical
method to identify fixed points of the map in A that correspond to periodic phase-locked
modes. The long dashes indicate tr_b plotted against ts_b and the short dashes indicate ts_m
plotted against tr_m. C. Dynamic Clamp set up for hybrid circuits. D. Phase-locking in a
hybrid circuit. Biological neuron has short spikes, model neuron has tall ones.

decay and the associated steady phase-locked mode is stable. As shown in
(Oprisan et al., 2004), the roots (or eigenvalues) λ depend on the slopes (indicated by ') of the first and second order phase resetting curves at the steady
locking point as follows:

$$\lambda^2 - \left\{ \left(f'_{1b}\left(\phi_b*\right) - 1\right)\left(f'_{1m}\left(\phi_m*\right) - 1\right) - f'_{2b}\left(\phi_b*\right) - f'_{2m}\left(\phi_m*\right) \right\}\lambda$$
$$+ f'_{2b}\left(\phi_m*\right)f'_{2m}\left(\phi_m*\right) = 0$$

where f_{ib} $'(\phi_b*)$ refers to the slope of the ith order PRC of the biological neuron
at the steady state phase ϕ_b* and f_{im} $'(\phi_m*)$ refers to the slope of the ith order PRC
of the model neuron at the steady state phase ϕ_m*.

Robustness to Noise: Theoretical Approach
Based on the Envelope for Noisy PRCs

We utilize the simplest circuit that we can design that still contains a real biological neuron to illustrate how the robustness to noise of a predicted locking can be determined. We used the Dynamic Clamp (Sharp et al., 1993) to reciprocally connect model and biological neurons (Figure 6.2C) by injecting a virtual conductance into the biological neuron from the model neuron, using the membrane potential in the biological neuron to calculate the postsynaptic voltage for the synapse from model to biological as well as the presynaptic potential for the biological to model synapse. The PRCs are generated (Figure 6.1) in an open loop configuration; then the observed closed loop network activity (Figure 6.2D) is compared to the predicted stimulus and recovery intervals for each neuron.

In seventy hybrid networks coupled by excitation (Sieling et al., 2009), some predictions were robust to noise, but others were not. Predictions that were not robust to noise involved a structural instability of the solution space in the presence of noise, as illustrated in Figure 6.3. The essential insight was that the noise in the measurement of the PRC (example shown in Figure 6.3C) produces a range of resetting values that can be observed when an input is received. The stimulus and recovery intervals needed for the graphical method presented in Figure 6.2B were calculated using the average phase resetting curve in the biological neuron (solid red curve in the example shown in Figure 6.3C). Plots of the recovery and stimulus intervals (Figures 6.3A1 and A2), however, can also be obtained by using the upper or the lower envelopes (dashed red curves in Figure 6.3C) that contain the experimentally observed data points. For robust predictions (Figure 6.3A1) using the envelopes instead of the average slightly shifted the fixed point, producing jitter in the phase-locking. In the special cases involving a structural instability of the solution space, the fixed point that resulted from using the average PRC disappeared (Figure 6.3A2) when the lower or upper envelope was used instead. Therefore, 1:1 phase-locking was predicted but not observed in the presence of noise, which can be viewed as causing the fixed point to flicker in and out of existence.

In addition to the graphical methods based on the existence and stability criteria, there is another way to predict network activity based on the PRC, which we call here an iterated map (Canavier et al., 1999; Netoff et al., 2005b; Sieling et al., 2010). Given the current phase of each oscillator (neuron) and its period, one can easily determine which neuron(s) will fire next. Given the phase resetting behavior of each neuron in response to the firing of every other

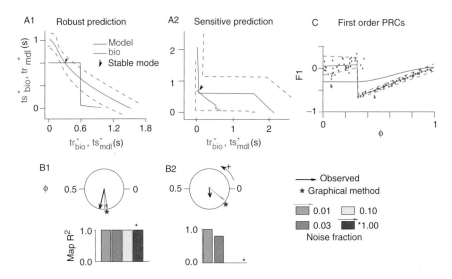

FIGURE 6.3 Iterated Map Results Capture Sensitivity of Predicted Phase-Locking to Noise A. Graphical method for identifying fixed points. A1. The curves intersect at the stable fixed point (arrowhead) whether the average (solid red) PRC or the upper and lower envelopes (red dashes) are used to calculate tr and ts. A2. The intersection only occurs for the curve based on the average PRC. B. The map was iterated with the level of noise actually observed in the PRC (red) or with a smaller fraction of noise (green is 1%). Circular statistics measured the length (R^2) of the average vector of the observed phase between bursts in the two neurons. B1. For the robust prediction, the phase vectors for the observed (black) and low (green) and actual (red) noise levels were similar to those for the graphical prediction (filled star) from part A. B2. For the sensitive case, only the lowest noise case (green) matched the graphical prediction (filled star). C. This example illustrates the noise inherent in measurement of PRCs in biological neurons (red dots).

neuron, one can then determine how the phases of each neuron are altered by each firing, so one can determine the future sequence of firing for all time, in the absence of noise. The determination of each firing event is considered one map iteration. The map may produce different firing patterns depending upon how it is initialized, because no fixed, predetermined firing order is assumed. The firing intervals can be specified by subtracting the starting phase from the ending phase, adding any resetting presumed to occur during the interval, and multiplying by the intrinsic period. The novel insight here was to randomize the phase resetting in the map by assuming a Gaussian distribution (with truncated tails) about the average PRC that characterized the actual experimentally observed noise. The width of this distribution was adjusted to reflect the full amount of observed noise or some smaller fraction. Under this protocol, the output of the iterated map could be analyzed using the same circular statistics (Drew and Doucet, 1991) applied to the experimental data from the hybrid circuits (Figure 6.3B.) The iterated map was robust to noise in the structurally stable case (Figure 6.3B1) and very sensitive to noise in the structurally unstable case (Figure 6.3B2) in agreement with the experimental data (compare red and black arrow lengths).

The implicit assumption usually made when PRC methods are applied to biological oscillators is that the noise inherent in biological systems does not qualitatively change the oscillatory activity of the network, but only adds jitter to the event times. On the contrary, our examination of networks coupled by reciprocal excitation revealed an example of a qualitative change in the dynamics of a nonlinear system. We discovered a way to predict whether a given amount of noise in the PRC would affect such a qualitative change in the phase-locking activity observed in a two neuron network.

Robustness to Heterogeneity: Approach
Based on the Envelope of the PRCs

Heterogeneity is implicit in our studies of hybrid circuits of one biological and one model neuron, because it is extremely unlikely that the two neurons would share the frequency or PRC shape exactly; as explained above, our methods are not restricted to homogeneous circuits. Nonetheless, the simplest cases in which to study synchronization frequently involve networks of identical, identically connected oscillators. In order for analyses of such idealized networks to generalize to populations of real neurons, the solutions obtained using a typical PRC to characterize each neuron type in the network must be robust to not only noise but also heterogeneity (Achuthan and Canavier, 2009b; Maran and Canavier, 2008; Oprisan et al., 2004; Sieling et al.,2009; Sieling et al., 2010). The success of the approach characterizing the qualitative susceptibility of a system to noise based on the structural stability of the PRC prediction method suggested a similar approach to heterogeneous circuits.

In order to examine how heterogeneity in frequency perturbs the solutions exhibited by a homogeneous network of two model neurons, we used a network comprised of two Morris-Lecar (ML) (Morris and Lecar, 1981) model neurons in the Type II membrane excitability (Izhikevich, 2007) regime, reciprocally coupled by inhibitory synapses (see Appendix for equations and parameters). In an identical and identically connected network antiphase locking was observed (see Fig. 6.4A1). The open circles represent the stimulus intervals (ts_i) observed when the differential equations for the closed circuit were integrated. The single open circle at each conductance value indicates that the two stimulus intervals were equal, as is the case for an exact antiphase mode. This solution depends on symmetry and was not robust to heterogeneity at weak coupling strength. For example, 1% heterogeneity in intrinsic frequencies produced phase walkthrough; the vertical column of circles in Figure 6.4A2 indicates that all possible phasic relationships were exhibited at a conductance strength of 0.01 mS/cm². A sharp transition to a 1:1 periodic locking was observed when the conductance was increased to 0.02 mS/cm². The antiphase is not exact, because the open circles corresponding to the two firing intervals are different and therefore do not overlay. A further increase in the coupling strength (Figure 6.4A2) however, causes the intervals to converge and approach the symmetric solution. With 5% heterogeneity, the bifurcation threshold between aperiodicity and periodic locking was increased to g_{syn} = 0.06 mS/cm² (Figure 6.4A3). Therefore coupling strength can compensate to some degree for heterogeneity in frequency. The PRCs (Figure 6.4B1) for 5% heterogeneity in frequency at the conductance strength indicated by the leftmost arrow in Fig. 4A3 (g_{syn} = 0.02 mS/cm²) produce phase walk through (Figure 6.4B2). The PRCs (Figure 6.4C1) for 5% heterogeneity in frequency at the conductance strength indicated by the rightmost arrow in Figure 6.4A3 (g_{syn} = 0.12 mS/cm²) produce a near antiphase (Figure 6.4C2) 1:1 phase-locking. This indicates the ability of stronger coupling to compensate for heterogeneity and restore, at least approximately, the symmetric solution.

The loss of the solution structure illustrated in Figure 6.4A2 and A3 has a sudden onset, like a bifurcation. A structural instability in the solution space was able to explain whether the predicted solution was robust to heterogeneity, just as it was able to account for whether a solution displayed robustness to noise. For a model neuron, noise introduces temporal variability in the phase resetting at a given phase. On the other hand, heterogeneity introduces spatial variability considering that each network component occupies some space in the frequency and PRC shape among network components of a given class. Figure 6.5A1 shows ts-tr plots for networks given in Figure 6.4A1. The antiphase solution shown in Figure 6.5A1 for an identical, identically coupled network results from symmetry, and is manifested by an intersection of the tr-ts curves on the 45 degree line in Figure 6.5A1 and B1 at coupling strengths of 0.02 mS/cm² and 0.12 mS/cm² respectively. The synchronous lockings are represented by the square symbols in Figure 6.5A1 and B1 corresponding to stimulus intervals of zero and the network period and are unstable due to the initial negative slope of the PRCs (Figure 6.4B1 and C1). At the weakest value of conductance, a 5% heterogeneity in frequency destroys the symmetric solution as shown by the failure of the ts-tr curves to intersect (Figure 6.5A2). In this case, no 1:1 locking is predicted (or observed, see Figure 6.4B2). This is a form

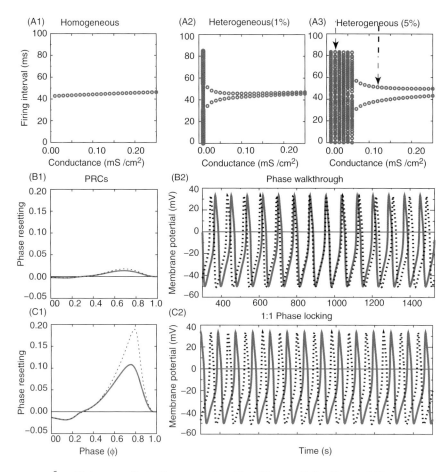

FIGURE 6.4 Heterogeneity in Frequency in a Two-Neuron Pulse Coupled Network
The network dynamics of two ML model neurons with inhibitory synaptic connectivity
in the Type II membrane excitability regime is shown as synaptic conductance and
heterogeneity is varied (see Appendix for the parameters used). (A1) Anti-phase
locking is exhibited by an identical and identically connected network. (A2) A 1%
variability in the intrinsic frequencies was introduced by setting $Istim_1 = 99.52\mu A/cm^2$
and $Istim_2 = 100.48\ \mu A/cm^2$. Phase-locking is only observed above a conductance
threshold. (A3) A 5% variability in the intrinsic frequencies was introduced by setting
$Istim_1 = 97.81\mu A/cm^2$ and $Istim_2 = 102.19\ \mu A/cm^2$. The synaptic conductance
threshold for phase-locking is increased compared to panel A2. (B1) PRCs
corresponding to 5% heterogeneity in intrinsic frequencies with $g_{syn} = 0.02\ mS/cm^2$
(left arrow in panel A3). (B2) Simulated network activity corresponding to 5%
heterogeneity in intrinsic frequencies with $g_{syn} = 0.02\ mS/cm^2$ and exhibiting a phase
walkthrough. (C1) PRCs corresponding to 5% heterogeneity in intrinsic frequencies
with $g_{syn} = 0.12\ mS/cm^2$ (right arrow in panel A3). (C2) Simulated network activity
corresponding to 5% heterogeneity in intrinsic frequencies with $g_{syn} = 0.12\ mS/cm^2$
and a near antiphase 1:1 locking.

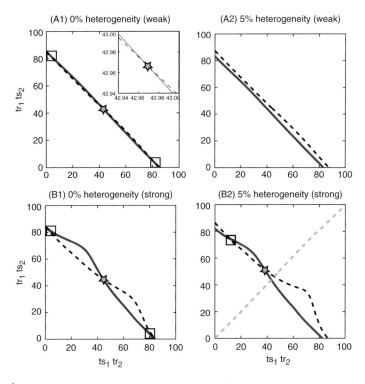

FIGURE 6.5 Prediction Method Based on PRC Reveals Structural Instability in the Solution Space. The ts-tr plots corresponding to two different synaptic conductance strengths for the identical neurons (left panels) and 5% heterogeneous in frequency (right panels) are shown here. (A1) Symmetric antiphase solution (star) for $g_{syn} = 0.02$ mS/cm^2 and 0% heterogeneity in frequency. Inset shows blow up around fixed point. Square indicates an unstable synchronous mode. (A2) Intersection point is lost for the same coupling strength as in A1 but with 5% heterogeneity in frequency. (B1) Symmetric antiphase solution (star) for $g_{syn} = 0.12$ mS/cm^2 and 0% heterogeneity in frequency. (B2) The intersection point (star) at the same conductance strength as in B1 is shifted to the left with 5% heterogeneity in frequency. In addition, an unstable near synchronous solution is reestablished (square). Any exact antiphase solution would lie on the 45 degree dotted line on which all intervals are equal.

of structural instability. An increase in conductance strength to 0.07 mS/cm^2 restores the intersection point, however, and a further increase to 0.12 mS/cm^2 moves the intersection point (Figure 6.5B2) towards the 45 degree line that marks the symmetric solution. This once again implies that increasing the conductance strength does compensate for heterogeneity.

The rationale for examining how heterogeneity perturbs solutions is that when analyzing real networks in vivo, the best one can do is to use PRC exemplars that only approximate the PRCs of component neurons. Variability is expected in the intrinsic properties that determine PRC shape, in connectivity, and in intrinsic frequency. Therefore, we need an estimate of the robustness of the solutions based on the prediction methods in order to determine their applicability. The methods illustrated in this chapter are expected to scale up to larger networks of N neurons, and to apply to other forms of heterogeneity rather than just to differences in intrinsic frequency (Oprisan et al., 2004; Sieling et al., 2009; Sieling et al., 2010).

Conclusions

One-to-one phase-locked activity in two neuron networks with reciprocal pulsatile coupling can be predicted using the PRCs generated with the perturbation that each neuron receives in a network. Here, we have extended this analysis to encompass predictions of the robustness of the lockings in the presence of temporal variability such as noise, and spatial variability in the presence of the inevitable heterogeneity between real neurons. The ability of coupling strength to compensate for variability suggests a mechanism for modulating the level of synchronization between neural ensembles by transiently modulating the coupling strength.

Acknowledgments

This work was supported by NIH grant NS 054281 under the CRCNS program.

REFERENCES

Achuthan S, Canavier CC (2009a). Phase resetting curves determine synchronization, phase-locking, and clustering in networks of neural oscillators. *J. Neurosci.* 29: 5218–5233.

Achuthan S and Canavier CC (2009b). Prediction of phase-locked neuronal network activity in the presence of heterogeneity and noise using phase resetting curves. *Soc. for Neurosci.* Abstr.

Acker CD, Kopell N and White JA (2003). Synchronization of strongly coupled excitatory neurons: relating network behavior to biophysics. *J. Comput. Neurosci.* 15: 71–90.

Bartos M, Vida I, Frotscher M, Geiger JRP and Jonas P (2001). Rapid signaling at inhibitory synapses in a dentate gyrus interneuron network. *J. Neurosci.* 21: 2687–2698.

Buszaki G (2006). *Rhythms of the brain.* New York: Oxford University Press.

Canavier CC (2005). The application of phase resetting curves to the analysis of pattern generating circuits containing bursting neurons. In: Coombes S and Bressloff P (eds) *Bursting: The Genesis of Rhythm in the Nervous System*. Series in Mathematical Neuroscience, World Scientific, Singapore, 175–200.

Canavier CC, Gurel Kazanci F, and Prinz AA (2009). Phase resetting curves allow for simple and accurate prediction of robust N:1 phase-locking for strongly coupled neural oscillators. *Biophys. J.*, 97: 59–73.

Canavier CC, Baxter DA, Clark JW and Byrne JH (1999). Control of multistability in ring circuits of oscillators. *Biol. Cybernetics* 80: 87–102.

Canavier CC, Butera RJ, Dror RO, et al (1997). Phase response characteristics of model neurons determine which patterns are expressed in a ring circuit model ofgait generation. *Biol Cybernetics* 77: 367–380.

de la Iglesia, H.O., T. Cambras, W.J. Schwartz, and Diez-Noguera, A. (2004). Forced desynchronization of dual circadian oscillators within the rat suprachiasmatic nucleus. *Curr. Biol.*, 14: 796–800.

Drew T and Doucet S (1991). Application of circular statistics to the study of neuronal discharge during locomotion. *J Neurosci. Methods*, 38: 171–181.

Dror RO, Canavier CC, Butera RJ, Clark JW and Byrne JH (1999). A mathematical criterion based on phase response curves for stability in a ring of coupled oscillators. *Biol.Cybern.*, 80: 11–23.

Fell J, Klaver P, Lehnertz K, Grunwald T, Schaller C, Elger CE, and Fernandez G (2001). Human memory formation is accompanied by rhinal-hippocampal coupling and decoupling. *Nature Neuroscience*, 4: 1259–1264.

Glass, L. and M.C. Mackey (1988). *From Clocks to Chaos: the Rhythms of Life*. Princeton, N.J: Princeton University Press.

Goel P and Ermentrout B (2002). Synchrony, stability, and firing patterns in pulse-coupled oscillators. *Physica D*, 163 (3–4): 191–216.

Hammond C, Bergman H and Brown P (2007). Pathological synchronization in Parkinson's disease: networks, models and treatments. *TINS* 30: 357–364.

Izhikevich EM (2007). *Dynamical systems in neuroscience: the geometry of excitability and bursting*. Cambridge, Mass.: MIT Press.

Llinas R. *I of the Vortex: From Neurons to Self*. Cambridge, Mass.: MIT Press.

Luo C, Canavier CC, Baxter DA et al (2004). Multimodal behavior in a four neuron ring circuit: Mode switching. *IEEE Transactions on Biomedical Engineering* 51: 205–218.

Maran SK, and Canavier CC (2008). Using phase resetting to predict 1:1 and 2:2 locking in two neuron networks in which firing order is not always preserved. *J Comput. Neurosci* 24: 37–55.

Morris C and Lecar H (1981). Voltage oscillations in the barnacle giant muscle fiber. *Biophys. J.*, 35: 193–213.

Netoff TI, Acker CD, Bettencourt JC and White JA (2005a). Beyond two-cell networks: experimental measurement of neuronal responses to multiple synaptic inputs. *J Comput. Neurosci.* 18: 287–295.

Netoff T, Banks M, Dorval A, Acker C, Haas J, Kopell N, and White J (2005b).
Synchronization in hybrid neuronal networks of the hippocampal formation.
J. Neurophysiol., 93: 1197–1208.

Oprisan, SA, Prinz, AA, Canavier, CC (2004). Phase resetting and phase-locking in
hybrid circuits of one model and one biological neuron, *Biophys. J.*, 87: 2283–2298.

Perez Velasquez JL, Galan RF, Dominguez LG, Leshchenko Y, Lo S, Belkas J and
Guevara Erra R. (2007). Phase response curves in the characterization
ofepileptiform activity. *Phys. Rev. E*, 76: 061912.

Pervouchine DD, Netoff TI, Rostein HG, White JA, Cunningham MO,Whittington MA
and Kopell NJ (2006). Low dimensional maps encoding dynamics in entorhinal
cortex and hippocampus. *Neural Comput.*, 18:2617–2650.

Rinzel J and Ermentrout GB (1998). Analysis of neural excitability and oscillations.
In C. Koch and I. Segev (Eds), *Methods in neuronal modeling from ions to networks.*
Cambridge, Mass.: MIT Press.

Rodriguez E, George N, Lachaux JP, Martinerie J, Renault B, and Varela F (1999).
Perception's shadow: Long distance synchronization of human brain activity.
Nature, 397: 430–433.

Sharp AA, O'Neil MB, Abbott LF and Marder EE (1993). Dynamic clamp computer
generated conductances in real neurons. *J. Neurophysiol.*, 69:992–995.

Sieling FH, Canavier CC and Prinz AA (2009). Predictions of phase-locking in
excitatory hybrid networks: Excitation does not promote phase-locking in pattern
generating networks as reliably as inhibition, *J. Neurophysiology*,102: 69–84.

Sieling FH, Canavier CC, Prinz AA (2010). Inclusion of noise in iterated firing time
maps based on the phase response curve, *Phys. Rev. E* 81, 1.

Singer W (1999). Neural synchrony: a versatile code for definition of relations. *Neuron,*
24: 49–65.

Stein SG, Grillner S, Selverston AI and Stuart DG, eds (1997). *Neurons, networks, and
motor behavior.* Cambridge, Mass: MIT Press.

Strogatz SH (2003). Sync: *How order emerges from chaos in the universe, nature, and daily
life.* New York: Hyperion.

Uhlhaas PJ and Singer W (2006). Neural synchrony in brain disorders: relevance for
cognitive dysfunctions and pathophysiology. *Neuron*, 52: 155–168.

Winfree A (1987). *The Timing of Biological Clocks.* New York: Scientific American Books.

Yuste R, MacLean JN, Smith J and Lansner A (2005). The cortex as a central pattern
generator. *Nature Rev. Neurosci.* 6: 477–483.

APPENDIX

The current balance equation for each Morris-Lecar model (ML model)
neuron is:

$$CdV/dt = -I_{Ca} - I_K - I_L - I_{syn} + I_{stim}$$

where the capacitance $C = 20\mu F/cm^2$, V is the cell membrane voltage in millivolts and t is time in milliseconds. The calcium current is given by $I_{Ca} = g_{Ca}m_\infty(V)(V-E_{Ca})$. The leak current is given by $I_L = g_L(V-E_L)$. The steady state activation is :

$$m_\infty(V) = 0.5\left[1 + \tanh\left\{(V - V_1)/V_2\right\}\right]$$

where $V_1 = -1.2$ mV and $V_2 = 18$ mV. The potassium current is given by $I_K = g_K w(V-E_K)$. The rate equation for the activation variable w in the expression for the potassium current is:

$$dw/dt = \varphi\left(w_\infty(V) - w\right)/\tau_w(V)$$

where φ was set to 0.04 with the steady state activation amplitude as:

$$w_\infty(V) = 0.5\left[1 + \tanh\left\{(V - V_3)/V_4\right\}\right]$$

and activation rate as:

$$\tau_\infty(V) = 1/\cosh\left\{(V - V_3)/2V_4\right\}$$

with $V_3 = 2$ mV and $V_4 = 30$ mV. The reversal potentials E_{Ca}, E_K and E_L were set to 120, −84 and −60 mV, respectively. The maximal potassium (g_K) and leak (g_L) conductances were set to 8.0 and 2.0 mS/cm^2, respectively. For calcium, the maximal conductance maximal (g_{Ca}) was set to 4.4 mS/cm^2 and I_{stim} was set at 100.0 $\mu A/cm^2$ for the homogeneous model neuron. Unless otherwise stated, the values for the various parameters for the Type II excitability regime were equal to those given above and were taken from Rinzel and Ermentrout (1998).

The synaptic current is given by $I_{syn} = g_{syn}s(V-E_{syn})$, where g_{syn} is the maximum synaptic conductance and E_{syn} is equal to −75 mV for inhibitory synaptic connectivity. The rate of change of the gating variable s is given by :

$$ds/dt = \alpha T\left(V_{pre}\right)(1-s) - s/\tau_{syn},$$

with $T(V_{pre}) = 1/[1 + \exp(-V_{pre}/2)]$, where V_{pre} is the voltage of the presynaptic cell, $\alpha = 6.25 ms^{-1}$ is the rate constant of the synaptic activation (Bartos et al. 2001), and τ_{syn} is the synaptic decay time constant and was set to 10 ms.

7

Understanding Animal-to-Animal Variability in Neuronal and Network Properties

Astrid A. Prinz, Tomasz G. Smolinski,
and Amber E. Hudson

Introduction

A large portion of this book describes and discusses *trial-to-trial* variability, i.e., variability in the responses of a given neuron to multiple presentations of a stimulus. In this chapter, we will focus on another type of variability, namely *animal-to-animal* variability of neuronal and network properties in identified neurons and circuits.

The term "identified neurons" refers to neurons that exist in an often fixed, and usually small, number of copies in every animal of a species and are identical or very similar from animal to animal in their overall morphology, innervation pattern, synaptic connections, electrical activity, response to inputs, and function within a circuit. Such identified neurons are predominantly found in invertebrates and their variability has been most extensively studied in the pyloric and gastric pattern-generating circuits of the crustacean stomatogastric ganglion (STG), which is why most of this chapter will focus on these neurons and circuits. Existing data from other nervous systems and decades of experience with lessons first learned in the STG and then generalized to other systems (Marder and Bucher, 2007) strongly suggest that the conclusions reached here will most likely be generally applicable to other, if not all, nervous systems and neuron types.

A thread running through this chapter will be the interplay of experimentation and computational modeling. On the one hand, animal-to-animal variability in neuronal and circuit properties poses challenging problems for the modeler that we will discuss below. On the other hand, comparing the variability of and relationships between neuron and network properties in living versus model neurons and circuits can lead to important insights and hypotheses regarding the functional significance of neuronal variability.

In the course of the chapter we will summarize recent results indicating that neuronal and network properties vary from animal to animal, but that correlations between cellular parameters exist both in biological and in model neurons.

Similar Neuron and Network Function from Variable Properties

That neurons of a given type vary in cell size, ion channel densities, synapse strengths, and other properties has been known for decades. Examples of such variability from different nervous systems and cell types are shown in Figure 7.1. As the figure illustrates, variability occurs both in the *parameters* of neural systems that underlie the generation of electrical activity (Figure 7.1A-D) and in the *output characteristics* of that activity (Figure 7.1C and G). For the remainder of the chapter, we will focus mostly on parameter variability. Typical parameter ranges found in neural systems show three-, four-, or five-fold variation in current amplitudes or membrane and synaptic conductance densities, and up to 10 mV shifts in ion channel activation thresholds. This level of variability exists even in identified invertebrate central pattern-generating neurons with their relatively stereotyped and reliable electrical activity, indicating that parameter variability does not necessarily translate into output variability. In other words, similar and functional electrical activity can be produced on the basis of widely varying cellular and synaptic parameter combinations (Marder and Goaillard, 2006).

Is animal-to-animal parameter variability in neuronal circuits a "bug" resulting from imprecise and stochastic operation of the molecular pathways that regulate properties such as ion channel and synaptic receptor densities? Or is it a "feature" that actually supports proper neuron and network function? Although this question has not been conclusively answered and remains an area of ongoing research, results from the study of how neurons and circuits homeostatically respond to perturbations in their activity suggest that it is the

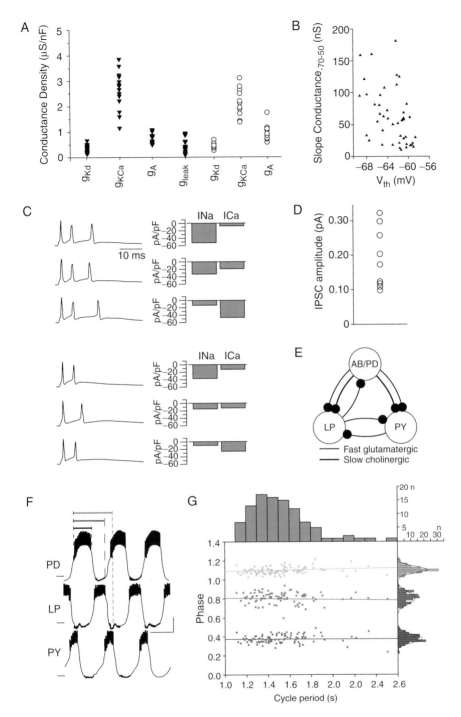

FIGURE 7.1 Animal-to-animal variability in neuronal and network properties
A) Conductance densities of ionic membrane currents in crab inferior cardiac (triangles)
and pyloric dilator neurons (circles). Each data point represents one animal. Adapted
from (Golowasch, et al. 1999; Goldman et al., 2000). B) Conductance amplitude and

FIGURE 7.1 (Continued) activation threshold variability of a potassium current in guinea pig ventral cochlear nucleus neurons. Slope conductance, defined as the slope of the current-voltage relationship between –70 mV and –50 mV, is used as a measure of conductance amplitude. Adapted from (Rothman and Manis, 2003). C) Action potential bursts and current amplitudes in mouse Purkinje neurons show variable current amplitudes in neurons with similar electrical activity. Adapted from (Swensen and Bean, 2005). D) Variability in inhibitory post-synaptic current (IPSC) amplitude at a synapse between identified leech heart interneurons. Each data point represents one animal. Adapted from (Marder and Goaillard, 2006). E) Simplified schematic of the crustacean pyloric pattern-generating circuit. AB/PD – anterior burster and pyloric dilator pacemaker kernel; LP – lateral pyloric neuron; PY – pyloric constrictor neuron. F) Voltage traces of PD, LP, and PY neurons in the pyloric motor pattern. Scale bars are 1 s and 10 mV. Definition of intervals PDon-PDoff (black), PDon-LPoff (dark gray), and PDon-PYoff (light gray) are indicated. E) and F) adapted from (Prinz et al., 2004). G) Distributions of cycle period and PDon-PDoff, PDon-LPoff, and PDon-PYoff phases in 99 lobster pyloric circuits. Phases are defined as interval duration divided by cycle period. Gray scale assignments are as in F). Adapted from (Bucher et al., 2005).

level and temporal patterning of electrical activity, rather than particular parameter values, that neurons are trying to maintain (Davis, 2006). Figure 7.2 shows changes in the densities of ionic membrane currents in STG neurons during homeostatic recovery of activity and in response to activity manipulation and demonstrates that membrane parameters are not fixed values, but rather, they are highly adjustable over the time course of hours. Since functional activity can be achieved with different parameter combinations, animal-to-animal variability of neuronal parameters could therefore be a consequence of the cells' homeostatic regulatory machinery being geared toward maintaining a particular level and type of activity, rather than particular values of membrane and synaptic properties.

Impact of Biological Variability on Model Construction

Beyond its potential biological implications for reliable network operation, neuronal parameter variability also has practical consequences for the construction of computational neuron and network models. Such models are intended to replicate experimentally observed cellular or circuit activity while simultaneously allowing the manipulation of experimentally not accessible parameters, and have become an important tool for neuroscientists (Prinz, 2006; Calabrese and Prinz, 2009). Given several-fold ranges of animal-to-animal variability in

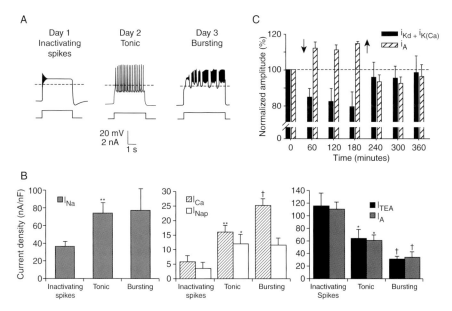

FIGURE 7.2 Conductance changes and activity homeostasis A) Recovery of bursting activity in isolated STG neurons. Neurons acutely isolated in culture initially are unable to generate bursts of action potentials in response to current injection and instead generate inactivating spikes. Over the course of days, bursting reminiscent of the neuron's in vivo activity is recovered. B) Densities of different membrane currents at three stages of activity recovery (inactivating spikes, tonic spiking, and bursting). Inward currents increase significantly during recovery (left, middle), while outward currents decrease (right). A) and B) adapted from (Turrigiano et al., 1995). C) Current amplitude changes in response to activity manipulation in STG neurons. Downward and upward arrows show onset and offset of rhythmic stimulation, respectively. Different K+ currents differentially and reversibly increase or decrease in response to rhythmic activity. Adapted from (Golowasch et al., 1999).

many biological parameters, what particular values should one chose for the equivalents of those parameters in a model? One approach would be to try to model a particular, individual neuron as a representative of a neuron type by using its particular, experimentally determined combination of parameter values in the model. Practically, this approach is almost never feasible due to the fact that it is – and probably always will be – virtually impossible to measure more than a small fraction of an individual neuron's cellular properties.

Another simple, and seemingly straightforward, choice of model parameters would seem to be the use of parameter values obtained by averaging measurements in an entire population of neurons of a given type. Unfortunately, years of painful experiences by model designers have shown that models constructed from averaged parameter values often fail to replicate the behavior of the neuron type they are intended to mimic, and often even fail to generate biologically plausible behavior at all, or to be dynamically stable. Figure 7.3 provides an explanation for this failure of averaged parameter values to generate functional behavior (Golowasch, Goldman et al., 2002). The problem lies in the fact that the distribution in parameter space of parameter combinations that generate functional neuron or network output – also called the neural system's "solution space" – is often complex (Achard and De Schutter, 2006) and can have convex features (Taylor, Hickey et al., 2006), such that averaging each parameter individually over a population of neurons can lead to a combination of averaged parameter values that itself is *not* part of the solution space (Golowasch, Goldman et al., 2002).

Interestingly, something akin to parameter averaging can occur in biological systems when there is tight electrical coupling between neurons of the same type, as is the case between the two pyloric dilator (PD) neurons and within the group of five to eight pyloric constrictor (PY) neurons in the STG. Tight electrical coupling in essence generates a coupled system that behaves

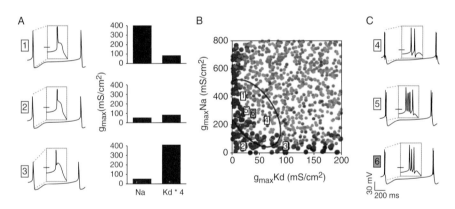

FIGURE 7.3 Failure of parameter averaging for model construction A) Voltage traces (left) and sodium and delayed rectifier potassium conductance densities (right) in three versions of a model neuron that generate virtually identical tonic spiking activity with different conductance combinations. Spike shapes are shown in insets. Scale bar from C) applies. B) Location of model versions with different electrical activity in the model conductance space. Spiking models with electrical activity as in A) are indicated by large dark dots. Lighter, smaller dots indicate models that generate bursts of spikes, as in C). Locations of models from A) and C) are indicated by numbers. Ellipse shows the 1 standard deviation (SD) covariance region around model 6. C) Voltage traces of models that lie within the covariance ellipse but generate bursting activity different from the tonic spiking shown in A). Model 6 is the model obtained by averaging the conductances of all tonically spiking models, but generates bursts of three spikes.

much like a larger neuron with the membrane conductances of the individual neurons acting in parallel. This effectively corresponds to a larger neuron with approximately the average of the original conductance densities for all ion channel types. Intriguingly, this biological parameter "averaging" may not run into the problem outlined in Figure 7.3, because at least in the case of the PD neurons in the STG, the two PD neurons in the same animal have been shown to have tightly correlated ion channel parameters to begin with (Schulz, Goaillard et al., 2006), and are thus likely already located in close proximity in parameter space.

Because models constructed on the basis of averaged parameter values are often not viable, other strategies for finding suitable model parameter sets become necessary. Among the approaches taken in the past (see (Prinz, 2007b) for a more detailed review and comparison of these methods) are (1) hand-tuning of model parameters based on the modeler's intuition of the relationship between parameters and model behavior, (2) optimization methods such as gradient descent that minimize the difference between model output and a target activity pattern, (3) evolutionary algorithms (see e.g., (Bäck, Fogel et al., 1997; Ashlock 2005)) that use methods inspired by natural selection to gradually "evolve" suitable model parameter sets over the course of multiple generations of model simulation, and (4) systematic exploration of a model by covering its parameter space with a regular grid or uniform random distribution of simulated parameter sets. The results of this latter type of parameter space exploration are often collected in so-called "model databases".

The four strategies outlined above tend to be used to address slightly different questions and generate different types of solution sets. Optimization methods such as hand-tuning and gradient descent (items 1 and 2 above) are often applied when the goal is to approximate the electrical behavior recorded from an individual neuron or circuit as a representative of its cell or circuit type. Almost by definition, they tend to converge quickly toward a single or a few viable solutions rather than map the entire solution space of a neural system. Evolutionary algorithms (item 3 above) are somewhat intermediate in that they can explore significant portions of the parameter space before converging on an "elite" population of solutions, although information about lower fitness individuals occurring early in the evolution process is often discarded, and the evolutionary algorithm neither guarantees to, nor is designed to, explore the entire solution space. In contrast, brute-force exploration of entire solution spaces and model database construction is often applied not with the purpose of matching one particular, "typical" individual, but instead is intended to locate the entirety of all parameter sets that generate behavior that falls within the biologically observed range (Prinz, 2007a). In the context of animal-to-animal variability, systematic parameter exploration therefore provides datasets that are uniquely suited for comparison with parameter sets assembled from a biological population of neurons of the same type. This will become clearer in the following section.

Model Databases Replicate Biological Variability

Model databases constructed by exploring a neuron or network model's parameter space allow for the selection of a subpopulation of parameter combinations that generate activity within the range of activities observed in the corresponding biological system, also termed the model's "solution space". An example of two such solutions for a model of the pyloric network in the crustacean STG is shown in Figure 7.4 (Prinz, Bucher et al., 2004).

Do model solution spaces and the parameter ranges they cover show variability similar to that found in the corresponding biological system (see Figure 7.1 for variability examples)? Figure 7.4 illustrates that, in many cases, they do. For example, in a model database constructed by exploring the cellular and synaptic parameter space of a model of the pyloric circuit in the STG (Prinz, Bucher et al., 2004), it was found that the solution space covered the entire range explored in the model database for all but one of the seven synapses in the circuit (Figure 7.4C). These conductance ranges spanned several orders of magnitude; from zero synaptic conductance to a maximal conductance value that was saturating in the sense that it would force the postsynaptic membrane potential to the synaptic reversal potential (increasing the synaptic conductance beyond this saturating value would have no bigger effect on the postsynaptic neuron). Similarly, the solution space of a single-cell model of the pyloric pacemaker kernel showed parameter ranges (characterized by the standard deviation divided by the mean) in the range of 0.3 to 0.5 (Prinz, Billimoria et al., 2003), comparable to the ranges found in the biological pacemaker neurons (Fig. 7.1) (Golowasch, Abbott et al., 1999; Goldman, Golowasch et al., 2000). A similar correspondence between parameter variability in a neuron type and its corresponding model neuron database has also been reported for mammalian globus pallidus neurons (Gunay, Edgerton et al., 2008).

Correlations of Neuronal Properties

Thus far we have discussed neuronal animal-to-animal variability only by examining the ranges covered by individual parameters. However, results from

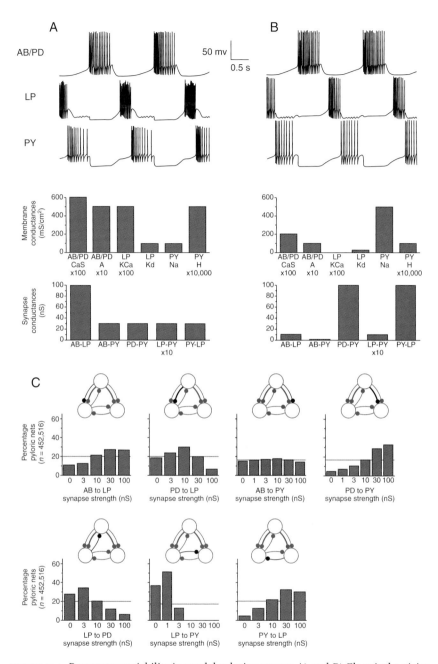

FIGURE 7.4 Parameter variability in model solution spaces A) and B) Electrical activity (top) and cellular and synaptic parameters (bottom) of two pyloric network models that generate similar and functional activity on the basis of widely different parameters. C) Distributions of the pyloric network model's solution space over the strengths of the synapses in the circuit. With one exception (synapse from LP to PY), all synapses cover the entire explored range of strengths, which encompasses several orders of magnitude. Adapted from (Prinz et al., 2004).

the modeling study (Golowasch, Goldman et al., 2002) presented in Figure 7.3 suggest that neuronal parameters may not vary independently from solution to solution, and recent experimental evidence obtained with a variety of independent methods shows that, indeed, there can be interdependences between multiple parameters and their variability. Most often, these interdependencies seem to take the form of linear correlations between pairs or higher numbers of parameters. This is illustrated in Figure 7.5 with data obtained from electrophysiological measurements of current amplitudes in identified STG neurons (Khorkova and Golowasch, 2007), and with single-cell PCR measurements of the mRNA levels coding for different ion channels, also in identified STG neurons (Schulz, Goaillard et al., 2007). The mRNA copy number has been established as a good proxy for ionic current amplitude for two out of three current types for which the relationship was examined (Schulz, Goaillard et al., 2006).

Several things are noteworthy about the neuronal parameter correlations that have been reported thus far based on experimental data:

1. All the correlations reported in the literature are linear relationships, i.e., fixed ratios between two or more conductances or mRNA levels. The only exception is an apparently logarithmic relationship that has been observed between specific pairs of ionic conductances of STG neurons in voltage clamp experiments (Jorge Golowasch, personal communication).

2. All linear relationships reported have positive slope, meaning that if one conductance is large, so is the other. Based on the available repertoire of intracellular regulatory cascades that could potentially underlie cellular parameter correlations, it is not clear why negative correlations do not appear to be implemented in biological neurons. For example, one could imagine two ion channel species under the control of the same transcription factor, with one being up-regulated and the other being down-regulated when the intracellular concentration of the transcription factor is increased (Gomez-Ospina, Tsuruta et al., 2006). Furthermore, negative correlations between specific pairs of conductances would appear to make physiological sense in the case of conductances with similar function, because an overabundance of one type of ion channel could be compensated for by a reduction in another channel type with similar properties.

3. Correlations between different cellular parameters are not limited to pairs of parameters. Rather, it appears than in some cases up to four parameters can be correlated to each other (see Figure 7.5B).

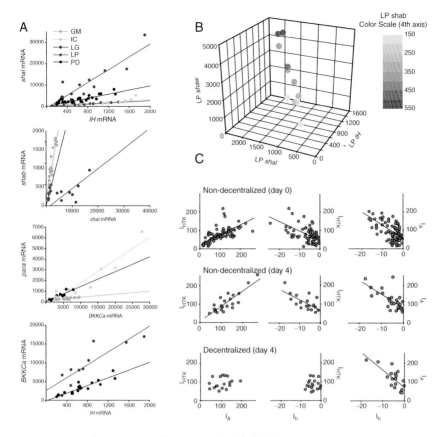

FIGURE 7.5 Conductance correlations in identified STG neurons A) Linear relationships between mRNA copy numbers of pairs of ion channel types in different cell types of the STG. GM – gastric mill neuron; IC – inferior cardiac neuron; LG – lateral gastric neuron. Ionic current types corresponding to the different mRNAs are: *shal* – transient potassium current I_A; *IH* – hyperpolarization-activated inward current I_h; *shab* – delayed rectifier potassium current I_{Kd}; *para* – sodium current I_{Na}; *BKKCa* – calcium-dependent potassium current I_{KCa}. B) The LP neuron shows a four-way correlation between *shaw, shal, shab,* and *IH* mRNA copy numbers. A) and B) adapted from (Schulz et al., 2007). C) Correlations between current densities (in nA/nF) in crab PD neurons before and after STG decentralization. I_{HTK} is a high-threshold potassium current. Two of three correlations present in the intact system are abandoned in response to decentralization. Adapted from (Khorkova and Golowasch, 2007).

4. Correlations vary from cell type to cell type even within the same species. For example, Figure 7.5A shows that the conductance of the transient potassium current (I_A) and that of the delayed rectifier potassium current (I_{Kd}) are correlated in LP (lateral pyloric), GM (gastric mill), and LG (lateral gastric) neurons in the STG, but not in PD and IC (inferior cardiac) neurons.

5. In cell types that share a correlation between a pair of conductances, such as that of the hyperpolarization-activated inward current I_h and I_A in LP, PD, IC, and LG neurons, the slope of the correlation can be different, as shown in Figure 7.5B. Points 4 and 5 together suggest that it may be the complement of conductance coregulation rules and the corresponding conductance ratios that underlie the specific electrical properties of an identified cell type (Schulz, Goaillard et al., 2007).

6. Conductance correlations may depend on the modulatory or activity state of a cell or circuit and may therefore not be constant throughout the lifetime of an animal. This is suggested by Figure 7.5C, which shows that STGs that have been deprived of neuromodulatory input and electrical activity by deafferentation abandon some of their coregulation rules while maintaining others (Khorkova and Golowasch, 2007).

The molecular basis for the parameter correlations illustrated in Figure 7.5 remains largely unknown. Possible mechanisms and molecular interactions that could establish and maintain parameter correlations could potentially occur at any stage of the intracellular machinery that leads from ion channel genes through transcription, translation, post-translational modification, and membrane insertion, to a functional channel in the neuronal membrane (Davis, 2006). The only case in which some light has been shed on the mechanisms underlying a conductance correlation is the correlation between I_A and I_h in PD neurons of the crab STG. In a series of elegant papers, Harris-Warrick and coworkers have established that PD neurons react to over-expression of the ion channel underlying I_A by proportionally up-regulating I_h (MacLean, Zhang et al. 2003), that over-expression of I_A, even in the form of a non-conducting mutant, is sufficient to trigger up-regulation of I_h, and that the effect is unidirectional, meaning that over-expression of I_h does not trigger up-regulation of I_A (Zhang, Oliva et al., 2003). Notably, a fixed ratio between the I_A and I_h amplitudes also exists in naïve PD neurons in which neither channel has been over-expressed (MacLean, Zhang et al., 2005). Together, these findings suggest that the correlation between I_A and I_h in PD neurons of the STG is the result of a regulatory structure substantially more complex than the simple co-control of two channels by the same transcription factor. What exactly underlies this and other parameter correlations remains subject to future investigation.

The notion—introduced earlier in this chapter—that similar neuronal or network activity can result from different cellular and synaptic parameter combinations has recently been challenged (Nowotny, Szucs et al., 2007). In that work, Selverston and co-workers have argued that cells and circuits that generate similar activity with different parameter combinations could be expected to react differently to the application of neuromodulators or pharmacological blockers that act on a subset of membrane conductances or synapses, because such modulatory or pharmacological intervention would unmask differences in the remaining cell or network properties that would lead to different electrical activity. In contrast, experimental data show that the pyloric circuit in the STG tends to react in an impervious way to neuromodulation or channel blocking (Szucs and Selverston, 2006).

The conductance correlations shown in Figure 7.5 suggest an intriguing possible resolution to this apparent conundrum. If pairs or higher numbers of ionic conductances can be co-regulated in neurons, why couldn't such co-regulation rules also exist between the membrane densities of ion channels and receptors for neuromodulators? In this scenario, relationships between membrane and synaptic properties and susceptibility to neuromodulator action could be coordinated in a way that would ensure proper and reliable response to modulators despite different cellular and synaptic properties (Marder and Goaillard, 2006). In the absence of experimental data showing such correlations this remains speculation, but future experiments examining possible relationships between cellular and network properties and susceptibility to modulation could address this question.

Parameter Correlations in Model Populations

As shown above, populations of functional model neurons and networks selected from model databases replicate the parameter variability seen in biological neurons and networks. Do they also exhibit parameter correlations such as those described in Figure 7.5? To answer this question, we analyzed a population of biologically realistic two-compartment models of the pyloric pacemaker neuron AB (anterior burster) for pair-wise correlations between maximal conductance values (Prinz, Smolinski et al., 2008; Smolinski and Prinz, 2009). This model population had previously been generated by exploring the twelve-dimensional maximal conductance space of the model around a hand-tuned, canonical model version (Soto-Treviño, Rabbah et al., 2005). Correlations between pairs of parameters reminiscent of those shown in Figure 7.5 were indeed found in the model population. One example is shown in Figure 7.6A, where a relationship between two currents, namely the fast transient calcium current I_{CaT} and I_{Kd}, in the model AB neuron is represented by a characteristic "ridge" with a clearly positive slope. Interestingly, and in contrast to the always positive conductance correlations found in biological neurons, model neuron populations can exhibit both positive and negative correlations (see Figure 7.7 for some examples).

As mentioned above, model populations needed for solution space analysis can be obtained not only through systematic parameter space exploration and database construction, but also through the use of evolutionary algorithms. Figure 7.6B shows a population of suitable AB models obtained with an evolutionary algorithm applied to the same pacemaker model whose parameter space was explored systematically in Figure 7.6A (Smolinski and Prinz, 2009). The section of parameter space accessible to the evolutionary algorithm in this case was substantially bigger than the space explored in Figure 7.6A, and went to upper limits that are several-fold larger than the maximal conductance values that are experimentally observed in living AB neurons. Remarkably, the evolutionary algorithm produced a model population that not only spanned close to the entire accessible (and in large parts physiologically unrealistic) parameter range, but also maintained the correlation seen in Figure 7.6A. Because the solution population in Figure 6B includes parameter combinations that are physiologically not realistic, additional constraints may need to be implemented if model exploration is intended to result in model populations that are truly comparable to biological populations of a given neuron type. For example, imposing metabolic constraints that would penalize excessive ionic current flows – and the need for energetically costly ion pump activity that comes with them – might have limited the evolution of model versions in Figure 7.6B to lower and more realistic conductance values.

Are Parameter Correlations Functionally Relevant?

If both experimental data from identified neuron types and model populations exhibit conductance correlations, how are the two related? Do biological neurons and their model counterparts show the same correlation structure, or are there correlations between specific parameter sets that occur in the living neurons but not in the models, or *vice versa*? These questions are closely related to the big-picture question of whether correlations between cellular parameters are functional – i.e., whether they promote or even ensure proper electrical activity of the neurons in question. A correlation between particular parameters that occurs both in the model population and in the biological neurons would appear to be adaptive in the sense that it might support the generation

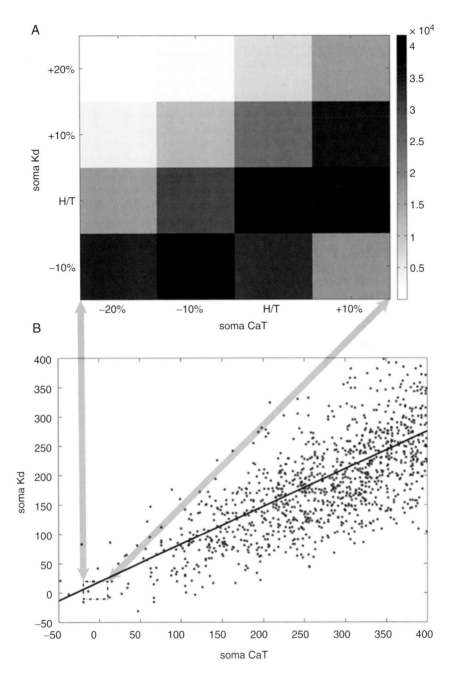

FIGURE 7.6 Example of a conductance correlation in the solution space of an AB pacemaker model neuron A) Density of suitable AB models for different values of two somatic membrane conductances based on parameter space exploration on a regular grid. Explored conductance values included the canonical, hand-tuned value (H/T) and deviations from it by up to +20% or -20%. Gray scale shows number of

FIGURE 7.6 (Continued) solutions in units of 10,000. B) Solutions obtained with an evolutionary algorithm for the same model neuron, but on a parameter range extending from -100% to +400% of the canonical conductance values. Line is a linear fit to the data. The extent of the parameter space covered in A) is indicated by a rectangle in B). Adapted from (Smolinski and Prinz, 2009).

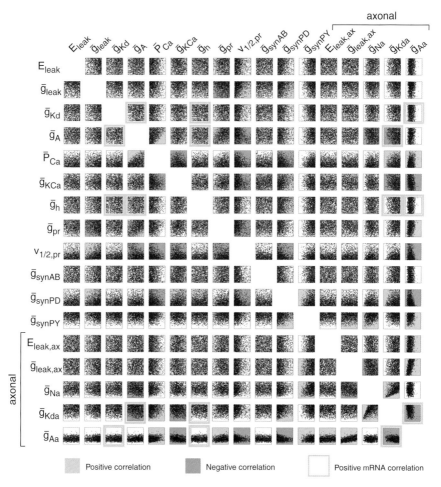

FIGURE 7.7 Conductance correlations in a population of 1,304 LP model neurons Each scatterplot corresponds to a pair of model parameters as indicated by the labels above and to the left of the matrix. Within each scatterplot, each point corresponds to one LP model version. Model parameter pairs with a positive correlation are shaded in light gray while pairs with a negative correlation are shaded in dark gray. The scatterplots of parameter pairs for which a positive correlation between channel mRNAs was found in living LP neurons (Schulz et al., 2007) are framed in gray. Adapted from (Taylor et al., 2009).

of functional cellular activity. In contrast, a correlation between parameters that is seen in the model population but is not implemented in the living neurons could be seen as a "missed opportunity", that is, a correlation that, if it had occurred in the living neuron, might have increased its chances of producing functional activity. Finally, a correlation that occurs in the biological neurons but has no counterpart in the model population invites speculation that it is an epiphenomenon of the specific intracellular regulatory cascades that have evolved in the neurons, but has no relation to functional activity.

With only very few experimental and modeling results on conductance correlations published thus far, the answers to the questions posed above are still inconclusive. We have already seen, however, that there appear to be fundamental differences between the types of correlations found in biological versus model neurons. As stated above, all correlations found in living neurons thus far are positive, whereas correlations with both positive and negative slopes are found in model studies. One example of such a study is shown in Figure 7.7, which shows the complete pair-wise correlation structure of a population of models of the LP neuron in the pyloric circuit (Taylor, Goaillard et al., 2009). This model population was generated by selecting models with functional activity from a database generated by covering the model's parameter space with a uniform, random distribution of simulations. Not only does the model population show both positive and negative correlations, as indicated in the figure, but there is also no overlap between the positive correlations found in the model population and those found in living LP neurons. Following the line of argument presented above, it would therefore seem that at least in the case of the LP neuron, parameter correlations implemented in the living neuron may *not* play a role in ensuring proper electrical function. An alternative explanation for the discrepancy between correlations found in the model and those found in the biological neuron could be that the model and the constraints used to select its functional parameter combinations were not physiologically realistic enough to accurately reproduce the biological neuron's properties and parameter correlations.

Summary and Conclusions

Even within identified neuron and circuit types with highly stereotyped electrical output and function, parameters can vary widely from animal to animal. This variability is reproduced by populations of model neurons or circuits selected from model databases. Parameters do not always vary independently, however; relationships between pairs or sets of neuronal parameters can take the form of linear correlations with positive slope. Such relationships also occur in model populations, but often do not coincide with the relationships seen in the corresponding biological neuron type. Furthermore, model populations also show linear parameter relationships with negative slope, a type of relationship thus far not seen in living neurons despite its functional plausibility and molecular feasibility.

Whether animal-to-animal variability of—and correlations between— neuronal and circuit properties are functionally important and what molecular regulation mechanisms underlie these correlations is currently not entirely clear. These questions are the subject of ongoing and future investigative efforts that should help us better understand the significance of variability in neuronal systems.

Acknowledgments

This work was supported by a Burroughs Welcome CASI award to AAP. We thank Adam Taylor and Anne-Elise Tobin for help with figures.

REFERENCES

Achard, P. and De Schutter, E. (2006). Complex parameter landscape for a complex neuron model. *PLoS Computational Biology, 2,* 794–804.

Ashlock, D. (2005). *Evolutionary computation for modeling and optimization.* NY: Springer.

Bäck, T., Fogel, D.B., and Michalewicz, Z., Eds. (1997). *Handbook of evolutionary computation.* NY: Taylor & Francis.

Bucher, D., Prinz, A.A. and Marder, E. (2005). Animal-to-animal variability in motor pattern production in adults and during growth. *J of Neuroscience, 25,7,* 1611–1619.

Calabrese, R. L. and Prinz, A.A. (2009). Realistic modeling of small neuronal networks. *Computational Modeling Methods for Neuroscientists.* DeSchutter, E., Ed. Cambridge, Mass.: MIT Press.

Davis, G. W. (2006). Homeostatic control of neural activity: From phenomenology to molecular design. *Annual Review of Neuroscience, 29,* 307–323.

Goldman, M. S., Golowasch, J., Marder, E. and Abbott, L.F. (2000). Dependence of firing pattern on intrinsic ionic conductances: Sensitive and insensitive combinations. *Neurocomputing, 32,* 141–146.

Golowasch, J., Abbott, L.F. and Marder, E. (1999). Activity-dependent regulation of potassium currents in an identified neuron of the stomatogastric ganglion of the crab Cancer borealis. *J of Neuroscience, 19,20,* Art. No.-RC33, 1–5.

Golowasch, J., Goldman, M.S., Abbott, L.F. and Marder, E. (2002). Failure of averaging in the construction of a conductance-based neuron model. *J of Neurophysiology*, *87*,*2*, 1129–1131.

Gomez-Ospina, N., Tsuruta, F. et al. (2006). The C terminus of the L-type voltage-gated calcium channel Ca(v)1.2 encodes a transcription factor. *Cell*, *127*,*3*, 591–606.

Gunay, C., Edgerton, J.R. and Jaeger, D. (2008). Channel density distributions explain spiking variability in the globus pallidus: A combined physiology and computer simulation database approach. *J of Neuroscience*, *28*,*30*, 7476–7491.

Khorkova, O. and Golowasch, J. (2007). Neuromodulators, not activity, control coordinated expression of ionic currents. *J of Neuroscience*, *27*,*32*, 8709–8718.

MacLean, J. N., Zhang, Y., Goeritz, M.L., Casey, R., Oliva, R., Guckenheimer, J. and Harris-Warrick, R.M. (2005). Activity-independent coregulation of I-A and I-h in rhythmically active neurons. *Journal of Neurophysiology*, *94*,*5*, 3601–3617.

MacLean, J. N., Zhang, Y., Johnson, B.R. and Harris-Warrick, R.M. (2003). Activity-independent homeostasis in rhythmically active neurons. *Neuron*, *37*,*1*, 109–120.

Marder, E. and Bucher, D. (2007). Understanding circuit dynamics using the stomatogastric nervous system of lobsters and crabs. *Annual Review of Physiology*, *69*, 291–316.

Marder, E. and J. Goaillard, M. (2006). Variability, compensation and homeostasis in neuron and network function. *Nature Reviews Neuroscience*, *7*,*7*, 563–574.

Nowotny, T., Szucs, A., Levi, R. and Selverston, A.I. (2007). Models wagging the dog: Are circuits constructed with disparate parameters? *Neural Computation*, *19*,*8*, 1985–2003.

Prinz, A. A. (2006). Insights from models of rhythmic motor systems. *Current Opinion in Neurobiology*, *16*,*6*, 615–620.

Prinz, A. A. (2007a). Computational exploration of neuron and neuronal network models in neurobiology. *Methods in Molecular Biology: Bioinformatics*. Crasto, C., Ed. Totowa N.J. Humana Press: 167–179.

Prinz, A. A. (2007b). Neuronal parameter optimization. *Scholarpedia*, *2*,*1*, 1903.

Prinz, A. A., Billimoria, C.P. and Marder, E. (2003). Alternative to hand-tuning conductance-based models: Construction and analysis of databases of model neurons. *J of Neurophysiology*, *90*,*6*, 3998–4015.

Prinz, A. A., Bucher, D. and Marder, E. (2004). Similar network activity from disparate circuit parameters. *Nature Neuroscience*, *7*,*12*, 1345–1352.

Prinz, A. A., Smolinski, T.G., Soto-Treviño, C. and Nadim, F. (2008). *Conductance coregulations in a 2-compartment model of the anterior burster (AB) neuron in the lobster pyloric pacemaker kernel.* Society for Neuroscience Annual Meeting, Washington, D.C.

Rothman, J. S. and Manis, P.B. (2003). Differential expression of three distinct potassium currents in the ventral cochlear nucleus. *J of Neurophysiology*, *89*,*6*, 3070–3082.

Schulz, D. J., Goaillard, J.M. and Marder, E. (2006). Variable channel expression in identified single and electrically coupled neurons in different animals. *Nature Neuroscience*, *9*,*3*, 356–362.

Schulz, D. J., Goaillard, J.M., and Marder, E. (2007). Quantitative expression profiling of identified neurons reveals cell-specific constraints on highly variable levels of gene expression. *Proceedings of the National Academy of Sciences of the United States of America, 104*, 13187–13191.

Smolinski, T. G. and Prinz, A.A. (2009). *Computational Intelligence in Modeling of Biological Neurons: A Case Study of an Invertebrate Pacemaker Neuron*. International Joint Conference on Neural Networks, Atlanta, Ga.

Soto-Treviño, C., Rabbah, P., Marder, E. and Nadim, F. (2005). Computational model of electrically coupled, intrinsically distinct pacemaker neurons. *J of Neurophysiology, 94,1*, 590–604.

Swensen, A. M. and B. P. Bean. (2005). Robustness of burst firing in dissociated Purkinje neurons with acute or long-term reductions in sodium conductance. *Journal of Neuroscience, 25,14*, 3509–3520.

Szucs, A. and Selverston, A.I. (2006). Consistent dynamics suggests tight regulation of biophysical parameters in.a small network of bursting neurons. *J of Neurobiology, 66,14*, 1584–1601.

Taylor, A. L., Goaillard, J.M. and Marder, E. (2009). How Multiple Conductances Determine Electrophysiological Properties in a Multicompartment Model. *J of Neuroscience, 29,17*, 5573–5586.

Taylor, A. L., Hickey, T.J., Prinz, A.A. and Marder, E. (2006). Structure and visualization of high-dimensional conductance spaces. *Jl of Neurophysiology, 96,2*, 891–905.

Turrigiano, G., Lemasson, G. and Marder, E. (1995). Selective regulation of current densities underlies spontaneous changes in the activity of cultured neurons. *Journal of Neuroscience, 15,5*, 3640–3652.

Zhang, Y., Oliva, R., Gisselmann, N., Hatt, H., Guckenheimer, J. and Harris-Warrick, R.M. (2003). Overexpression of a hyperpolarization-activated cation current (I-h) channel gene modifies the firing activity of identified motor neurons in a small neural network. *J of Neuroscience, 23,27*, 9059–9067.

8

Dynamical Parameter and State Estimation in Neuron Models

Henry D. I. Abarbanel, Paul H. Bryant, Philip E. Gill,
Mark Kostuk, Justin Rofeh, Zakary Singer,
Bryan Toth, and Elizabeth Wong

Introduction

In exploring networks of neurons, the electrophysiology of the nodes (the neurons) and the links (synaptic or gap junction connections) provide two of the three essential ingredients for initiating analysis of the network. The third is the functional connectivity of the network. We have developed a method for network analysis that allows parameters and states of the nodes and of the links of the network to be accurately estimated from observations of membrane voltages. We call this analysis method (Creveling et al, 2008) "dynamical parameter estimation" (DPE) because it allows a dynamical look into properties of biological nervous systems in a quantitative manner using only voltage observations coupled with a mathematical model of the network. In that sense, it can replace the pharmacological manipulations usually required for the analysis of channel properties in establishing neuron models. It can also establish the connectivity of a network with the same ingredients.

The key to the development of DPE is the notion, suggested some years ago, of estimating parameters in a nonlinear model by synchronizing the output of experimental observations of a system with a model of the system (Pecora et al, 1990; Parlitz et al, 1996; Dedieu et al., 1997; Maybhate and Amriktar, 1999; Pikovsky et al., 2001; Broecker et al., 2001; Broecker et al., 2002; Sakaguchi, 2002; Tokuda et al, 2002; Voss et al., 2004; Konnur, 2003; Huang, 2004). As we explain in the next section, these formulations of the parameter estimation problem utilize a standard least-squares metric that suffers from various numerical difficulties (Voss et al., 2004) Additionally, many current papers, of which (Yu et al., 2007; Yu et al. 2006; and Abarbanel et al,. 2008) are typical, employ *ad hoc* update rules for the model network and synchronization coupling parameters. The comparison metric is typically a form of least-squares evaluation of the difference between measured data and the model equivalent of the data. This metric suffers from having a very complex surface in the space of network parameters arising from the possibility of chaos in the network (Voss et al., 2004).

We analyze these difficulties and suggest a formulation of the parameter and state estimation problem that avoids them. As it happens, the resulting optimization problem is equivalent to the well-studied, long-standing problem of the optimal tracking of a trajectory. In our case, the "trajectory" is the observed voltage measurement $V_{data}(t)$ and the optimization problem is to control a model that is developed for the biophysical goal of quantifying the description of the experimental system. We require that the model output equivalent to the observed voltages track the observation, i.e., synchronize with it. We use this requirement to estimate the model parameters, along with a cost for the control.

A first step in the formulation of DPE is to establish a balanced synchronization between the data and the model to ensure that experimental data is transmitted to the model efficiently and accurately. This synchronization also ensures that the coupling is not so strong that the model is simply entrained by the data and the model is overwhelmed by the connection to the data. This balance is explored in Abarbanel et al., 2008, and briefly described here for clarity. The key idea is the need to couple the data to the model sufficiently strongly to provide stability on the synchronization manifold (where observed data equals model output) but not so strongly that entrainment of the model by the data stream is induced. This also removes the plethora of local minima that are seen when using least-squares metrics (Voss et al., 2004) to stabilize the synchronization manifold of the data and the model.

In this paper we do not explore the use of DPE in determining parameters and states using observed data. Our goal is more limited: to demonstrate within a series of neuron models that model parameters from "data" generated with a known set of parameters can be recovered using DPE as we formulate and explain it here. Thus, we use our artificial data to determine how well DPE is working when we, in fact, know both the parameters used in generating the data as well as the state variables of the "data" system that are not experimentally observable; we call these "twin experiments". In our examples of neuron models, one typically can observe dynamical variables such as membrane voltages, but cannot observe the activation and inactivation variables for voltage gated ion channels. Nonetheless, providing the model and DPE approach with the data voltage $V_{data}(t)$ alone is shown to allow accurate estimation of the unobserved state variables as well as the system parameters.

There is a history of interesting approaches to parameter estimation for neurobiological models of neurons and networks of neurons, and, of course, an equally intense exploration in many other fields. In neuroscience one can point to the recent papers (Bhalla and Bower, 1993; Foster et al., 1993; Vanier and Bower 1999; Tabak et al., 2000; Prinz et al., 2003; Prinz et al. 2004; Hayes et al. 2005; Huys et al., 2006; Haufler et al, 2007) and the recent paper of Tien and Guckenheimer (2007). The paper (Haufler et al., 2007) uses the idea of synchronization of data with a model, although it does not address some of the problems with this approach we examine here. Our goal is more in the spirit of some of the earlier papers cited that look at parameter estimation in models of neurons and networks. We present a general framework within which one can use any specific knowledge of particular models or neuron types.

After a discussion of the formulation of DPE, this paper considers the application of the method to some individual neuron models. We begin with the familiar Hodgkin-Huxley (HH) model found in textbooks on neurophysiology. Johnston and Wu (1994) discuss both the model and the manipulations usually required to establish the model parameters from observational data. This is a four-dimensional model of a neuron that can exhibit chaotic behavior (Guckenheimer and Oliva, 2002). We apply our methods to parameter regimes where the attractor is a rest state or a periodic limit-cycle oscillation,and not those where chaotic oscillations are possible. This parameter regime describes many neurobiological settings. The chaotic regimes pose no particular difficulties for the DPE approach, as it was developed for such systems. However, for the HH neuron these chaotic regimes do not correspond to biophysically interesting parameters.

Our second example is the two degrees-of-freedom Morris-Lecar (ML) model (Morris and Lecar, 1981; Fall et al., 2002).(See Chapter 12). The ML neuron cannot express chaos in its time development, but it allows us to illustrate the use of DPE in the determination of parameters entering nonlinearly into a neuron model through the kinetic equations for voltage gated channels.

The ML model has both a rest state for small and large applied DC current and an oscillating, spiking, state for a range of intermediate currents. We show that the use of stimulation protocols taken directly from familiar current clamp ideas for the determination of neuron parameters in a laboratory work here as well. Current clamp twin experiments on the model neuron show that all parameters of the model—those that enter the model linearly and those that enter nonlinearly—may be determined using our method.

In investigating the effect of additive noise on the measurements presented to our parameter and state estimation procedure, we observed that the estimated state was much closer to the noise-free data than to the noisy data that were provided. This "cleaning" of a signal was apparently known to radio engineers in the former Soviet Union as early as the 1950s and 1960s (Rabinovich, 2008), though we have not been able to find a specific reference to their work. We did find a compilation of papers from a group at Moscow State University that does refer to this phenomenon for nonlinear dynamical systems with a limit cycle oscillation[1] In an Appendix, we discuss this noise-reduction feature of our method and extend the discussion to chaotic nonlinear oscillators. The example presented there is not connected to neurobiology.

The methods described here have much broader applications than neurobiology. Our formulation of DPE applies to all models described by differential equations or discrete time maps. Our goal in developing DPE, however, has been to provide a quantitative tool for exploring networks. This paper discusses only the analysis of nodes at networks, and we will report on its use in networks in the near future (Kostuk and Abarbanel, to appear).

Formulation of the Method: Dynamical Parameter Estimation (DPE)

Data

The dynamical problem we wish to solve can be formulated in the following manner: We are observing a network of neurons connected by synaptic and gap junction couplings. The state of the system is described by the dynamical variables, or degrees of freedom, $\mathbf{x}(t) = [x_1(t), x_2(t), \ldots]$. In addition there are fixed parameters in the system. There may also be external forcing or external inputs to the network, which are identified explicitly, when present.

---

[1] For work related to the noise reduction for amplitudes, not phases, in nonlinear limit cycle oscillators, see the papers in Kuznetsov, P. I., R. L. Stratonovich, and V. I. Tikhonov, *Non-Linear Transformations of Stochastic Processes*, Pergamon Press, London (1965); translated by J. Wise and D. C. Cooper.

The $\mathbf{x}(t)$ are all required to determine the full state of the network, but typically only one or a few of the components of $\mathbf{x}(t)$ can be observed. In quite general discussions of the parameter estimation problem at hand, one often takes as an observable variable a scalar function of the state: $h(\mathbf{x}(t))$. In the applications to neurobiology of interest to us, we know that the easily measured state variables are the membrane voltages of neurons in the network. In particular, for our discussion of the model formulation, we assume only one voltage $V_{data}(t)$ can be measured, and we call that observed variable $x_1(t)$.

We measure $x_1(t)$ and pass that information, along with explicit information about any injected currents, to our model of the neurobiological network. In a current-clamp protocol, this would include the specifics about the current introduced into the neuron over a fixed time interval. With this information in hand, we can begin the analysis we call "dynamical parameter estimation".

We want to build a model of the data generating network and, using our observations of $x_1(t)$, accurately estimate the parameters, typically unknown, in the formulation of the network. In DPE we also estimate the unobserved state variables $\mathbf{x}_\perp(t)$, and, naturally, we also want the model variable equivalent to $x_1(t)$ to be accurately estimated.

The DPE formulation could include partial differential equations discretized in space appropriately. While this poses real computational challenges, it does not alter the general framework we present in this discussion. This means intracellular diffusion processes could be included, for example. This paper does not address how we create the model from biophysical and neurobiological principles. We also do not address questions associated with the fact that any model we do construct will be wrong in some manner.

Model

We now formulate a model of the observed network using what anatomical and physiological evidence we possess and whatever biophysical model construction ideas we choose to be relevant. We represent the dynamical variables of the model as $\mathbf{y}(t) = [y_1(t),\, y_2(t),\, ...,\, y_D(t)] = [y_1(t),\, \mathbf{y}_\perp(t)]$. The model will involve unknown fixed parameters $\mathbf{p} = [p_1,\, p_2,\, ...,\, p_L]$. In a neurobiological network these fixed parameters may be maximal conductances, reversal potentials, and numerical parameters entering the kinetic coefficients for the activation and inactivation dynamics of the channel.

We identify $y_1(t)$ as equivalent to the observed $x_1(t)$; again, in neurobiology, it is likely to be a membrane voltage. We wish to find a set of parameters that are the same as those in the underlying, but unknown, equations for the network, and we wish to provide accurate estimates for the $\mathbf{y}(t)$ which are 'near' the $\mathbf{x}(t)$: $\mathbf{y}(t) \approx \mathbf{x}(t)$. Since we have observed only $x_1(t)$, we cannot ever be certain, except in the kind of exercise we carry out in this paper, where we actually know both the $\mathbf{x}(t)$ equations and the $\mathbf{y}(t)$ equations, that our estimates of the unobserved $\mathbf{y}_\perp(t) \approx \mathbf{x}_\perp(t)$ are accurate. The same is true of the estimated parameters. Our artificial situation where we know precisely the source of our data should be seen as a testing ground for the DPE method. Perhaps one should think of the work in this paper where we generate the data and then analyze how well DPE is able to reproduce what we know as a "proof of concept" of the method. In applying DPE to laboratory data acquired with a certain set of stimulus protocols, we would verify the model by asking how well it predicts set of additional experiments with different stimuli.

Since one cannot know, in the setting where only experimental observations $x_1(t)$ are available, whether we have also properly captured the time dependence of the other state variables, one needs to develop a set of verification and validation methods for testing the model once the parameters have been estimated and we have established that $y_1(t) \approx x_1(t)$. We do not address this important question in this paper as we do so elsewhere (Abarbanel et al., 2009), and here we have the details of the system that generated both $x_1(t)$ and the unobserved $x_\perp(t)$ and can directly verify that $y_\perp(t) \approx x_\perp(t)$.

An issue of concern when applying methods for parameter estimation using synchronization of experimental data and a model of the experimental network is that the data may lie on the system attractor so information about all degrees of freedom associated with the negative Lyapunov exponents bringing orbits to the attractor is lost. We show in the neuron models discussed here, however, that transient data, which do carry information lost when an orbit has reached the attractor, is enough for determination of the parameters. Transient data result from perturbations to the dynamical system as it evolves along its attractor, so perturbations induced by the experimenter, as in the current clamp protocol, are critical. This approach now avoids a long standing concern about identifying model parameters and state variables solely on the system attractor. Further, it is an important nexus with our interest in neurobiological applications as essentially all data and functional actions of nervous systems take place in transient regimes.

With all that said, our model takes the form

$$\frac{dy_1(t)}{dt} = F_1(y_1(t), \mathbf{y}_\perp(t), \mathbf{p})$$

$$\frac{d\mathbf{y}_\perp(t)}{dt} = \mathbf{F}_\perp(y_1(t), \mathbf{y}_\perp(t), \mathbf{p}). \tag{1}$$

Except when the data is generated, as here, by a specific model known to us $F(y,p)$ can never be exactly correct. Any attempt to seek solutions of the model $y(t)$ matching the data $y(t) \approx x(t)$ can only be correct in the sense of generalized synchronization (Rulkov, et al, 1995; Abarbanel, et al., 1996; Tang and Heckenberg, 1997).

The data are sampled discretely in time, and we take the sampling to be performed at every time interval τ starting at an initial time $t_0 = 0\tau$. Time is thus discrete $t = t_m = t_0 + m\tau$ with $m = 0, 1, 2,\ldots, N$ until the final time $T = t_0 + N\tau$ that data collection is completed. Our data is then $x_1(t_m = t_0 + m\tau) = x_1(t_m)$, for m=0, 1,..., N.

If we report the solution to the model equations (1) at intervals τ so $y(t = t_0 + m\tau) = y(t_m)$, then to compare the quality of synchronization of the time-series, we traditionally would evaluate the cost function $C(p)$

$$C(\mathbf{p}) = \frac{1}{2(N+1)} \sum_{m=0}^{N} (x_1(t_m) - y_1(t_m))^2,$$

using the data and the model output. It is natural to expect that when the parameters in the model equal those of the source of the observed data, this cost function $C(\mathbf{p})$ will be a minimum.

This requires us to evaluate the zeros of $\partial C(\mathbf{p})/\partial \mathbf{p}$, and this leads directly to the source of the numerical challenges noted above and discussed at some length in the review article (Voss et al. 2004).

Returning for notational simplicity to the continuous time form of $C(\mathbf{p})$

$$C(\mathbf{p}) = \frac{1}{2T} \int_0^T dt(x_1(t) - y_1(t))^2,$$

we see that we must study the properties of

$$\frac{\partial C(\mathbf{p})}{\partial \mathbf{p}} = \frac{1}{T} \int_0^T dt \, \frac{\partial y_1(t)}{\partial \mathbf{p}} (y_1(t) - x_1(t)).$$

Noting that $\partial y_1(t)/\partial \mathbf{p}$ satisfies the following coupled, driven linear equations along with $\partial y_\perp(t)/\partial \mathbf{p}$

$$\frac{d}{dt}\left(\frac{\partial \mathbf{y}(t)}{\partial \mathbf{p}}\right) = \frac{\partial \mathbf{F}(\mathbf{y},\mathbf{p})}{\partial \mathbf{y}}\left(\frac{\partial \mathbf{y}(t)}{\partial \mathbf{p}}\right) + \frac{\partial \mathbf{F}(\mathbf{y},\mathbf{p})}{\partial \mathbf{p}},$$

we see that the Jacobian matrix $\mathbf{DF(y,p)}=\partial\mathbf{F(y,p)}/\partial\mathbf{y}$ that enters here is precisely the one that leads to chaos in nonlinear systems. Consider the differential equation associated with "sensitivity to initial conditions"

$$\frac{d}{dt}\left(\frac{\partial\mathbf{y}(t)}{\partial\mathbf{y}(0)}\right)=\frac{\partial\mathbf{F(y,p)}}{\partial\mathbf{y}}\left(\frac{\partial\mathbf{y}(t)}{\partial\mathbf{y}(0)}\right),$$

and recall that this Jacobian iterated along the orbit $\mathbf{y}(t)$ may possess positive global Lyapunov exponents which are the hallmark of chaotic behavior. Unregulated, this chaotic behavior will lead to decorrelation of any connection between the observations $x_1(t)$ and the model output $y_1(t)$, and this is the source of the complex dependence on parameters of $C(\mathbf{p})$

We need a way to induce the correlation or equality or synchronization $x_1(t) \approx y_1(t)$ both to efficiently pass information from the data to the model and to minimize our metric $C(\mathbf{p})$. A strategy for this was suggested by several authors. The idea in these papers is to couple the data stream $x_1(t)$ into the model equations in a manner that would synchronize the model output $y_1(t)$ with the data. The suggested manner for this coupling is

$$\frac{dy_1(t)}{dt} = F_1(y_1(t),\mathbf{y}_\perp(t),\mathbf{p})+k(x_1(t)-y_1(t))$$

$$\frac{d\mathbf{y}_\perp(t)}{dt} = \mathbf{F}_\perp(y_1(t),y_\perp(t),\mathbf{p}), \qquad (2)$$

with k an appropriate, constant coupling. This passes information from the data to the model and, when k is large enough, leads to the synchronization of the data and the model. The manner in which this is expected to work is that the Jacobian $\mathbf{DF}(y,p)$ which may have led to the presence of a positive Lyapunov exponent for the solutions to Equation (1) is now altered to $\mathbf{DF}(y,p)-K$ where $K_{11} = k$ and all other elements are zero. This new Jacobian matrix when iterated along an orbit of Equation (2) yields a conditional Lyapunov exponent (CLE) (Pecora and Carroll, 1990) as the solutions are conditioned on the properties of the data $x_1(t)$ coupled into the equation for $y(t)$. If a Lyapunov exponent associated with $\mathbf{DF}(y,p)$ is positive, and the largest CLE of $\mathbf{DF}(y,p)-K$ is negative, then the synchronization manifold $y(t)=x(t)$ is stabilized, and one might expect that the complex behavior in parameters space of $C(\mathbf{p})$ would be eliminated.

It might appear unusual that the equations (2) are actually different from the model as the term $k(x_1(t)-y_1(t))$ is present, and thus the dynamics of $\mathbf{y}(t)$

will be different from the model. Fortunately, in the implementation of DPE discussed below, the way in which this occurs leads naturally to $k \to 0$ as the optimization proceeds.

This raises an issue of some importance in our work. We seek to synchronize the data and the model. It is not generally true that providing one state variable, here $x_1(t)$, and asking that it match the equivalent model variable $y_1(t)$ will lead to synchronization of the other variables. An example is given by (Pecora and Carroll, 1990) in their work on synchronization of chaotic systems. We must ask then whether in any particular problem, the synchronization error $C(k) = (1/2T)\int_0^T dt(x_1(t) - y_1(t))^2$ in fact goes to zero for large k. In Figure 8.1 we show this quantity for two different Hodgkin-Huxley models, each of which has been coupled to a data stream $x_1(t)$. We see that in each case, synchronization occurs for a moderate value of $k \approx 2-3$, but for different k in each case.

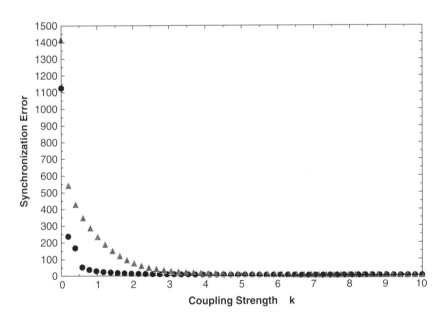

FIGURE 8.1 For two Hodgkin-Huxley Models with states $x(t)$ and $y(t)$; a term $k(x_1(t) - y_1(t))$ is added to the differential equation for $y_1(t)$. Solving for $y(t)$ we evaluate the synchronization error $x_1(t) - y_1(t)$ and plot it as a function of k. The synchronization error for two distinct HH models is shown. In the region of $k \approx 2-3$ synchronization sets in. For k smaller than this, the synchronization manifold $x_1(t) = y_1(t)$ is unstable and a positive conditional Lyapunov exponent is present.

The two models differ only in the selection of an injected DC current, and each undergoes a limit cycle oscillation of a different frequency.

To illustrate the regularity (or irregularity) of a cost function as a function of a model parameter, we have solved a simple three dimensional model of an RF oscillator (see the Appendix for the equations of this chaotic oscillator) having a parameter called η for various values of k; k=0.0, 1.9 and 11.4. These are shown in Figure 8.2. We evaluated the least squares error function $C(k,\eta,N)$ for different values of k,η and number of data points N. The value of η used in the calculation was η=6.2723. For k=0 where there is no coupling of the data into the model, we see from Figure (2) that $C(k$=0$,\eta,N)$ has no minimum near η=6.2723 and as N grows, namely the length of the data signal extends longer into time elapsed from it initiation, there appear many, irregular local minima in the dependence on η. This arises as the instability associated with a positive conditional Lyapunov exponent λ>0 manifests its influence on the error function as errors grow at a rate $e^{\lambda t N}$. As we increase k we see the synchronization error both become smooth in its dependence on η, flatter as a function of η, and smaller in magnitude.

It is clear that the absence of a coupling term such as $k(x_1(t) - y_1(t))$ can lead to complicated structure of a cost function $C(\mathbf{p})$ in parameter space (Voss et al., 2004)and that complexity can be cured by k large enough to yield stability of the synchronization manifold. As is beginning to appear in Figure 8.2, k can be too large as well. In fact, if we increase k in Equation (2), the coupling term soon comes to dominate the contribution $F_1(y_1(t), \mathbf{y}_\perp(t), \mathbf{p})$, namely the model itself, unless $|x_1(t) - y_1(t)| \approx 1/k$. When that occurs, the cost function becomes of order $1/k^2$ and is small in magnitude, reducing the size of the derivatives $\partial C(\mathbf{p})/\partial \mathbf{p}$. When the latter are too small, it becomes numerically difficult to determine its zeroes which is where we must search for model parameters to match those in the data.

To address this issue it would appear that a *balance* in the choice of coupling is required. The most natural option is to add a penalty to the cost function that requires the largest CLE to be slightly negative, but near zero as a function of k and $\mathbf{p}$. This just guarantees synchronization and assures us that k is not too small. As it happens, since the largest CLE behaves as $-k$ for large k, it also leads to a penalty of order k^2 in that regime.

Other ideas on how to balance the synchronization and the dynamical role of the coupling suggest that if the coupling k were time dependent $k \rightarrow u(t)$, then the fact that the synchronization manifold has varying stability over the attractor, namely the attractor is not homogeneous in state space, can be addressed through different values of the coupling along a trajectory.

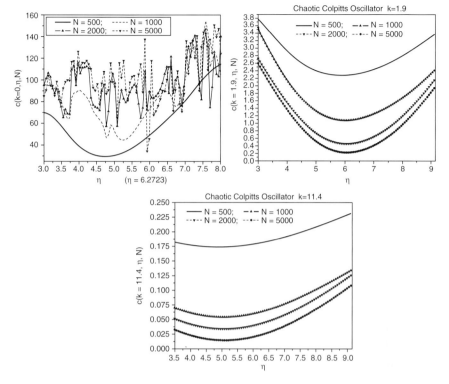

FIGURE 8.2 Two Colpitts oscillators (see the Appendix) are coupled with a term $k(x_1(t) - y_1(t))$ in the differential equation for $y_1(t)$ The least-squares error (cost) function $C(k,\eta,N) = \dfrac{1}{N}\sum_{l=1}^{N}(x_1(l) - y_1(l))^2$ is plotted as a function of the parameter η in the model equation (state variables $y(t)$), the strength of the coupling k and the number of terms in the sum. The minimum of $C(k,\eta,N)$ should determine η; the value in the input data is $\eta = 6.2723$. Upper Left Panel For $k = 0$ (no coupling) the cost function develops complex multiple local minima that interfere with the determination of the parameter η. This phenomenon is discussed in a recent review [11]. This structure comes from the positive Conditional Lyapunov exponent of the $y(t)$ system; that is, the instability of the synchronization manifold $x_1(t) = y_1(t)$. (Upper-Right Panel) As k increases and the two oscillators synchronize, the behavior in η becomes smooth. (Bottom Panel) As k increases further, the value of $C(k,\eta,N)$ decreases and the derivatives with respect to η, required to determine the minimum of the function all decrease and impair locating the minimum.

When we put these suggestions together we have a dynamical state and parameter estimation approach we call DPE:

Given data from an experimental observation $x_1(t)$ and a model for the orbits $\mathbf{y}(t)$ of the system being observed with one component of the model, $y_1(t)$, corresponding to the measured variable $x_1(t)$, **minimize**

$$C(\mathbf{y}, u, \mathbf{p}) = \frac{1}{2T} \int_0^T \{(x_1(t) - y_1(t))^2 + u(t)^2\},$$

subject to the model equations of motion

$$\frac{dy_1(t)}{dt} = F_1(y_1(t), \mathbf{y}_\perp(t), \mathbf{p}) + u(t)(x_1(t) - y_1(t))$$

$$\frac{d\mathbf{y}_\perp(t)}{dt} = \mathbf{F}_\perp(y_1(t), \mathbf{y}_\perp(t), \mathbf{p}), \tag{3}$$

to find the parameters $\mathbf{p}$, the states $\mathbf{y}(t) = [y_1(t), \mathbf{y}_\perp(t)]$, and the control $u(t)$. If we had the luxury of measuring more than one variable in the data acquisition, we would introduce a control coupling similar to $u(t)$ for each such observation, and the scalar $u(t)$ would be replaced by a vector of those control couplings.

Because of the form of the cost function, as we achieve synchronization $\mathbf{x}_1(t) \approx y_1(t)$, the control $u(t)$ is driven to zero, and we recover, *de facto*, the model equations we desire.

This formulation of the parameter and state estimation problem does not specify the control $u(t)$. It also leaves open the issue of how to implement the search in parameter space to find those $\mathbf{p}$ that minimize the cost (or objective) function. Some authors including ourselves (Abarbanel et al, 2008) have suggested *ad hoc* differential equations for $u(t)$, and/or let the parameters become time dependent (i.e., $\mathbf{p} \rightarrow \mathbf{p}(t)$) by introducing equations for $d\mathbf{p}(t)/dt$ that drive the parameters to a fixed point, perhaps with the local synchronization error $(x_1(t) - y_1(t))^2$ driven to zero at the fixed point as well. Each of these suggestions provides an interesting manner in which to perform the multidimensional search in the space of states $\mathbf{y}(t)$, controls $u(t)$ and parameters $\mathbf{p}$ required to locate the desired minimum of $C(\mathbf{y}, u, \mathbf{p})$. However, all choices for $d\mathbf{p}(t)/dt$ or $du(t)/dt$ are somewhat arbitrary from the point of view of the physical or biological system under investigation.

As it happens, the DPE approach is equivalent to a form of optimal trajectory tracking (Kirk, 2004; Bryson et al., 1969) formulated decades ago and analyzed quite thoroughly, along with the development of well tested software for implementing the method and solving the optimization problems associated with it. In a simple description, this recognizes that the data are, in fact, sampled at only a finite set of times, t_m, here separated by the sampling time τ, starting at an initial time $t_0 = 0$ and continuing through $t = t_0 + m\tau$; m=0, 1,..., M to $t_M = t_0 + M\tau = T$. The cost function becomes

$$C(\{\mathbf{y}(t_m)\}, \{u(t_m)\}, \mathbf{p}) = \frac{1}{2(M+1)} \sum_{m=0}^{M} \{(x_1(t_m) - y_1(t_m))^2 + u(t_m)^2\},$$

a function of the $D(M+1)$ state variables $\mathbf{y}(t_m)$, m=0, 1,..., M, the $D_C(M+1)$ control variables $u(t_m)$, and the L parameters $\mathbf{p}$. ($D_C = 1$ in our formulation.) The differential equations become equality constraints relating the state variables at $t = t_m$ to those at $t = t_{m+1}$. In the direct method a search is made in the (possibly) large $(D + D_C)(M+1) + L$ -dimensional space, imposing the equality constraints as well as some form of continuity or smoothness on the controls $u(t)$. The mathematical literature addresses the virtues and challenges of using the direct method (Gill et al., 2005; Barclay et al. 1998). Suffice it to say that in our application, the data are sampled finitely; $x_1(t)$ is, in fact, known only at t_m. Further, the role of the control $u(t)$ is to impose synchronization locally on the attractor of the dynamical system.

We implement the direct method as a solution option for DPE using the numerical package SNOPT (Gill et al., 2005). In the descriptions of SNOPT one discovers that the advantage of searching in the large dimensional space indicated, in addition to the finite sampling of the data, is that all optimization methods are variants of Newton's method, which involves the solution of large systems of linear equations. In the space of state and control variables, these equations are sparse, which implies that efficient, well-test numerical methods may be employed.

SNOPT does not dictate the interpolation, the method for smoothing the controls $u(t_m)$, or the integration method that connects $\mathbf{y}(t_m)$ with $\mathbf{y}(t_{m+1})$:$\mathbf{y}(t_m) \to \mathbf{y}(t_{m+1})$. The user must select these. Here we use a Hermite cubic interpolation scheme for the $u(t_m)$ and Simpson's rule for $\mathbf{y}(t_m) \to \mathbf{y}(t_{m+1})$. We have not yet explored other integration or interpolation schemes.

Neuron Models

The Standard Hodgkin-Huxley Model

The standard Hodgkin-Huxley (HH) model has four dynamical variables: membrane voltage $V(t) = y_1(t)$, and three activation and inactivation variables for the Na and K voltage-gated channels: $m(t) = y_2(t)$; $h(t) = y_3(t)$; $n(t) = y_4(t)$.

These are explored in many textbooks (Johnson et al, 1994; Beuter et al, 2003; Koch, 2004). In our notation these equations are written as

$$\frac{dy_1(t)}{dt} = p_1\{p_2 y_2(t)^3 y_3(t)(p_3 - y_1(t)) + p_4 y_4(t)^4 (p_5 - y_1(t))$$
$$+ p_6(p_7 - y_1(t)) + I_{app}(t)\} + u(t)(x_1(t) - y_1(t))$$

$$\frac{dy_2(t)}{dt} = \alpha_m(y_1(t))(1 - y_2(t)) - \beta_m(y_1(t))y_2(t)$$

$$\frac{dy_3(t)}{dt} = \alpha_h(y_1(t))(1 - y_3(t)) - \beta_h(y_1(t))y_3(t)$$

$$\frac{dy_4(t)}{dt} = \alpha_n(y_1(t))(1 - y_4(t)) - \beta_n(y_1(t))y_4(t)$$

where the kinetic coefficients $\alpha_X(V)$ and $\beta_X(V)$, $X=\{m,h,n\}$, are given by

$$\alpha_m(V) = \frac{p_8(p_9 - V)}{e^{(p_9 - V)p_{10}} - 1}; \qquad \beta_m(V) = p_{11}e^{-Vp_{12}}$$

$$\alpha_h(V) = p_{13}e^{-Vp_{14}}; \qquad \beta_h(V) = \frac{p_{15}}{e^{(p_{16} - V)p_{17}} + 1}$$

$$\alpha_n(V) = \frac{p_{18}(p_{19} - V)}{e^{(p_{19} - V)p_{20}} - 1}; \qquad \beta_n(V) = p_{21}e^{-Vp_{22}}$$

Altogether we have twenty-two parameters (with values given in Table 8.1), four state variables, and a control $u(t)$. In our calculations we selected the external applied current $I_{app}(t)$ and did not attempt to determine it as part of the optimization, although this is possible.

We generated "data" by integrating the equations with no control ($u(t)=0$) and $I_{app}(t)$ selected from a piece of the oscillation of a chaotic system. The parameters are independent of the applied current, and this kind of $I_{app}(t)$ moves the orbits off the autonomous system attractor to explore the full phase space of the system. This generated $x_1(t)$ (the "observed" membrane voltage) as well as $x_2(t)$, $x_3(t)$, $x_4(t)$ which cannot be observed.

The time series $x_1(t)$ was used in a numerical optimization search using SNOPT to determine the parameters as well as all of the state variables $\mathbf{y}(t)$ and the control $u(t)$, via minimization of the DPE cost function

$$C = \frac{1}{2T}\int_0^T dt[(x_1(t) - y_1(t))^2 + u(t)^2],$$

TABLE 8.1 HH Model: "Data" Parameters and Estimated Parameters.

Parameter	Data	τ=0.05 ms	τ=0.025 ms	τ=0.01 ms	$I_1 = 18.63$ $\mu A/cm^2$	$I_1 = 12.47$ $\mu A/cm^2$
$p_1\ cm^2/\mu F$	1.0	0.9303	1.0002	1.003757	1.0054	1.00450
$p_2\ mS/cm^2$	120.0	70.37	120.91	120.14126	125.36995	102.0289
$p_3\ mV$	115.0	127.83	115.01	115.0057	114.988	114.93126
$p_4\ mS/cm^2$	36.0	24.08	35.64	36.22558	35.2232	37.9208
$p_5\ mV$	−12.0	−12.05	−12.002	−12.0198	−12.0032	−12.0206
$p_6\ mS/cm^2$	0.3	0.239	0.3007	0.29405	0.29814	0.296999
$p_7\ mV$	−10.613	−8.769	−10.621	−10.508	−10.5998	−10.5853
$p_8\ mS^{-1}$	0.1	0.0642	0.0995	0.09989	0.09887	0.10936
$p_9\ mV$	25.0	21.6	24.877	24.8852	24.6860	27.0965
$p_{10}\ mV^{-1}$	0.1	0.0706	0.1001	0.100317	0.100879	0.09779
$p_{11}\ mS^{-1}$	4.0	6.00	4.001	3.9913667	3.99034	3.95311
$p_{12}\ mV^{-1}$	0.05555	0.0707	0.05542	0.055469	0.05573	0.05830
$p_{13}\ mS^{-1}$	0.07	0.0877	0.06974	0.0692276	0.067133	0.056587
$p_{14}\ mV^{-1}$	0.05	0.075	0.04964	0.05008349	0.05090	0.0948413
$p_{15}\ mS^{-1}$	1.0	1.001	1.0029	0.998656	1.0029	0.97478
$p_{16}\ mV$	30.0	29.632	30.141	30.028406	29.8754	30.3088
$p_{17}\ mV^{-1}$	0.1	0.1297	0.09933	0.09967	0.09890	0.10932
$p_{18}\ mS^{-1}$	0.01	0.0150	0.01006	0.0099501	0.010186	0.009366
$p_{19}\ mV$	10.0	15.00	9.946	10.29004	10.8077	9.1553
$p_{20}\ mV^{-1}$	0.1	0.1297	0.09933	0.098503	0.098519	0.1007235
$p_{21}\ mS^{-1}$	0.125	0.122	0.1248	0.12492	0.12397	0.12449
$p_{22}\ mV^{-1}$	0.0125	0.00625	0.012445	0.012535	0.013079	0.0124115

Chaotic $I_{app}(t)$ for various sampling times τ=0.05, 0.025, 0.01ms. Also Current Clamp Protocol (τ=0.01ms): $I_1 = 12.47\ \mu/cm^2$A would lead to a Fixed Point in the HH Dynamics. $I_1 = 18.63\mu/cm^2$ A would lead to Limit Cycle Oscillations in the HH Dynamics.

subject to the equations of motion for $\mathbf{y}(t)$, including the control term $u(t)(x_1(t) - y_1(t))$, equation.

To examine the sensitivity of our estimation procedure to the sampling rate of the data, we selected τ=0.05 ms (or sampling at 20kHz), τ=0.025 ms (or sampling at 40kHz), and τ=0.01 ms (or sampling at 100kHz). Following that we applied a current clamp protocol with two amplitudes of the current pulse. The results of the SNOPT optimization in these cases are given in Table 8.1.

We conclude from these calculations that the sampling rate of the data does matter in distinguishing model parameters. Undersampling may not permit one to identify the parameters accurately. Although we did not know *a priori* which sampling time would be needed, it appears that τ=0.02 ms and shorter will provide an adequate look at the variations in waveforms and allow a sufficient distinction. This means sampling data at 50 kHz or faster, and that is not usual for neurobiological experiments., so it is important to note that only 4000 data points at that sampling rate were used, and acquisition of 40 ms of data may not be a challenge even at a sampling rate of 100 kHz or higher. In assessing the SNOPT (or other optimization method) implementation of DPE, it seems clear that one should evaluate the parameters for a sequence of sampling times and look for a regime where the output becomes independent of τ.

Similarly we examined whether the estimated parameters in this HH model were independent of the input applied current. We changed the applied current protocol to that of a standard current clamp pulse with low current until some fixed time, a higher DC current I_1 for a chosen length of time, then return to the low current. We performed two current clamp calculations with the low current chosen as zero and the upper current selected as $I_1 = 18.63\mu A/cm^2$ and then as $I_1 = 12.47\mu A/cm^2$. In the first case, the neuron would undergo periodic limit-cycle oscillations at that current. In the second case, the neuron would remain at rest, but at a higher resting potential than with I=0.

In three of our calculations, done at different τ, we arrived at the same parameters when the sampling rate was high enough (τ=0.025 and 0.01 ms). Similarly, for the two current clamp calculations, the estimated parameters were remarkably good for each pulse amplitude. In the current clamp cases, we found better estimates of the parameters when the current was high enough to lead to an oscillatory state (limit cycle) of the neuron. We argue that this arises because one must move the model trajectories off their attractor and allow them to explore their full phase space, and a larger plateau current will accomplish this.

Indeed, this is an important consideration. It seems clear that if we attempted to estimate the parameters of an HH model, or any other dynamical system, when we observed that model system at a fixed point alone, we would not succeed; there must be many solutions to that problem. Observation of a point in a many (here four) dimensional space is inadequate. In a geometrical sense, what might be a good guideline is that perturbations to the model (and the data system) that move its orbits well off the attractor and out into the phase space of the system should be better than perturbations leaving the system close to its fixed points. The details of the transient motions in phase space distinguish one parameter setting from another, as the orbits, as indicated in the

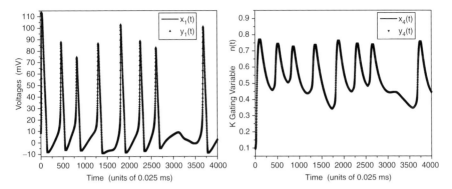

FIGURE 8.3 Comparison of the input model, voltage $x_1(t)$ and the SNOPT output $y_1(t)$; also comparison of the known, but not transmitted to the model, $x_1(t)$ and the SNOPT output $y_1(t)$) Left $x_1(t)$ and $y_1(t)$ (mV). (Right) $x_4(t)$ and $y_4(t)$, $\tau = 0.025$ ms $I_{app}(t)$, the injected current into the neuron is taken from the oscillations of a chaotic system.

Introduction, may well be sensitive to small changes in parameters. This view may also explain the success, once the sampling time was small enough, of using a signal from a chaotic generator in $I_{app}(t)$ to assist in the estimation procedure.

The Morris-Lecar Model

Our second example is the Morris-Lecar model, comprised of two dynamical equations for the membrane voltage $V(t)$ and a potassium activation variable $w(t)$ (Morris and Lecar, 1981; Fall et al., 2002). It was originally developed to describe an experimental study of the excitability of the giant muscle fiber of the huge Pacific barnacle, *balanus nubilis*. The dynamical variables in the model are the membrane voltage $y_1(t)$ and the K$^+$ activation variable $y_2(t)$. Parameters are chosen as well as an $I_{app}(t)$ and the following ordinary differential equations are solved for the data $V(t) = x_1(t)$ and $w(t) = x_2(t)$.

$$\frac{dx_1(t)}{dt} = p_{12}(p_9 m_0(x_1(t))(p_5 - x_1(t)) + p_{10} x_2(t)(p_6 - x_1(t))$$
$$+ p_{11}(p_7 - x_1(t)) + I_{app}(t))$$

$$\frac{dx_2(t)}{dt} = \frac{w_0(x_1(t)) - x_2(t)}{\tau(x_1(t))}.$$

where

$$m_0(V) = \frac{1}{2}\left(1 + \tanh\left(\frac{(V - p_1)}{p_2}\right)\right); \qquad w_0(V) = \frac{1}{2}\left(1 + \tanh\left(\frac{(V - p_3)}{p_4}\right)\right);$$

$$\tau(V) = p_8/\cosh\left(\frac{(V - p_3)}{2p_4}\right).$$

The parameters in the "data" source for $x_1(t)$ were selected as $p_1 = -1.2mV$, $p_2 = 18.0mV$, $p_3 = 2mV$, $p_4 = 30mV$, $p_5 = 120mV$, $p_6 = -84mV$, $p_7 = -60mV$, $p_8 = 0.04$, $p_9 = 4.4mS/cm^2$, $p_{10} = 8mS/cm^2$, $p_{11} = 2mS/cm^2$, and $p_{12} = 0.05cm^2/\mu F$.

The resulting $x_1(t)$ was coupled into the equation for $y_1(t)$

$$\frac{dy_1(t)}{dt} = p_{12}(p_9 m_0(y_1(t))(p_5 - y_1(t)) + p_{10} y_2(t)(p_6 - y_1(t))$$
$$+ p_{11}(p_7 - y_1(t)) + I_{app}(t)) + u(t)(x_1(t) - y)_1(t)$$

$$\frac{dy_2(t)}{dt} = \frac{w_0(y_1(t)) - x_2(t)}{\tau(y_1(t))}.$$

We first performed two current clamp twin experiments in which $I_{app}(t)$ was 0 until $t=50$ ms, then I_1 for 50 $ms \le t \le 220$ ms. We selected $I_1 = 75\mu A/cm^2$ for one calculation. At this value of the injected current, the ML model has a

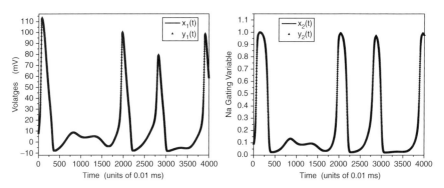

FIGURE 8.4 Comparison of the input, model, voltage $x_1(t)$ and the SNOPT output $y_1(t)$ also comparison of the known, but not transmitted to the model, $x_2(t)$ and the SNOPT output $y_2(t)$. Left $x_1(t)$ and $y_1(t)$ (mV). Right $x_2(t)$ and $y_2(t)$, $\tau = 0.025$ ms $I_{app}(t)$, the injected current into the neuron is taken from the oscillations of a chaotic system.

TABLE 8.2 ML Model: "Data" Parameters and Estimated Parameters

Parameter	Data	$I_{app}(t) = \mu A/cm^2$	$I_1 = 75\mu A/cm^2$	$I_1 = 115\mu A/cm^2$
$p_1 = V_1$ mV	−1.2	−1.20002	−1.11	−1.13
$p_2 = V_2$ mV	18.0	17.999	18.33	18.219
$p_3 = V_3$ mV	2.0	2.0008	2.80	2.64
$p_4 = V_4$ mV	30.0	30.0008	31.22	30.93
$P_5 = E_{Ca}$ mV	120.0	120.0011	120.85	120.68
$p_6 = E_K$ mV	−84.0	−83.9999	−84.25	−84.27
$p_7 = E_L$ mV	−60.0	−59.9998	−59.94	−59.93
$p_8 = \phi$ $(ms)^{-1}$	0.04	0.040000	0.04113	0.0407
$p_9 = g_{Ca}$ mS	4.4	4.3998	4.434	4.411
$p_{10} = g_K$ mS/cm²	8.0	8.0000	8.07	8.05
$p_{11} = g_L$ mS/cm²	2.0	1.99997	2.03	2.02
$p_{12} = 1/C_M$ cm²/μF	0.05	0.04999	Fixed at 0.05	Fixed at 0.05

Current Clamp Protocol: $I_1 = 75\ \mu A/cm^2$ would lead to a Fixed Point in the ML Dynamics. $I_1 = 115\mu A/cm^2$ would lead to Limit Cycle Oscillations in the ML Dynamics

fixed point or a constant resting voltage. A second current clamp experiment was performed with $I_1 = 115\mu A/cm^2$, at which current level the ML neuron undergoes periodic limit cycle oscillations.

After this current clamp protocol, we investigated another applied current $I_{app}(t) = 220(1 - cos(0.02t)e^{-0.005t})\mu A/cm^2$. The parameters in the ML model should be independent of $I_{app}(t)$. Table 8.2 shows the results of each injected current protocol on the determination of the parameters in the ML model.

Instrumental Noise in Hodgkin-Huxley Models

Additive Noise: Uniformly Distributed and Gaussian Distributed

All of the calculations we have reported until now have used a data signal $x_1(t)$ that was transmitted to a model system with no noise. To explore the effect of "instrumental" noise, namely additive noise on the data signal we added to $x_1(t)$ a random number at each time step. This means we took $x_1(t) \to x_1(t) + A\zeta(t)$ where the values of ζ at every time step were drawn from a probability distribution. We examined two such distributions: (1) numbers uniformly distributed the interval $[-1,1]$, and (2) numbers drawn from a gaussian distribution with variance equal unity: $P(x) = \dfrac{1}{\sqrt{\pi}}e^{-x^2}$. The average of these noise signals is zero,

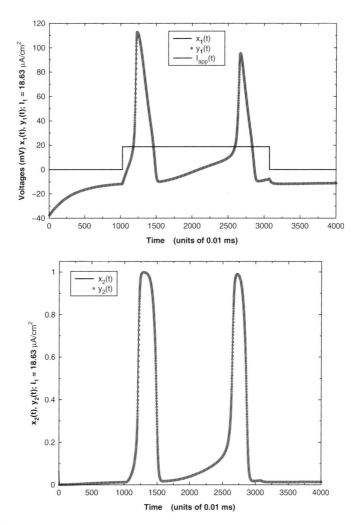

FIGURE 8.5 Comparison of the input, model, voltage $x_1(t)$ and the SNOPT output $y_1(t)$ also comparison of the known, but not transmitted to the model, $x_2(t)$ and the SNOPT output $y_2(t)$. Top $x_1(t)$ and $y_1(t)$ (mV). Bottom $x_2(t)$ and $y_2(t)$. The input current was a current pulse with plateau current $I_1 = 18.63 \mu A/cm^2$.

and the variances are is $\dfrac{A^2}{3}$ for uniformly distributed noise and A^2 for gaussian noise. We selected uniformly distributed noise so there would be no outliers on the tail of a distribution, and we selected gaussian noise since that is commonly observed, but the precise form of the noise contamination of the signal $x_1(t)$ is not significant for us.

TABLE 8.3 HH Model: "Data" Parameters and Estimated Parameters

Parameter	Data	S/N = ∞	S/N = 30 dB	S/N = 20 dB	S/N = 10 dB
p_1 cm^2/µF	1.0	1.00357	0.9978	1.0311	1.5
p_2 mS/cm^2	120.141	120.91	117.58	143.571	145.076
p_3 mV	115.0	115.0057	114.958	115.134	113.244
p_4 mS/cm^2	36.0	36.226	35.38	44.723	31.559
p_5 mV	−12.0	−12.0198	−12.097	−11.920	−12.66
p_6 mS/cm^2	0.3	0.29405	0.296	0.247	0.158
p_7 mV	−10.613	−10.508	−10.176	−11.80	−45.0
p_8 mS^{-1}	0.1	0.09989	0.0994	0.1127	0.0788
p_9 mV	25.0	24.977	24.8852	24.396	8.014
p_{10} mV^{-1}	0.1	0.10032	0.1014	0.1215	0.55
p_{11} mS^{-1}	4.0	3.9914	4.001	3.983	2.17
p_{12} mV^{-1}	0.05555	0.055467	0.055556	0.0539	0.020
p_{13} mS^{-1}	0.07	0.0692	0.06703	0.15	9.0492
p_{14} mV^{-1}	0.05	0.050	0.05338	0.0449	0.025
p_{15} mS^{-1}	1.0	0.99866	0.9993	0.8741	0.572
p_{16} mV	30.0	30.028	31.079	6.764	9.662
p_{17} mV^{-1}	0.1	0.0995	0.09764	0.1169	0.075
p_{18} mS^{-1}	0.01	0.00995	0.01013	0.007191	0.0150
p_{19} mV	10.0	9.401	10.290	11.90	40.25
p_{20} mV^{-1}	0.1	0.098503	0.0950	0.1093	0.1021
p_{21} mS^{-1}	0.125	0.12492	0.1231	0.1103	0.081
p_{22} mV^{-1}	0.0125	0.012535	0.01368	0.01896	0.0557

Chaotic $I_{app}(t)$ for τ=0.01 ms. Uniformly distributed noise was added to the data signal $x_1(t)$ with signal to noise ratios of ∞ (no noise), $30dB$, $20dB$, and $10dB$. We also examined noise at a 50 dB S/N level (not shown) and found the results indistinguishable from no noise at all. ($S/N = ∞$ dB).

Using a sampling time τ = 0.01 ms where we found accurate results for the noise-free estimation of states and parameters, we added noise with different values of A to the signal $x_1(t)$ presented to the model system. To give a quantitative measure to the magnitude of the noise relative to the signal, we evaluated the standard deviation of the noise free signal

$$< x_1 > = \frac{1}{T}\int_0^T dt x_1(t)$$

$$\sigma_{signal}^{2} = \frac{1}{T}\int_{0}^{T} dt(x_1(t) - < x_1 >)^2,$$

and defined a signal to noise ratio as

$$S/N = 10\log_{10}\left\{\frac{3\sigma_{signal}^{2}}{A^2}\right\}, \text{ for uniformly distributed noise}$$

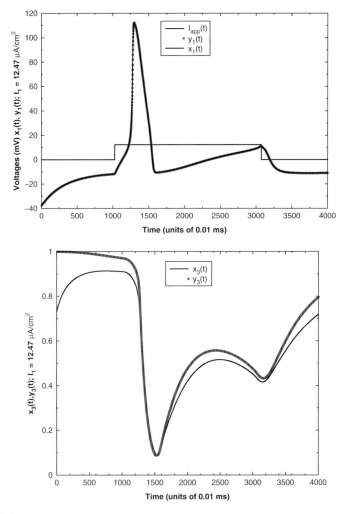

FIGURE 8.6 Comparison of the input, model, voltage $x_1(t)$ and the SNOPT output $y_1(t)$ also comparison of the known, but not transmitted to the model, $x_3(t)$ and the SNOPT output $y_3(t)$. Top $x_1(t)$ and $y_1(t)$ (mV). Bottom $x_3(t)$ and $y_3(t)$. The input current was a current pulse with plateau current $I_1 = 12.47\mu A/cm^2$.

$$S/N = 10\log_{10}\left\{\frac{\sigma_{signal}^2}{A^2}\right\}, \text{ for gaussian distributed noise}$$

Using the noisy input at signal to noise ratios of 30 dB, 20 dB, and 10 dB, we evaluated the parameters and the state variables using SNOPT as our optimization algorithm. In the figures we show the input voltages $x_1(t)$, and $x_{1-clean}(t)$ with and without noise as well as the output voltage $y_1(t)$ and the estimates of the activation and inactivation variables $y_2(t)$, $y_3(t)$, and $y_4(t)$ along with the values known to us $x_2(t)$, $x_3(t)$, and $x_4(t)$. The quality of the estimates of the unmeasured dynamical variables as well as of the parameters can be seen in these Figures and Table 8.3, and, as one should expect, they degenerate gracefully as the signal to noise ratio decreases. At S/N of 50 dB (not shown) and 30 dB, the noise is 0.5% or 5% of the RMS signal value, and we expect robustness of the estimation methods. When one has S/N = 10 dB, then the noise amplitude is 55% of the signal, and the interference is substantial.

In Figure 8.15 we show the normalized RMS errors for the estimation of the voltages and activation and inactivation variables for various levels of signal to noise ratio for each of the two distributions of noise we considered. We evaluated the RMS error between the estimated state variable $y_a(t)$, a=1, 2, 3, 4 and the known results $x_a(t)$, a=1, 2, 3, 4 ($x_1(t)$ has noise added to it)

$$RMS_{x_a,y_a} = \sqrt{\frac{1}{K}\sum_{k=1}^{K}(x_a(t_k) - y_a(t_k))^2},$$

for estimates at K time points, and we normalized these by the magnitudes of the average over the known clean data

$$<x_{a-clean}> = \frac{1}{K}\sum_{k=1}^{K}x_{a-clean}(t_k).$$

Noise Reduction by Dynamical Systems

In each of the cases we examined the voltage output signal $y_1(t)$ very accurately tracks the clean data signal $x_{1-clean}(t)$ for all values of S/N we examined including S/N = 0 dB (not shown). The output of SNOPT in its estimate of $y_1(t)$ is much cleaner than the input data voltage: the noisy $x_1(t)$!

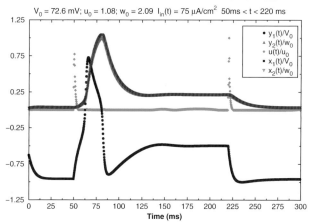

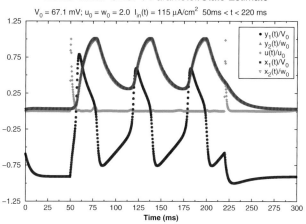

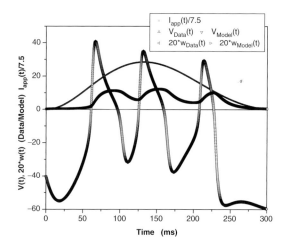

FIGURE 8.7 Estimating Parameters and the Unobserved state variable $x_2(t) = w(t)$ when the Morris-Lecar equations are perturbed by a current pulse protocol.

FIGURE 8.7 (Continued) (Top Panel) and (MiddlePanel), and (Bottom Panel) when the perturbation is selected as $I_{app}(t) = 220(1 - \cos(0.02t)e^{-0.005t}) \frac{\mu A}{cm^2}$. In the upper panels we exhibit the voltages $x_1(t)$ of the data source and $y_1(t)$ of the model, the activation variable of the data source $x_2(t)$ and of the model $y_1(t)$ as well as the control coupling $u(t)$. All of these are scaled to be visible in the graph. In the lower panel we scale the voltages $x_1(t)$ and $y_1(t)$ by a factor of forty.

How can this be? There are two factors at work here, in our evaluation:

♦ The SNOPT algorithm uses a temporal Hermite cubic interpolation formula to impose smoothness on the state and control variables. This includes having to estimate the derivative values at the endpoints of each integration interval of length τ, and these are minimized as the SNOPT procedure is carried out. This provides a smoothing of the output accounting, partially, for the reduction in the noise contamination of the output $y_1(t)$.

♦ The previous item is associated with the algorithm used to carry out the optimal tracking problem of DPE. There is another mechanism **intrinsic** to the nonlinear dynamics of this problem that was pointed out to us by M. I. Rabinovich (2008) as having been found by R. L. Stratonovich in the 1950s and 1960s through his research on nonlinear amplifiers used in radio communications.

We have not been able to locate a precise literature reference to this analysis, but a collection of papers from the group at Moscow State University, including Stratonovich, is available . Basically the argument is as follows:

The nonlinear equations of motion of our model, implemented as equality constraints by the SNOPT algorithm, have an attractor with negative Lyapunov exponents associated with motions off the attractor, one zero exponent for motion along the attractor, and, perhaps some positive Lyapunov exponents associated with chaotic behavior, if present (Abarbanel, 1996). The solutions to our model $y(t)$ define the attractor and from any initial condition $y(t=0)$ orbits will be drawn to the attractor. An injection of a signal, such as $x_1(t)$, while being driven to the attractor by a term $u(t)(x_1(t) - y_1(t))$ in the differential equation for $y_1(t)$, is also perturbed off the attractor by the instrumental noise. These perturbations are drawn back to the attractor by the intrinsic dissipative properties of the dynamics, and thus reduced in amplitude. Effectively, the noise on perturbations transverse to the attractor, and since we are imposing $x_1(t) \approx y_1(t)$, perturbations transverse to the synchronization manifold, are damped out. Perturbations along the attractor where the Lyapunov exponent is zero will not be reduced. The latter are phase disturbances that will show up as significant in long time series. Since we only utilize very short time series (for our calculations with τ=0.01 ms, we use only 40 ms of data) these phase perturbations do not become large.

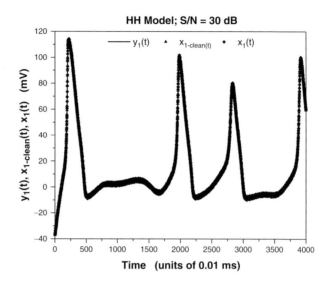

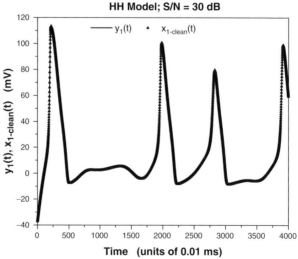

FIGURE 8.8 The noise free data signal $x_{1-clean}(t)$, the voltage presented to the model $x_1(t) = x_{1-clean} + A\eta(t)$, and the output of the SNOPT estimation algorithm $y_1(t)$. A is selected so that the signal to noise ratio is S/N = 30 dB. The output $y_1(t)$ is a very good approximation to the uncontaminated data signal $x_{1-clean}(t)$. The calculation uses $\tau = 0.01 ms$. (Top) Comparison of the three voltages $x_{1-clean}(t), x_1(t)$, and the SNOPT estimate $y_1(t)$ (Bottom) Comparison of the clean signal $x_{1-clean}(t)$ and the estimate $y_1(t)$.

Needless to say, this feature of nonlinear systems is welcome in the application of DPE to experimental data. It tells us that the model acts as a nonlinear filter to reduce the effects of noise in our task of estimating parameters and states. If the potential instability of the synchronization manifold were not cured, as we have noted, by our control term $u(t)(x_1(t) - y_1(t))$, then this fortuitous by product of our DPE approach might not have been available. This is further discussed in the Appendix to this paper.

Discussion

We have formulated the problem of estimating parameters in a dynamical model of neurobiological systems using the idea of synchronizing an observed data stream to the model output through a coupling in the model differential equations. In this paper we have examined features of single neuron model of Hodgkin-Huxley (HH) type to explore the robustness of the estimation method. In these examples we, of course, know the details of the "data" source so we are able to verify the accuracy of the method and to establish how the method is able to estimate dynamical variables of the system that may not be observed. As noted earlier, one may consider this exercise to be a "proof-of-principle" for the technique.

The method, called dynamical parameter estimation, or DPE, starts with a dynamical model of the system, comprised of a single neuron or a network of neurons, in which there are unknown parameters. We assume only one dynamical variable has been measured; for neurobiological examples this is the membrane potential time course for the neuron or for one of the neurons of a network. Calling this observation $x_1(t)$ we pass this and explicit knowledge of any external forcing of the experimental signal with injected current, for example, to the model for the full dynamics described by a state vector $\mathbf{y}(t) = [y_1(t), y_2(t), ..., y_D(t)] = [y_1(t), \mathbf{y}_\perp(t)]$. We identify the membrane voltage as $y_1(t)$. To the differential equation for $y_1(t)$ we add a local coupling term $u(t)(x_1(t) - y_1(t))$, and we have discussed the implication of large and small $u(t)$. Unknown parameters and unobserved states are estimated using a cost (or objective) function

$$\frac{1}{T}\int_0^T dt((x_1(t) - y_1(t))^2 + u(t)^2),$$

which is to be minimized subject to the differential equations

$$\frac{dy_1(t)}{dt} = F_1(y_1(t), \mathbf{y}_\perp(t), \mathbf{p}) + u(t)(x_1(t) - y_1(t))$$

$$\frac{d\mathbf{y}_\perp(t)}{dt} = \mathbf{F}_\perp(y_1(t), \mathbf{y}_\perp(t), \mathbf{p}), \tag{4}$$

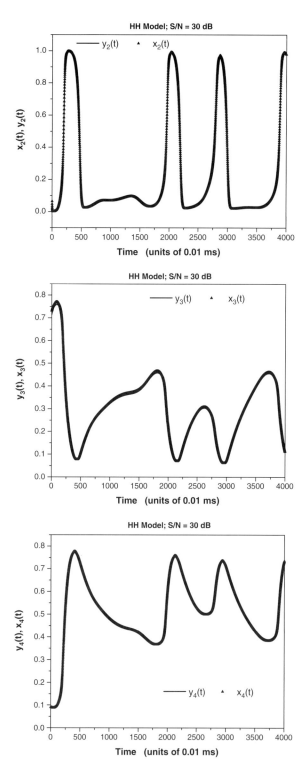

FIGURE 8.9 At a S/N = 30 dB with $\tau = 0.01\,ms$, (top Panel) we show the unobserved Na activation variable $x_2(t)$ and its estimate using SNOPT, $y_2(t)$;

FIGURE 8.9 (Continued) (Middle Panel) the unobserved Na inactivation variable $x_3(t)$ and its estimate using SNOPT $y_3(t)$; (Bottom Panel) and the unobserved K activation variable $x_4(t)$ and its estimate using SNOPT $y_4(t)$.

imposed as equality constraints. The optimization is over all the state variables at the discrete times $t_m = t_0 + m\tau$; $m=0, 1,..., M=T$, over the control at these same times, and over the fixed parameters $\mathbf{p}$.

The role of the term $u(t)^2$ in the cost function is two-fold: it bounds the size of the coupling $u(t)$ during the optimization as well as forcing the coupling to small values when synchronization $x_1(t) \approx y_1(t)$ has been accurately achieved. When the solution to this optimization problem is achieved, we expect that $y_1(t) \approx x_1(t)$, $\mathbf{y}_\perp(t) \approx \mathbf{x}_\perp(t)$ and $u(t)$ is small; of course, we also expect the estimated parameters $\mathbf{p}$ are close to those in the experimental system. Because $u(t) \approx 0$ at the end of the optimization, we have confidence that the parameters apply to the actual system of interest represented by the state variables $\mathbf{y}(t)$.

We applied the DPE procedure to a standard HH model (Johnson and Wu, 1994; Beuter et al., 2003; Koch, 2004) and showed that under presentation of various different applied currents, the twenty-two parameters in the model as well as the state variables $\mathbf{y}(t)=[V(t),m(t),h(t),n(t)]$ were accurately estimated when the sampling time was small enough. In this problem, we required $\tau \approx 0.01$ ms or smaller. Since the fixed parameters, representing maximal conductances, reversal potentials and numerical coefficients in the kinetic equations for the activation and inactivation variables, are independent of the applied current, it is a useful consistency check to perform the numerical estimation for a set of different injected currents. Here we explored two: (1) standard current pulses associated with a current clamp protocol, and (2) a waveform selected from the oscillations of a chaotic system. The key ingredient in these injected currents, we believe, is that each kicks the orbit $\mathbf{y}(t)$ off the attractor for the model system and allows it to wander through the full phase space of the model system. In this way we explore transients as well as attractor dynamics, both of which are sensitive to the specific parameters values of the "data." Indeed, as we explore parameter space through the numerical optimization procedure, distinguishing among the many parameter combinations seen through the optimization iterations is critical.

Our first result in this paper was a criticism of the familiar least squares method as a cost function to be minimized to estimate model parameters. This represents a departure from past investigations that addresses problems with the least squares method as they arise in investigations of nonlinear systems. Our suggestions cure those problems, though there may be other cures beyond

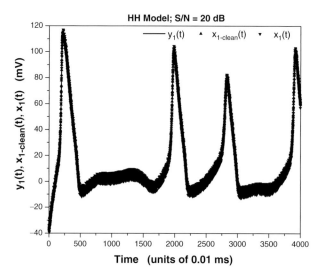

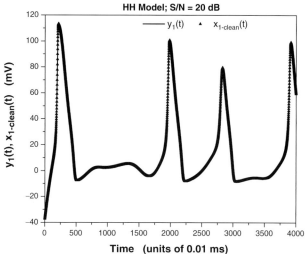

FIGURE 8.10 The noise free data signal $x_{1-clean}(t)$, the voltage presented to the model $x_1(t) = x_{1-clean} + A\eta(t)$, and the output of the SNOPT estimation algorithm $y_1(t)$. A is selected so that the signal to noise ratio is S/N = 20 dB. The output $y_1(t)$ is a very good approximation to the uncontaminated data signal $x_{1-clean}(t)$. The calculation uses $\tau = 0.01\,ms$. (Top) Comparison of the three voltages $x_{1-clean}(t)$, $x_1(t)$, and the SNOPT estimate $y_1(t)$. (Bottom) Comparison of the clean signal $x_{1-clean}(t)$ and the estimate $y_1(t)$.

those we have suggested here. Once one has made this departure from standard least squares estimation, how one implements the parameter search in the new context is a question remaining open. Many of the papers we noted earlier (Bhalla and Bower, 1993; Foster et al, 1993; Vanier and Bower,1999; Tabak et al., 2000; Prinz et al, 2003; Prinz et al, 2004; Hayes et al, 2005; Huys et al., 2006) were devoted to methods for parameter searches within the standard framework, and those investigations will be very helpful in pursuing DPE. The paper (Haufler et al, 2007) does connect data to a model using a synchronization method (Pecora and Carroll, 1990; Parlitz et al, 1996; Dedieu and Ogorzalek, 1997; Maybhate and Amriktar, 1999; Pikovsky et al., 2001; Broecker and Parlitz, 2001; Broecker et al., 2002; Sakaguchi, 2002; Tokuda et al., 2002; Voss et al., 2004; Konnur, 2003; Huang, 2004.but it does not address the balancing needed on the size of the coupling.

We selected the numerical optimization procedure called SNOPT (Gill et al., 2005; Barclay et al, 1998) as our technique for searching through state and control and parameter space for an optimal estimation of these, and we adopted one way, Simpson rule integration and Hermite cubic spline smoothing, to implement SNOPT. We have not explored other integration routines yet nor have we examined other smoothing methods to date.

We also explored the application of DPE to the estimation of parameters and states in the reduced HH like model introduced by Morris and Lecar (1981). Using a current clamp protocol and another injected current waveform, we were again able to accurately estimate the parameters and states of this system. Injected currents that bumped the system off its attractors, either a fixed point or a periodic limit cycle orbit, were essential to the quality of the success of the SNOPT estimation.

All experimental signals are contaminated by noise, and we investigated the robustness of our DPE procedure, implemented with SNOPT, to one form of noise: additive noise in the experimental signal $x_1(t) \rightarrow x_1(t) + A\zeta(t)$, where we took $\zeta(t)$ to be either uniformly distributed or gaussian. In using DPE to estimate the model states $\mathbf{y}(t)$ as well as the parameters of our HH model, we observed that the estimated signal $y_1(t)$ was much closer to the noise free signal $x_1(t)$ than to the noisy signal $x_1(t) \rightarrow x_1(t) + A\zeta(t)$ received by the estimation algorithm. We identified the dynamical origin of this, and noted that radio engineers in the former Soviet Union were apparently aware of this five decades ago, at least in the case of nonlinear limit cycle oscillators (See footnote). The appendix to this paper is devoted to exploring this noise reduction capability in a three dimensional chaotic system unrelated to the neurobiological focus of the main body of the paper.

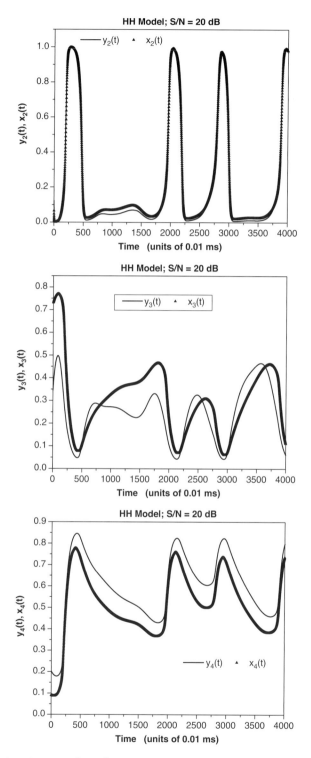

FIGURE 8.11 At a S/N = 20 dB with $\tau = 0.01\,ms$, (Top Panel) we show the unobserved Na activation variable $x_2(t)$ and its estimate using SNOPT, $y_2(t)$;

FIGURE 8.11 (Continued) (Middle Panel) the unobserved Na inactivation variable $x_3(t)$ and its estimate using SNOPT $y_3(t)$; (Bottom Panel) and the unobserved K activation variable $x_4(t)$ and its estimate using SNOPT $y_4(t)$.

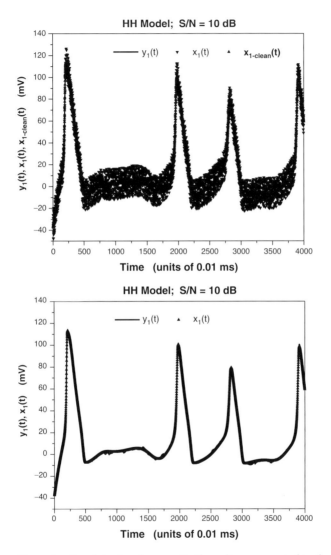

FIGURE 8.12 The noise free data signal $x_{1-clean}(t)$, the voltage presented to the model $x_1(t) = x_{1-clean} + A\eta(t)$, and the output of the SNOPT estimation algorithm $y_1(t)$. A is selected so that the signal to noise ratio is S/N = 10 dB. The output $y_1(t)$ is a very good approximation to the uncontaminated data signal $x_{1-clean}(t)$. The calculation uses $\tau = 0.01 ms$. (Top) Comparison of the three voltages $x_{1-clean}(t)$, $x_1(t)$ and the SNOPT $y_1(t)$. (Bottom) Comparison of the clean signal $x_{1-clean}(t)$ and the estimate $y_1(t)$.

Acknowledgments

We are very appreciative of M. I. Rabinovich for pointing out to us results of Stratonovich and colleagues apparently known to all workers in nonlinear dynamics in the former Soviet Union, and somehow not communicated effectively elsewhere. This work was partially funded by a grant from the National Science Foundation, NSF PHY0097134, and by a grant from the National Institutes of Health, NIH R01 NS40110-01A2. The first author is partially supported by the NSF sponsored Center for Theoretical Biological Physics at UCSD. The research on numerical optimization was partially funded by National Science Foundation grant NSF DMS-0511766.

REFERENCES

Abarbanel, H. D. I. (1996). *Analysis of observed chaotic data.* New York: Springer-Verlag.

Abarbanel, H. D. I., Creveling, D., Farsian, R., Kostuk, M. (2009). "Dynamical state and parameter estimation," *SIAM Journal of Applied Dynamical Systems,* Vol. 8, No. 4, 1341–1381.

Abarbanel, H. D. I., Creveling, D., Jeanne, J. (2008). "Estimation of parameters in nonlinear systems using balanced synchronization," *Physical Review E,* 016208.

Abarbanel, H. D. I., Rulkov, N. F., M. M. Sushchik. (1996). "Generalized synchronization of chaos: The auxiliary system approach," *Physical Review E,* 53, 4528.

Barclay, A., Gill, P. E., Rosen, J. B. (1998). In R. Bulirsch, et al., Eds, *Variational calculus, optimal control, and applications.* Vol. 124 of *International Series on Mathematics,* 207–222. Basel, Boston, and Berlin: Birkhäuser.

Beuter, A., Glass, L., Mackey, M. C., Titcombe, M. S., Eds. (2003). *Nonlinear dynamics in physiology and medicine.* Springer Verlag.

Bhalla, U., Bower, J. (1993). "Exploring parameter space in detailed single neuron models: Simulations of the mitral and granule cells of the olfactory bulb," *J. Neurophys., 69,* 1948–1965.

Broecker, J., Parlitz, U., Ogorzalek, M. (2002). "Nonlinear noise reduction," *Proceedings of the IEEE, 90,* 898–918.

Broecker, J. and Parlitz, U. (2001). "Efficient noncausal noise reduction for deterministic time series," *Chaos, 11,* 319–326.

Bryson, A. E., Jr. and Ho, Y-C. (1969). *Applied optimal control; optimization estimation and control.* Waltham, Mass.: Blaisdell Pub. Co.

Creveling, D., Gill, P. E. and Abarbane, H. D. I. (2008). "State and Parameter Estimation in Nonlinear Systems as an Optimal Tracking Problem," *Physics Letters A, 372,* 2640–2644.

Dedieu, H. and Ogorzalek, M. J. (1997). *IEEE Transactions, Circuits and Systems I, 44,* 948.

Fall, C. P, Marland, E. S., Wagner, J. M. and Tyson, J. J. (2002). *Computational Cell Biology,* New York: Springer-Verlag.

Foster, W., Ungar, L. and Schwaber, J. (1993). "Significance of conductances in Hodgkin-Huxley models," *J. Neurophys., 70*, 2502–2518.

Gill, P. E., Murray, W. and Saunders, M. A. (2005). "SNOPT: An SQP algorithm for large-scale constrained optimization," *SIAM Review, 47*, 99–131.

Guckenheimer, J. and Oliva, R. (2002). "Chaos in the Hodgkin–Huxley model," *SIAM Journal on Applied Dynamical Systems, 1*, 105–114.

Haufler, D., Morin, F., Lacaille, J. C. and Skinner, F. K. (2007). "Parameter estimation in single-compartment neuron models using a synchronization-based method," *Neurocomputing, 70*, 1605–1610.

Hayes, R., Byrne, J., Cox, S., and Baxter, D. (2005). "Estimation of single-neuron model parameters from spike train data," *Neurocomputing, 65*, 517–529.

Huang, D. (2004). "Synchronization-based estimation of all parameters of chaotic systems from time series," *Physical Review E, 69*, 067201.

Huys Q. J., Ahrens, M. B. and Paninski, L. (2006). "Efficient estimation of detailed single-neuron models," *J Neurophysiol, 96*, 872–90.

Johnston, D. and Miao-Sin Wu, S. (1994). *Foundations of Cellular Neurophysiology.* Cambridge, Mass.: MIT Press/Bradford Books.

Kantz, H. and Schreiber, T. (2003). *Nonlinear time series analysis.* 2nd Edition. Cambridge: Cambridge University Press.

Kirk, D. E. (2004). *Optimal control theory: An introduction.* Englewood Cliffs, N.J.: Prentice-Hall. (1970). Reprinted Mineola, N.Y.: Dover Publications.

Koch, C. (2004). *Biophysics of computation: information processing in single neurons.* New York: Oxford University Press.

Konnur, R. (2003). Synchronization-based approach for estimating all model parameters of chaotic systems, *Physical Review E, 67*, 027204.

Kostuk, M. and Abarbanel, H. D. I. Dynamical Parameter Estimation in Small Neurobiological Networks. to appear.

Maybhate, A. and Amriktar, R. E. (1999). "Use of synchronization and adaptive control in parameter estimation from a time series," *Physical Review E, 59*, 284.

Morris, C. and Lecar, M. (1981). "Voltage oscillations in the barnacle giant muscle.," *Biophys. J., 71*, 3030–3045.

Parlitz, U., Junge, L., Lauterborn, W. and Kocarev, L. (1996). "Experimental observation of phase synchronization," *Physical Review E, 54*, 2115.

Pecora, L. M. and Carroll, T. L. (1990). "Synchronization in chaotic systems," *Physical Review Letters, 64*, 821–824.

Pikovsky A., Rosenblum, M., and Kurths, J. (2001). *Synchronization. A universal concept in nonlinear sciences.* Cambridge: Cambridge University Press.

Prinz, A. A., Billimoria, C. P. and Marder, E. (2003). "Alternative to hand-tuning conductance-based models: Construction and analysis of databases of model neurons," *J. Neurophysiol., 90*, 3998–4015.

Prinz, A. A., Bucher, D. and Marder, E. (2004). "Similar network activity from disparate circuit parameters," *Nature Neuroscience, 7*, 1345–1352.

Rabinovich, M. I., private communication, 2008.

Rulkov, N. F., Sushchik, M. M., Tsimring, L. S., and H. D. I. Abarbanel. (1995). "Generalized synchronization of chaos in directionally coupled chaotic systems," *Physical Review E*, **51**, 980.

Sakaguchi, H. (2002). "Parameter evaluation from time sequences using chaos synchronization," *Physical Review E*, **65**, 027201.

Strang, G. (1986). *Introduction to applied mathematics*. 175, Wellesley-Cambridge Press.

Tabak, J., Murphey, C. R. and Moore, L. E. (2000). "Parameter estimation for single neuron models," *J. Comput. Neurosci.*, *9*, 215–236.

Tang, D. Y. and Heckenberg, N. R. (1997). "Synchronization of mutually coupled chaotic systems," *Physical Review E*, *55*, 6618–6623.

Tien, J. H. and Guckenheimer, J. (2007). "Parameter estimation for bursting neural models," *J. Comput. Neurosci.*, e-print 13 November 2007.

Tokuda, I, Parlitz, U., Illing, L.,Kennel, M. B. and H. D. I. Abarbane. (2002). "Parameter estimation for neuron models," Proceedings of the 7th Experimental Chaos Conference, San Diego, California.

Vanier, M. C., and Bower, J. M. (1999). "A comparative survey of automated parameter-search methods for compartmental neuron models," *J. Comput. Neruosci.*, *7*, 149–171.

Voss, H. U., Timmer, J. and Kurths, J. (2004). "Nonlinear System Identification from Uncertain and Indirect Measurements," *International Journal of Bifurcation and Chaos*, **14**, 1905–1933.

Yu, W., Chen G., Cao J., Lü J., and Parlitz U. (2007). "Parameter identification of dynamical systems from time series," *Physical Review E*, *75*, 067201.

Yu, D., Righero, M. and Kocarev, L. (2006). "Estimating topology of networks," *Physical Review Letters*, *97*, 188701.

APPENDIX

Noise Reduction by Dynamical Systems

This Appendix has nothing specifically to do with the application of our DPE method to neuron models. We were rather surprised, however, by the noise reduction of input signals by our model dynamical systems, so we thought it important to investigate this matter on its own. Our comments apply to applications in neurobiological systems, but they also stand on their own.

When solving the optimization problem posed as our DPE method when additive, or instrumental, noise is present, we observed that the output $y_1(t)$ is close to the noise-free data $x_1(t)$ rather than close to the noisy data $x_1(t) + noise$ when the latter is the input to the model. We suggested this came from the presence of negative conditional Lyapunov exponents in our estimation calculation using SNOPT, and that these negative CLEs brought the noisy data back to the synchronization manifold $x_1(t) - y_1(t)$ in a manner that removes the fluctuations, due to the additive noise, off this manifold.

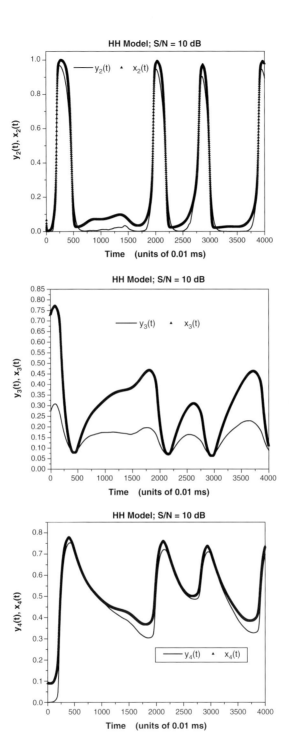

FIGURE 8.13 At a S/N = 10 dB with $\tau = 0.01\,ms$, (Top Panel) we show the unobserved Na activation variable $x_2(t)$ and its estimate using SNOPT, $y_2(t)$; (Middle Panel) the unobserved Na inactivation variable $x_3(t)$ and its estimate using SNOPT $y_3(t)$; (Bottom Panel) and the unobserved K activation variable $x_4(t)$ and its estimate using SNOPT $y_4(t)$.

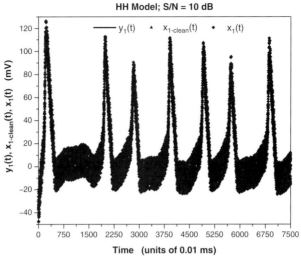

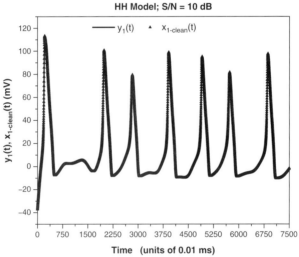

FIGURE 8.14 Noise reduction by action of the Hodgkin-Huxley model. We ask, for a fixed coupling $k(x_1(t) - y_1(t))$ in the equation for $y_1(t)$ between the voltage of a HH neuron $x_1(t)$ and the voltage $y_1(t)$ of a receiver HH neuron, with k large enough to lead to synchronization of the HH neurons (see Figure 1) what reduction in noise level is seen when the input signal is $x_1(t) = x_{1-clean} + A\eta(t)$. k is 4.1 in this calculation. A is chosen so the signal to noise ratio is 10dB. $\tau = 0.01\,ms$. (Top Panel) Comparison of the clean signal $x_{1-clean}(t)$, the noisy input signal $x_1(t)$, and the output of the receiver HH neuron $y_1(t)$. (Bottom Panel) Comparison of the noise free transmitter neuron voltage $x_{1-clean}(t)$ and the receiver HH neuron voltage $y_1(t)$. The increase in signal to noise ratio from this passage of the noisy signal through the HH models is about 13-15 dB or a factor of 25 or so in reduction of noise on the contaminated signal.

A consequence of this observation, apparently known to Soviet scientists through the work of Stratonovich and others (Rabinovich, 2008)in the 1950s and 1960s, when the model or receiver system expressed a limit cycle, is that when the signal $x_1(t)$ is chaotic, then until the synchronization coupling in the equation for $y_1(t)$, $u(t)(x_1(t) - y_1(t))$ stabilizes the motion on the synchronization manifold, the positive Lyapunov exponents will enhance the noise effects, and then when stability of the synchronization manifold has been achieved, noise reduction will occur once more. We have not found any references in the literature to the use of chaotic systems for this kind of dynamical noise reduction.

To investigate this, we analyzed a simple three-dimensional chaotic system called the Colpitts oscillator. The equations of motion for the state variables $x(t) = [x_1(t), x_2(t), x_3(t)]$ are

$$\frac{dx_1(t)}{dt} = \alpha x_2(t)$$

$$\frac{dx_2(t)}{dt} = -\gamma(x_1(t) + x_3(t)) - q x_2(t)$$

$$\frac{dx_3(t)}{dt} = \eta(x_2(t) + 1 - e^{-x_1(t)}).$$

For fixed $\gamma=0.08$, $q=0.7$, and $\eta=6.3$. For $\alpha_D \geq 3$, chaotic behavior was exhibited. The "data" $x_1(t)$ was collected for $\alpha=5.0$.

The time series $x_1(t)$ was passed to another copy of the Colpitts oscillator after adding noise uniformly distributed in the interval $[-A, A]$: $x_{1-noise}(t) = x_1(t) + A\eta(t)$ where $\eta(t)$ is uniformly distributed in $[-1,1]$.

The equations of the receiver system $y(t) = [y_1(t), y_2(t), y_3(t)]$ are the same with $x \rightarrow y$ and $k(x_{1-noise}(t) - y_1(t))$ added to the equation for $y_1(t)$. We selected $A=1.55$ which corresponds to a signal to noise ratio $S/N = 10 log_{10}(3\sigma_{Colpitts}^2/A^2)$ of 20 dB. In the upper left panel of Figure 8.16 we show the average least squares difference between the output signal $y_1(t_m = t_0 + m\tau)$ and the noisy input $x_{1-noise}(m)$

$$\frac{1}{N} \sum_{m=1}^{N} (y_1(m) - x_{1-noise}(m))^2,$$

and the average least squares difference between the output signal $y_1(t_m = t_0 + m\tau)$ and the noise-free input $x_1(m)$

$$\frac{1}{N} \sum_{m=1}^{N} (y_1(m) - x_1(m))^2,$$

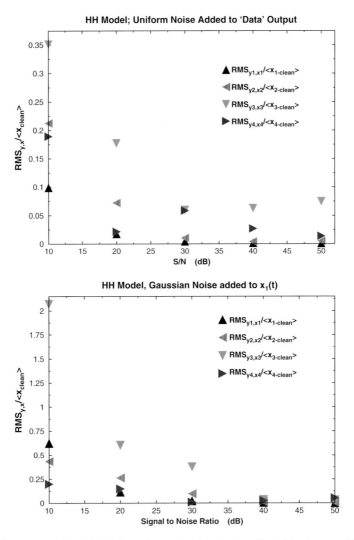

FIGURE 8.15 Normalized RMS Error for estimation of State Variables in the HH model when Additive Noise is present in the-"Data"-Top Panel Uniformly Distributed Noise, Bottom Panel Gaussian Noise.

as a function of k. We see that for small k the difference between the output $y_1(t)$ and either the noise-free signal $x_1(t)$ or the noisy signal $x_{1-noise}(t)$ is amplified by the positive Lyapunov exponents of the chaotic system, when $k \approx 0.2$ or larger, these least squares differences become quite small. In the upper right panel of the Figure we zoom in on the behavior for $k \geq 0.2$, we see that the least squares error between the output signal and the noisy data is larger by a factor of about 20 than the least squares error between the clean signal $x_1(t)$

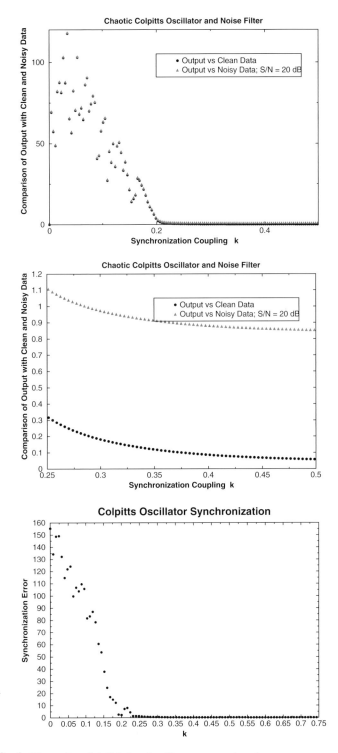

FIGURE 8.16 (Upper Panels) Colpitts Oscillator comparison between output $y_1(t)$ and input noisy signal with S/N = 20 dB and clean, noise free data. (Top) Least squares

and the output $y_1(t)$. Indeed, the difference in these variations is $A^2/3 = 0.800$ with A=1.55. This what is expected when $y_1(t) \approx x_1(t)$.

In the bottom panel of Figure 8.16, we plot the synchronization error of two Colpitts oscillators as a function of their coupling. When this is a large number, it indicates the two oscillators have not synchronized, and the largest CLE of the receiver oscillator for transverse perturbation of the synchronization manifold $\mathbf{y}(t) = \mathbf{x}(t)$ is positive. At the same value of k where synchronization occurs, $k \approx 0.2$, the output signal $y_1(t)$ moves close, on the average over the time series, to the clean signal $x_1(t)$. This tells us that when the synchronization manifold stabilizes because all CLEs are negative, passing the noisy signal $x_{1-noise}(t)$ through the receiver will lead to a reduction in the noise on the signal. For smaller k the noise is enhanced. In our case the noise reduction was about 13 dB.

Part 3: Neuronal Variability and Cognition

9

Capturing "Trial-to-Trial" Variations in Human Brain Activity
From Laboratory to Real World

Akaysha C. Tang, Matthew T. Sutherland,
and Zhen Yang

Part One: Variability and Context

Ubiquity of Variations

Variations in the patterns of human behavior under seemingly identical conditions can be observed across a diverse range of human activities. Glenn Gould's performance of the same Goldberg's Variations at the beginning and near the end of his career differed significantly. Professional basketball players cannot guarantee the success of every long shot in their career. During an uneventful week, one does not rise with the same feeling of freshness and alertness. Children raised in the same family can become distinct individuals displaying little resemblance to their siblings with respect to attitudes and capabilities. The same traumatic event does not result in the development of post-traumatic stress disorder (PTSD) in every individual. Facing the same school challenge, some students rise to the situation, while others fall apart. The same food can evoke opposite responses at the beginning or the end of a meal. A first drive along an unfamiliar road can be perceived as amazingly long, while the drive seems surprisingly short the second time around. A worker on an assembly line intends to repro- duce the same action sequence, yet mistakes are made on repetitions. In labo- ratory experiments, a subject is instructed to respond as fast as possible to the onset of a stimulus, yet the response time is not identical over repeated trials. It is obvious that across what appear to be repeated "trials" of similar events, the unique context of *each instance* serves as a source of variability creating a wide range of human experiences.

Causal Inference and Removal of Context

The scientific method as taught in today's academic institutions has as its explicit goal the establishment of causal relations between two variabless; let's call them X and Y (Rosenthal and Rosnow, 2008; Rosnow and Rosenthal, 2008). The simplest, and also a limited, way of evaluating causality has been to observe Y under an experimental (E) and a control (C) condition, each of which corresponds to one level of X. Students, thus trained, hope to support causality by demonstrating a sufficiently large difference *on average* between the E and C conditions across many units of sampling. Using this framework, variation across sampling units is considered noise to be "overcome" by a sufficiently large effect of X via averaging. Implicit in this approach to causality is the assumption that the **only** worthy finding is in the form of a *general* law that X causes Y, regardless of the context.

A more sophisticated way of establishing causality while considering con- text in a limited number of dimensions is via the method of n-way analysis of variance (n-way ANOVA) (Fisher 1962). Using this framework, the causal relation between X1 (factor 1) and Y is context-dependent upon particular levels of multiple variables X2, X3,…, Xm (factors 2, 3,…, m). If the causal relation between X1 and Y is dependent upon particular configurations of X1, X2, and Xm levels, then the n-way *interaction effects* should be sufficiently large in com- parison to the variation of sampling units within each of the conditions. Thus, variability across the sampling units within each of the conditions is once again treated as noise to be removed via averaging. The specific context under which the observation of each sampling unit is made is once again not only ignored but removed.

In both cases, in pursuit of causality from X to Y, one would forgo the opportunity to characterize the remaining variation across the sampling units along unspecified dimensions and forgo the attempt to understand their possi- ble functional significance. Side effects of this intense focus on establishing causality between known variables may be: (1) a false sense of generalizability of the causal relation, (2) a lack of sensitivity to the possibility of context-dependency outside of the manipulated dimensions, and (3) a strongly held misconception that all interaction effects between multiple variables X1, X2,... Xm are trivial extensions of the effects due to X1, X2,... or Xm *alone*, i.e., interaction effects can be inferred from experiments where only a *single* variable Xi is manipulated.

The significance of such unintended side effects is a prevailing tendency, which often goes undetected, to overgeneralize, that is, generalizing a causal relation, initially found within a very narrow range of circumstances, to situations involving different contexts (Kagan, 1996).

Return of Context and Alternative Forms of Inquiry

Against the background of this mainstream approach to scientific inquiry, the significance of context, within which causal relations should be investigated, has been slowly receiving attention. When the skin of the sea slug *aplysia* is stimulated by a constant force, the population of single neurons within the abdominal ganglion show highly variable patterns of responses from one touch to another such that a given single neuron may or may not participate in responding on a particular trial of stimulation (Wu et al., 1994). When *aplysia* displays a decrease in the gill withdrawal response, not all of the neurons decrease their firing rate—some show increased, while others show decreased firing (Falk et al., 1993). A simple averaging across neurons showing opposite response patterns would lead to the false conclusion that no change in firing rates during a habituated gill withdrawal response was present.

When a rodent neocortical neuron, maintained in isolation, is stimulated by a fixed stimulus of fluctuating current injection, the temporal pattern of the resulting spike train appears to be rather stable. Yet trial-to-trial variations in spike-timing of neocortical neurons can be up to 20 ms (Mainen and Sejnowski, 1995) and under the influence of major neuromodulators, such trial-to-trial variations may further increase (Tang et al., 1997). As it turns out, a spike timing difference of a few milliseconds can result in qualitative differences in how synapses adjust their strength according to experience. If the presynaptic neuron's firing precedes that of the post-synaptic neuron, the synapse is strengthened and if the order reverses, the synapse is weakened (Markram et al., 1997). This appears to be the case not only *in vitro* but also *in vivo* (Fu et al., 2002). The criticality of relative timing of events indicates that the impact of one event cannot be determined by that event alone and that the context plays a critical role.

At the level of large ensemble network activity, an electroencephalography (EEG) study showed that behavioral reaction times are correlated with trial-to-trial variations in the phase relation between the presentation of a visual stimulus and on-going EEG oscillations (Makeig et al., 2002). This finding suggests that the precise phase context is important for subsequent sensory-motor integration. Such a finding is considered "suggestive" because the phase relation was not manipulated as an independent variable but instead, merely co-varied with the dependent variable, reaction time. Findings of similar sorts are often criticized for "being merely correlational" and hence dismissed by some investigators. In a memory study, variations in the on-going EEG immediately before the presentation of an item to be remembered have been shown to affect how well the item will be recalled later (Otten et al., 2006). Once again, trial-to-trial variations in the on-going EEG offered the critical context within which variations in memory formation could be explained.

Together, these two studies demonstrate that on-going EEG context can not only affect the immediate sensory processing but also influence subsequent memory formation. Although the origin of these trial-to-trial variations cannot be ascertained within these experiments themselves and the causal relation between the context and the processing outcomes are suggested via "correlational" instead of "experimental" data, the findings nevertheless offer significant value as they serve to characterize cognitive processes in relation to their rich context.

Part Two: Capturing the Context of Brain State

The Context of Cognition

Perception, action, emotion, and thoughts occur within the rich context of our immediate environment and our past history. Such a rich context lies within a world of unlimited dimensions, in which individual human lives differ in their infinite subtleness. One way to understand the effect of such a rich context is to isolate one dimension or a few dimensions at a time and investigate their specific impact using the "experimental" methods that afford strong causal inferences. An alternative approach is to consider first that the brain is the center of information processing; thus, its state at or near the time of such processing must provide highly relevant contextual information for predicting outcomes, as was illustrated in the two previously described EEG studies. Therefore, an alternative form of inquiry may be to begin with identifying reliable associations between the outcomes of information processing and the moment-to-moment measure of brain states in dimensions higher than those manageable by typical factorial designs used in experimental approaches.

Measuring Brain State with High-Density EEG

EEG is a mature technique for measuring electrical brain activity non-invasively from sensors directly attached to the scalp (Niedermeyer and Lopes da Silva, 2004). The development of high-density electrode arrays in the form of a cap brought this old technology into the arena of brain imaging (Holmes et al., 2005). With its millisecond temporal resolution, EEG outranks functional magnetic resonance imaging in its capability of discriminating neural events that differ by a few milliseconds. The introduction of two blind source separation (BSS) methods to the analysis of high-density EEG data (Makeig et al., 1997; Tang, et al., 2005) makes the intractable problem of source localization with EEG tractable. For example, using the well-characterized human primary somatosensory cortex (SI)'s response to median nerve electrical stimulation as a "benchmark", the cross-subject variability of the estimated SI location is within only a few millimeters (Tang et al., 2005; Sutherland and Tang, 2006). Such tight spatial clustering across different subjects is at least comparable, if not surpassing, what is attainable with magnetoencephalography (MEG) (Mauguiere et al., 1997)

From a Sensor-Based to a Source-Based Language for Brain-State Characterization

Prior to the introduction of BSS methods, the language available for describing brain states was based on the readings from EEG sensors. An EEG researcher may describe a pathological pattern of brain activity in terms of the left frontal (F5) *electrode* for example (Rugg and Coles, 1995). A potential problem with this language is that the activity recorded at that frontal electrode is by no means a reflection of only frontal lobe neural activity. The same electrode may be influenced by electrical activity originating from posterior parietal lobe as well as activity associated with eye movement and eye blinks. Thus, it could be argued that without an effective method to translate the sensor-based description to a functional-neural-source-based description, one simply does not have an adequate language for characterizing the functionally relevant context of brain states.

A second problem with this sensor-based language is that over repeated recording sessions and across different subjects, the precise location of the sensors relative to the underlying neural structures would be highly variable.

Because the neocortical tissues are folded, a small change in electrode location can cause a large change in what signal sources are being recorded at a given electrode. Using such a sensor-based language, it is possible that the F5 sensor could end up measuring activity from different brain regions across different recording sessions with the same individual or between two different individuals.

With the aid of BSS methods, now it appears possible to overcome these problems by the arrival of a new language that describes the brain state in terms of millisecond-to-millisecond variations in brain electrical activity originating from *functionally distinct* and *anatomically specific* brain regions.

Part Three: Recovering Neuronal Sources Using SOBI—Validations and Proper Usage

If new technical advances are available, why is it the case that the evolution from a sensor-based to a source-based language has been so incredibly slow since its initial introduction? While there are many barriers to the rapid adoption of any new language, one key barrier here may be a relative lack of validation that would convince the long-time users of the old language that this new language: (1) does offer something different from other previously described methods, such as principle component analysis (PCA); (2) does provide signals from functionally distinct and anatomically specific brain regions; (3) has a clear internal logic that can be communicated to its users; and (4) comes with an "instructional booklet" that provides streamlined processing and a declaration of all key parameters critical for its proper usage.

Because algorithm developers tend to focus on the mathematics of the algorithms and speak a language that is unfamiliar to the typical EEG user, and because each data domain has its own unique issues critical for the algorithms' proper usage, there has been an unfulfilled need for methodological papers that connect the world of algorithms to the world of neuroscience and clinical science application. Below, we will summarize how we have attempted to deal with these issues through our own experience with one particular BSS algorithm, the second-order blind identification (SOBI) algorithm (Belouchrani et al., 1993; Belouchrani et al,. 1997).

Validating Using a Common Noise Source

The word "validation" in the world of source modeling typically means validation using simulated source data that are generated using a known source model with various assumptions made about characteristics of the true neuronal sources. A source separation algorithm is often considered validated if the simulated sources are properly recovered. This approach wins on the merit of knowing the signal generators but loses on the drawback that the model sources may not adequately represent the real neuronal sources; therefore, the validity of the algorithm for separating real neuronal sources cannot be inferred necessarily from the successful separation of sources contained in the simulated data.

We attempted to overcome this drawback by taking advantage of a known source from a typical EEG experiment. That is, the so-called noisy- or bad-sensor. It is considered known because the location of the noisy-sensor can be verified independently from the source separation algorithm by visual inspection of the raw data, channel by channel. This is how EEG researchers identify the "bad" sensors independent of any source separation algorithms. For example, in Figure 9.1 (Tang et al., 2005), we know the spatial location of the noisy-source because visual inspection of a brief 200 ms window of continuous EEG waveforms indicates that one particular sensor (boxed) contains an unusually high amount of 60 Hz noise. This known bad-sensor location matches the location of a SOBI-recovered source (Figure 9.1B) that contains predominately 60 Hz waveforms (Figure 9.1 C, blue waveform). Notice the contrast between the recovered source waveforms and those from the raw sensor (Figure 9.1C, red), which is a mixture of 60 Hz activity and other brain-related signals as well as signals from other possible noise sources. These observations serve to confirm that SOBI is indeed able to separate out signals associated with at least one bad sensor correctly.

Now one may ask, what about more than one simultaneously present bad sensor, and what if some noise sources are shared among multiple electrodes as a result of unintended bridging among neighboring electrodes due to excessive gelling? To simulate this situation, we artificially created noisy-sources across multiple electrodes by simultaneously touching the interior of the electrodes with a blunt needle. Figure 9.2 shows that the recovered source locations matched the known locations where the noise was intentionally "injected," and the time courses from the recovered sources also matched those directly recorded at the touched sensors (Tang et al., 2005). Therefore, SOBI is able to simultaneously recover multiple overlapping noise sources.

Distinct SOBI Results in Comparison to PCA

PCA is an algorithm most commonly used for dimension reduction when working with high-dimensional data. Applications of BSS algorithms and PCA

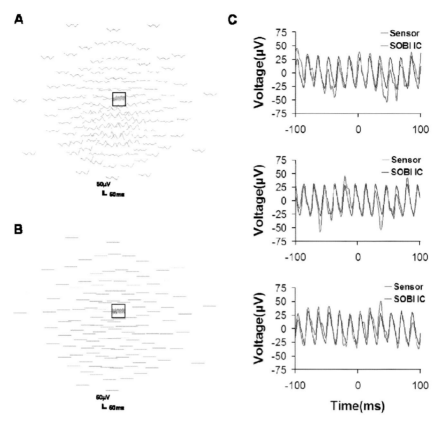

FIGURE 9.1 SOBI isolation of a noisy sensor (AB) Comparison of the known location of the noisy sensor (A) and the spatial location of a SOBI component (B) also referred to as a SOBI-recovered source, in sensor space projection maps (indicated by boxed locations). (C) Comparison of the time courses of the known noisy sensor (red) and the SOBI-recovered noise source (blue) across three arbitrarily chosen epochs.

to EEG data both involve the use of linear transformations of signals from the original *sensor space* to a space defined by a new set of axes. We investigated whether the axes identified by SOBI differ from those identified by PCA. Once again we take advantage of the known 60 Hz noise-source (Figure 9.3AB, Tang et al., 2005). PCA is often available as a built-in option within commercially available EEG data analysis software and easily generates components containing 60 Hz signals, but the "purity" of the PCA-recovered 60 Hz source is questionable, as the power spectra of a PCA-recovered source indicated the presence of non-60 Hz signals within this recovered source) (Figure 9.3C). In contrast, the power spectra of the SOBI-recovered noisy-source showed a clear narrow peak centered at 60 Hz (Figure 9.3D). Therefore, while SOBI does

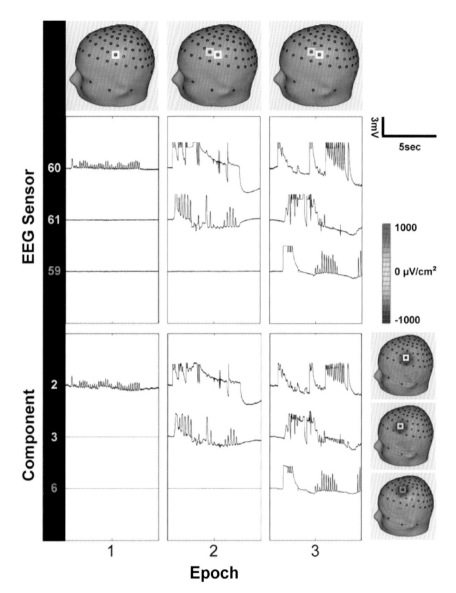

FIGURE 9.2 SOBI isolation of multiple artificially created noise sources (Top) Location and time course of three temporally overlapping noise sources. Colored boxes indicate the sensor locations where noise was injected. (Bottom) Location and time course of the SOBI-recovered noise components. Colored boxes indicate the center of activation on the current source density (CSD) maps from each of the SOBI components. The numbers on the left give the corresponding sensor and component IDs. Notice the similarity, both spatially and temporally between the known and SOBI-recovered artificial noise sources.

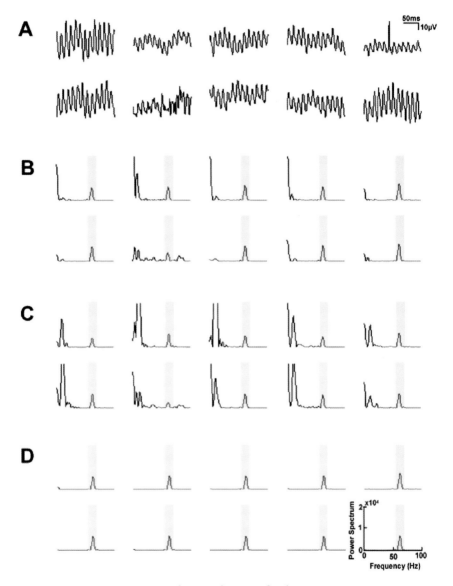

FIGURE 9.3 Comparing SOBI with PCA The case of isolating 60 Hz noise. (A) Ten randomly selected epochs of unprocessed EEG sensor data from the known 60 Hz noisy-sensor. (B) Power spectra of the ten epochs in A. (CD) Power spectra of the PCA-(C) versus SOBI-recovered (D) 60 Hz noise source (projected at the same sensor as in A). Note that D contains only a single peak around 60 Hz while C contains signals in other frequency ranges.

an excellent job at isolating this type of noise source, PCA is not able to isolate it well.

It should be noted that the recovery of such noise sources does not need *any* manual page-by-page pre-processing prior to SOBI application if the EEG data are collected using normally functioning amplifiers. In contrast to InfoMax ICA which requires pre-cleaning of data (Delorme and Makeig, 2004), all SOBI separation results presented in this chapter are a result of direct application of SOBI to raw unfiltered, nonepoched, nonbaseline corrected, continuous EEG data.

Validating SOBI-Recovered Neuronal Sources

The most common concern that EEG users have about sources recovered by BSS methods has to do with whether the *recovered*-sources do in fact capture neuronal activity associated with specific physiologically meaningful and neu-roanatomically relevant brain regions and whether such recovered source signals are contaminated by signals originating from elsewhere. A related concern has to do with the use of the phrase "independent component (IC)" derived from the ICA literature. Brain researchers have trouble believing that neural activity from different brain regions is truly independent. Thus, it is easy to dismiss the entire BSS approach on this ground.

Particularly relevant to this concern, is the fact that SOBI differs from other ICA methods in at least one aspect—it is designed for recovering *corre-lated* sources (Belouchrani et al,. 1997) and it does not call itself an ICA algo-rithm, nor does it refer to its recovered sources as "independent components". To examine whether SOBI does recover correlated neuronal sources, we use data from an experiment involving somatosensory stimulation to provide both correlated (paired left and right) and un-correlated (left or right alone) sensory inputs to the left and right primary somatosensory cortices (Left and Right SI). The correlated sensory stimulation, coupled with the effective interhemispher-ical influence between the two homologous brain regions, guarantees that the to-be-recovered neuronal signals originating from the left and right SI are correlated, thus offering a challenging benchmark for SOBI's ability to recover neuronal sources that have correlated activities. Similar points can be made with experiments involving a mixture of unilateral and bilateral visual stimula-tion (McKinney et al., 2003).

From EEG data collected from correlated neuronal sources using mixed left, right, and bilateral median nerve stimulation, SOBI decomposition resulted in the recovery of two SOBI-components that corresponded to the left and right SI. This correspondence was established via both principled spatial

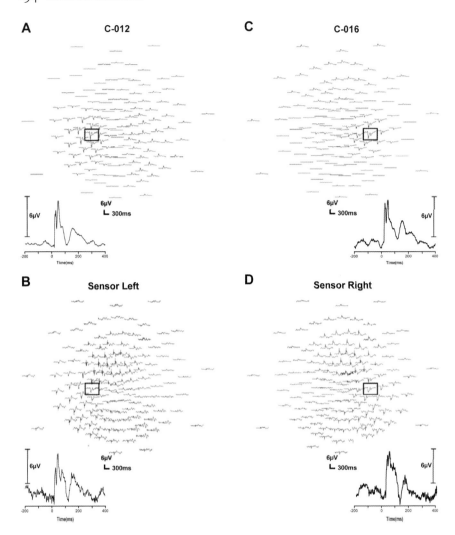

FIGURE 9.4 SOBI isolation of neuronal sources: Temporal characteristics. (AC) SOBI-recovered left (C-012) and right (C-016) SI showed characteristic SI response to median nerve stimulation (MNS). Boxes indicate the sensor location where the largest responses were observed (SEPs displayed in the inserts). (BD) Sensor space projections of the SEPs from the unprocessed EEG sensor data. Note the more diffused activation in the unprocessed sensor data by contralateral stimulation and the "noisier" SEPs ($n = 400$ trials).

and temporal criteria as discussed in detail elsewhere (Tang, et al., 2005; Sutherland and Tang, 2006). Briefly, the SOBI-recovered SI components showed, in the temporal domain, characteristic SI responses to median nerve stimulation (Figure 9.4) and in the spatial domain, a corresponding single dipole solution that accounted for >95% of the variance in the component's

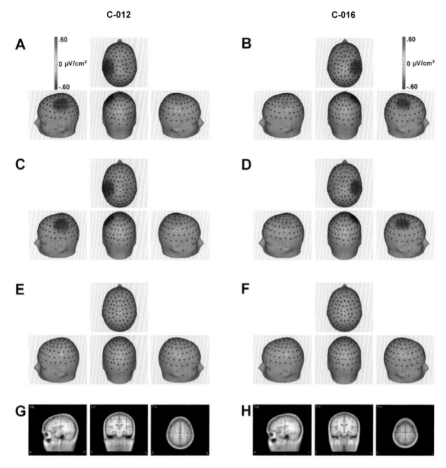

FIGURE 9.5 SOBI isolation of neuronal sources: Localization. (AB) CSD maps of the SOBI-recovered left (C-012) and right (C-016) SIs. (CD) CSD maps generated from an equivalent current dipole (ECD) model with the best least-squares fit to the data. (EF) CSD maps of the model residuals. (GH) ECD locations for the SOBI-recovered left and right SI, respectively, shown against the structural MRI of a standard brain (left is shown on the right).

spatial projections across the sensors (Figure 9.5). The benefit in the temporal domain is a clearly improved signal to noise ratio (SNR) (Figure 9.6A) and, in the spatial domain, is the ability to conclude that the waveform in the time domain originates from a specific region within the brain as opposed to concluding that the waveform is merely a signal recorded at a particular sensor (Figure 9.5). The latter does not address the question of how a specific brain structure corresponds with a specific function.

As both the left and right SI can influence each other via inter-hemispheric connections and share common input during bilateral stimulation, some

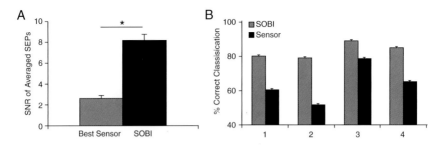

FIGURE 9.6   Benefits of using SOBI SEPs computed from the SOBI recovered SIs showed greater SNR (A) and lower cross-subject variability (B) than those from the raw sensor data measured at the "best sensor."

degree of correlation between their activation time courses should be expected. Had SOBI incorrectly imposed independence, then one might expect to find the activity of the SOBI-recovered left and right SI sources to show *a lack* of expected correlation. To check for this possibility, we examined the coherence plots (Delorme and Makeig, 2004) between the two recovered left and right SI components (Figure 9.7 left). Increased correlations between the two SIs does occur for a brief period shortly after the stimulus onset and within specific frequency bands, as one would expect to happen between two brain regions sharing both inputs and interconnections. As a control, similarly generated coherence plots for a SOBI-recovered SI and a noise-source showed no such frequency- and time-dependent increase in correlation (Figure 9.7 right).

Benefit of Using SOBI-Recovered Sources: Capturing
Trial-to-Trial Variability in Neural Response

A major challenge in investigating contextual effects, particularly trial-to-trial variations, is the presumed poor SNR in single-trial EEG data. This assumption is not unreasonable and can be confirmed by every experienced EEG researcher who has viewed large amounts of raw sensor-based data. This assumption is also reflected in the common practice of signal averaging across trials and sometimes across nearby electrodes showing similar response patterns in order to improve SNR. If SOBI can indeed parse the mixture of signals contained in the EEG sensors into their separate sources of origin, then the SNR of each *recovered source* may be sufficiently increased to allow classification of single-trial responses, specifically to determine whether a given trial involved left, right, or bilateral stimulation.

Using a neural network classifier, we compared classification success rates between two types of inputs: small segments (20 ms) of SOBI recovered

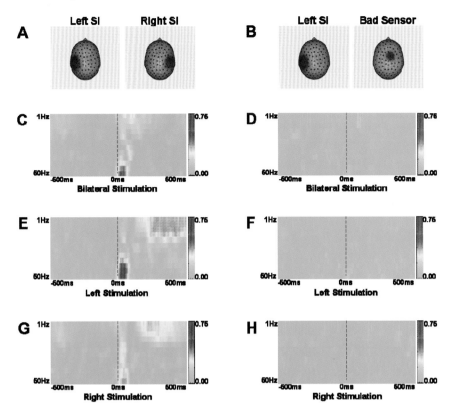

FIGURE 9.7 SOBI isolation of correlated neuronal sources: SOBI-recovered SIs preserved the expected correlations. (AB) CSD maps of SOBI-recovered sources. (Left) The coherence plots between the two recovered left and right SI components. (Right) The coherence plots between one SOBI-recovered SI and a noise source, where no correlations were expected. Coherence plots are shown for (CD) bilateral stimulation, (EF) left stimulation, and (GH) right stimulation.

SEPs from the left and right SIs and the same length of data from the raw waveforms recorded at the so-called "best-sensor" location. Classification success rate for SOBI components was significantly higher in comparison to that from the sensor-based measures (Figure 9. 6B). Furthermore, the cross-subject *variability* in classification performance was significantly reduced when source-based measures were used (Figure 9. 6B) (Tang et al., 2006), thus potentially reducing the sample size needed and cost of a given study. This benefit should have significant clinical implications in the context of drug testing. Therefore, SOBI recovered neuronal source signals provide a clear advantage over those of the sensors in characterizing trial-to-trial variations in brain responses.

A Short SOBI Primer

What does using SOBI for analyzing high-density EEG data involve? If we can assume that the data are collected with properly calibrated amplifiers[1], then the steps are rather simple. First, make sure that the number and range of temporal delays are properly set (Tang et al., 2005). Typically, a set of commonly used default values can be adopted without modification. The effects of varying these parameters on recovering benchmark neuronal sources have been documented (Tang et al., 2005). Second, make sure that the input to SOBI is continuous, as opposed to *epoched*, EEG data. When concatenated, *epoched EEG* "trials" would *create* abrupt changes in voltage at the boundary of the epochs that did not exist in the original continuous data. Third, make sure that input to SOBI is not filtered or manually "cleaned" by "chopping out" windows of EEG data. Cutting out a window of data would create artificial boundaries similar in effect as that of concatenated epochs of data and filtering would remove useful information that could be otherwise used by SOBI to properly distribute signal variations to its proper sources, including both neuronal and noise sources. Use of a single instead of a wide-range of temporal delays, concatenation of epoched EEG data, and unnecessary pre-cleaning, are erroneous practices likely committed by novice users of SOBI in preparation for source separation.

Internally, what SOBI does is conceptually very simple. To recombine signals from different EEG sensors into signals originating from a source is mathematically equivalent to changing the axes within which the high-dimensional EEG data are described. The original axes are the sensors and resulting axes are sources. SOBI makes the transition from the sensor (electrode) based axes to the source-based axes via an iterative process that minimizes the *sum* of squared correlations between every pair of new axes at all temporal delays. Because it is the *sum* of many squared correlations across different temporal delays that is being minimized, as opposed to having every squared correlation minimized, it is possible for SOBI to find the final set of axes that "tolerate" some degree of correlation at a few temporal delays.

In comparison to other BSS algorithm, SOBI uses a relatively small number of parameters, which are the temporal delays described above. The setting of these temporal delays are not random and can be selected based on the expected temporal delays among the neuronal sources to be separated (Tang et al., 2005). Once these delays are set, there is no randomness in the SOBI process in the sense that only one set of source solutions will be found once the delay parameters are set. This contrasts with InfoMax ICA, whose

---

[1] Inappropriately calibrated amplifiers may generate waveforms containing "steps" due to amplifier saturation.

final set of source solutions are averaged across N neural networks, each of which starts with a set of randomly selected weights. Each network has to be trained and this training requires the setting of additional parameters, e.g. learning rate and other parameters describing the function of "neurons" in these neural networks. This lack of randomness in the SOBI process, not only makes the interpretation of the final solution more clear and straightforward but empirically offers efficiency in finding the final solution. In the case of recovering the left and right SI components using SOBI, as few as 20–40 iterations were sufficient to recover the components corresponding to the SI sources described in Figures 9. 4 and 9.5. Additional iterations do not lead to further improvement in the resulting source localizations, at least in the case of recovering SI (Figure 9.8).

SOBI outputs a square matrix W, the unmixing matrix. Using this matrix, the time course of the recovered signals can be computed by matrix multiplication (Figure 9.9, Step 2) (Sutherland and Tang, 2006) and the spatial

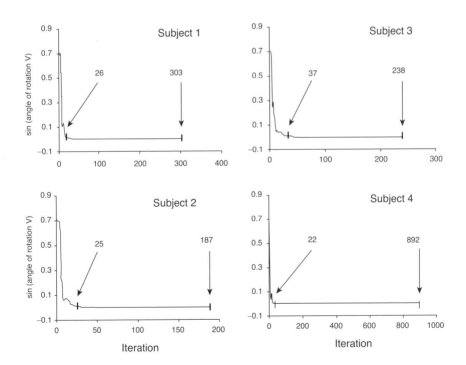

FIGURE 9.8 SOBI source separation is deterministic and fast. The recovery of the SIs in four subjects shown in Figure 9.6 took only a few tens of iterations. The numbers above the arrows indicate the number of iterations needed to reach asymptotic performance in source localization accuracy. Further iterations did not produce significantly different source locations or waveforms.

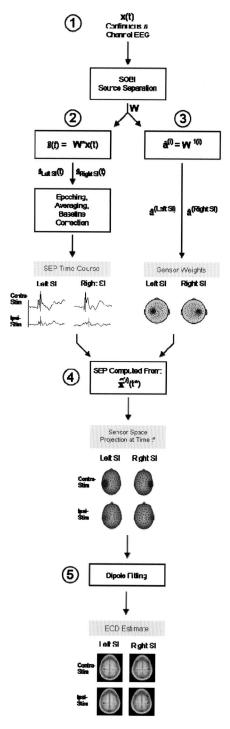

FIGURE 9.9 A schematic illustration of recovering neuronal sources using SOBI. (1) The continuous EEG sensor data, x(t), was supplied as input to the SOBI algorithm. The output of SOBI is an unmixing matrix, W. (2) Identifying the candidate SI components

FIGURE 9.9 (Continued) using temporal information: The continuous time course of the ith component, $\hat{s}_i(t)$, is given by the ith row of $W*x(t)$. From $\hat{s}(t)$, left and right stimulation-triggered averages, can be computed for each SOBI component. Components that correspond to left- and right-SI, $\hat{s}_{Left-SI(t)}$ and $\hat{s}_{Right-SI(t)}$, can be easily identified by characteristic waveforms in the SEPs following contralateral stimulation. (3) Identifying the candidate SI components using spatial information: The sensor-weight map of the ith component is determined by $\hat{a}^{(i)}$, the ith column of W^{-1}; $\hat{a}_{(Left-SI)}$ and $\hat{a}_{(Right-SI)}$ are two easily identifiable weight maps that correspond to the estimated left- and right-SI sources. (4) The sensor space projection of a candidate SI component's average SEP is computed from $x^{\wedge(i)}(t)=\hat{s}_i(t)*\hat{a}^{(i)}$; (5) Location and strength of the candidate left- and right-SI components can be determined with BESA using the sensor space projection of contra- and ipsilateral SEPs as inputs.

projection of each recovered source can be obtained from the inverse of W (Figure 9.9, Step 3). From the time course, single-trial as well as averaged event-related potentials (ERPs) can be computed. From the spatial projection, dipole-based or distributed source modeling can be applied to localize the sources to specific brain regions (Scherg, 1990; Hamalainen, et al. 1993; 1987; Ioannides et al., 1990). The benefit in the temporal domain is an improved SNR in the averaged ERPs and clearly discernable single-trial ERPs; the benefit in the spatial domain is the circumvention of the intractable inverse problem by reducing the number of possible solutions for each given recovered source.

Part Four: From the Laboratory to the Context of Real World

External Validity of a Scientific Finding

Brain imaging studies are often conducted in laboratory settings under restricted conditions. In most cases, it is not clear to what extent these findings can generalize to real world situations. As the peer review process focuses nearly exclusively on the internal validity of a study, issues of generalization, i.e., external validity, are simply assumed or left to the hands of newspaper reporters. The meaning and relevance of a laboratory finding in the real world can only be established, not merely speculated upon, via a new type of experiment that relaxes most, if not all, major laboratory constraints and removes major laboratory-related artifacts. In this section, we will present results from several studies that attempt to extract high-temporal resolution electrical signals from specific brain regions under conditions of free and continuous eye movement without the requirement of repetitive stimulus presentation and without the requirement of a task that entails specific responses.

Separating Sensor Noise, Eye-Movement, and Neuronal Sources under Natural Context

In human experiments involving the use of scalp recorded EEG, one common characteristic of laboratory experiments is the presentation of a target stimulus against a relatively impoverished background. This is for the purpose of maximizing the chance of detecting neural responses to the specific stimulus against background brain activity. This impoverished background produces minimal variation; therefore the context thus provided is bound to differ from those occurring in real-world situations, where sensory stimulation is continuously streaming instead of discretely presented and originating from multiple unknown sources instead of a few known ones.

The second common characteristic is the requirement for minimal eye movements during EEG recording due to the large ocular artifact produced by such eye movement that affect signals recorded across many sensors. Participants are often instructed to fixate and withhold blinks. This requirement entails additional mental effort and diverts attention to something other than the processing intended in its natural context.

Aside from these deviations from the natural context, in order to remove remaining ocular artifacts, a large amount of data is often discarded. This is the case even when using some BSS algorithms. For example, it has been recommended that before using InfoMax ICA, manual cleaning of the raw EEG data be performed (Delorme and Makeig, 2004). Such manual artifact removal would fail if EEG data are collected during continuous eye movement because there would be no clear on- and off-set of eye movement related signal, thus it would be impossible to remove this source of "noise" by removing particular time windows.

We applied SOBI to data collected under the challenging conditions of free-viewing with continuously varying visual scenes involving sustained eye movement and natural blinks. In a simulated warship commander task, the operator is to monitor, track, and discriminate a wave of incoming airplanes and text-display panels, and make decisions about whether to treat the airplanes as friends or shot them down as enemies. There is no preplanned operator action, and every operator will perform this game freely and differently, with the only shared instruction being to shoot down enemy planes and avoid firing upon friends. There is no repetition of visual scenes and, consequently, no repetition of context from one moment to the next during the task.

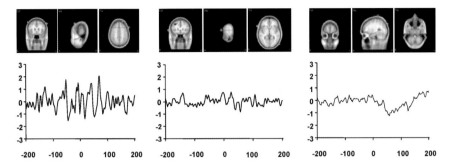

FIGURE 9.10 SOBI isolation of sensor related noise sources in a "real world" task situation where the subject was playing a video game in an electrically noisy office environment and with minor head and body movement. Three examples of SOBI noise-components. ECDs are superimposed on a standard structural MRI showing the origins of the signals are the EEG sensors.

Under these challenging conditions, SOBI was able to separate not only noise signals associated with "bad sensors" (Figure 9.10) but also signals associated with eye movement (Figure 9.11), visual processing (Figure 9.12), and frontal-lobe activity (Figure 9.13) (Tang et al., 2006). It is worthwhile to point out that these data were collected with a 64-channel EEG system in an electrically noisy office environment without any shielding. The "events" used to generate the ERPs were button-presses proceeding either a waiting period or proceeding a display of English text that entails visually-based language processing. It is remarkable that visual evoked potentials (VEPs) originating from posterior visual cortex (Figure 9.12) can be cleanly isolated from signals associated with continuous eye movements (Figure 9.11) even though the VEP waveforms and lateral eye-movements (towards the text panel) overlapped in time. Furthermore, the SNR is sufficiently high that the VEPs can be discerned even at the single-trial level.

Separating Distinct Neuronal Sources without the Requirement of Task Performance

The third common characteristic of laboratory-based EEG research is the need for participants to perform some form of a perceptual, motor, or cognitive task[2]. The requirement of task performance sets limitations on the population

---

[2] With the exception of sleep research.

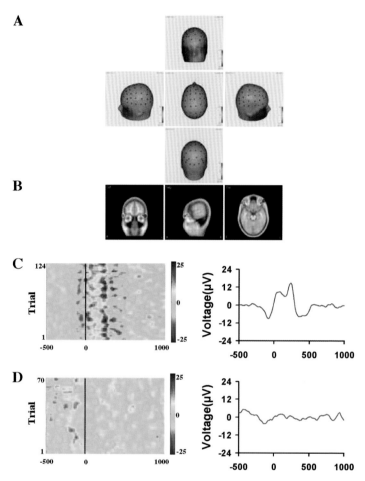

FIGURE 9.11 SOBI isolation of an ocular "artifact" associated with continuous free eye movement in the same "real world" task situation as in Figure 9.10. (A) CSD scalp map. (B) ECD model. (CD-left) single-trial ERP display. (CD-right) averaged ERPs generated with two contrasting events (COMM, WARN) that differ in the patterns of eye movement as well as in the type and amount of cognitive process. Notice that the ERPs of this SOBI component captures the expected differences in eye movement patterns (C) COMM event: the pressing of one of the many numbered communication buttons, which is preceded by holding a number in working memory, moving the eye from a moving target anywhere on the screen to the array of buttons, and identifying the button whose number matches the one in working memory and is followed by horizontal eye movement to text display box and reading of the text; D) WARN event: the pressing of the WARN button, which is preceded by an eye movement to the WARN button at a fixed location and followed by a 3 sec waiting period.

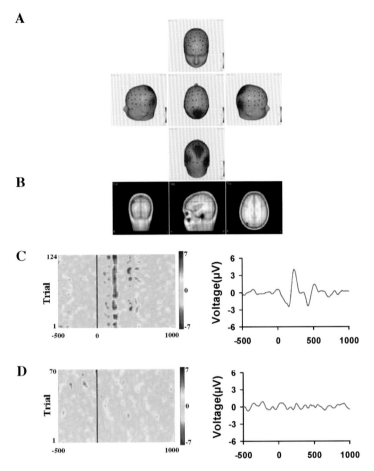

FIGURE 9.12 SOBI isolation of a visual source in the same "real world" task situation as in Figure 9.10. Despite the presence of continuous, free eye movement and the large eye-movement related signals shown in Figure 9.11, this component has a sensor space projection well accounted for by a pair of dipoles located in the posterior parietal cortex (AB) and has an ERP waveform characteristic of a VEP (CD). All parts arranged as in Figure 9.11.

of research participants whose brain activity can be studied, thus reducing the external validity of the intended research findings. For example, individuals suffering from autism or Parkinson's disease, or who are in a coma, either have difficulties or are completely incapable of acquiring and performing laboratory tasks. Infants and young children are more than likely to share the same problem, due to limitations associated with physical and mental maturation.

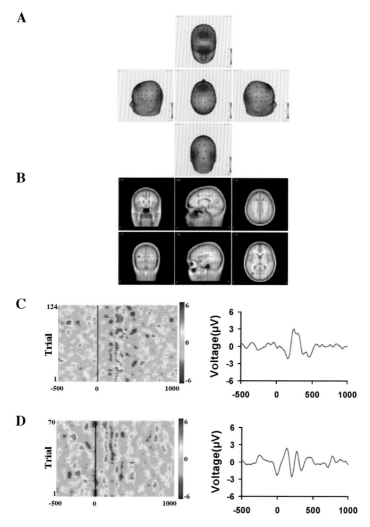

FIGURE 9.13 SOBI isolation of a distributed and synchronized anterior- posterior (SAP) network in the same "real world" task situation as in Figure 9.10. Despite the presence of continuous, free eye movement and the large eye-movement related signals shown in Figure 9.11, this component has a sensor space projection well accounted for by two pairs of dipoles located in both the frontal (anterior) cortex and the posterior parietal cortex (AB). All parts arranged as in Figure 9.11.

Therefore, the capacity to isolate neural source signals from functionally distinct brain regions in a *task-free* manner would be critical for studying information processing within these special populations. Such a capacity would also enable sleep researchers to characterize brain states in terms of sources instead of sensor signals.

Applying SOBI to approximately ten minutes of continuous EEG data collected while a participants was at "rest," we were able to identify a set of SOBI components that localized to brain regions along both the dorsal and ventral visual pathways (Figure 9.14, Sutherland and Tang, 2006). This demonstrates that it is possible to separate sources using SOBI without the requirement of an explicit task. In a study in which a larger sample of participants were asked to rest with eyes closed, rest with eyes open, or passively view a video, SOBI was able to isolate neuronal sources: (1) in the absence of any explicit task performance; (2) in the absence of any discrete "trials" of stimulation; and (3) in the presence of free eye movement (Figure 9.15, shown only frontal and posterior sources). These findings demonstrate that with the aid of SOBI, a task-free approach to EEG data assessment is viable for the monitoring of developmental, aging, and disease conditions as well as treatment progressions.

Matching Neuronal Sources from One Session to Another—within Subject Reliability Across Time

In order to use SOBI-recovered sources to characterize brain state change as a result of development, disease progression, and treatment effects, one needs to be able to match neuronal *sources* recovered from one session to those recovered from another. In other words, one needs to establish within-subject, cross-session reliability in finding the neural sources that correspond to the same neuroanatomical structures. We evaluated SOBI's ability to repeatedly identify the same neural sources within each subject across a time window of up to one month.

In a longitudinal study involving three testing sessions taking place one week and four weeks from the initial testing session, participants experienced a few minutes of resting with eyes closed, resting with eyes open, watching a silent video, and thinking about the video. No explicit task performance or behavioral responses were required. Subjects were once again free to move their eyes or blink. We applied SOBI to continuous EEG data collected within each session. Neural sources were recovered from posterior visual cortex and frontal cortex within each session and across sessions these sources could be matched (Figure 9.16) (Tang et al,. 2007).

To researchers of child development, aging, diseases, and treatment, this ability will help to reduce the variations and uncertainties associated with differences in electrode placement across time and consequently allow better characterization of changes in brain function in health and in disease.

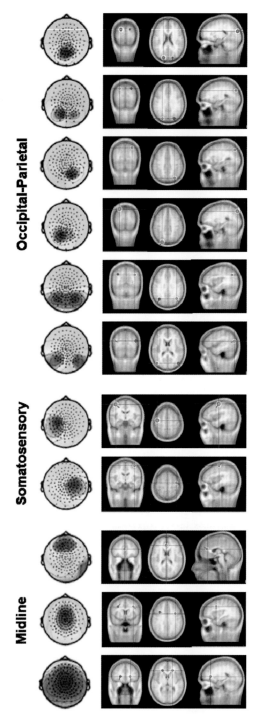

FIGURE 9.14 SOBI isolation of a family of neuronal sources from a single subject using ~ 10 min EEG recorded while the subject was at "rest". Scalp maps (left) and ECD locations (right).

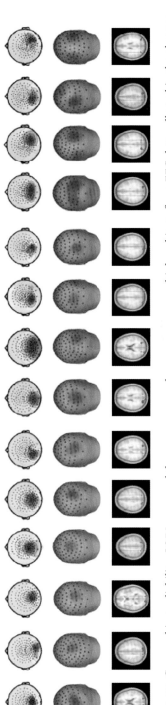

FIGURE 9.15 Cross-subject reliability: SOBI recovered the same neuronal sources across multiple subjects from EEG data collected in the absence of an explicit task. Scalp maps (Row 1), CSD (Row 2), and ECD locations (Row 3) of anterior components (top) and posterior components (bottom).

209

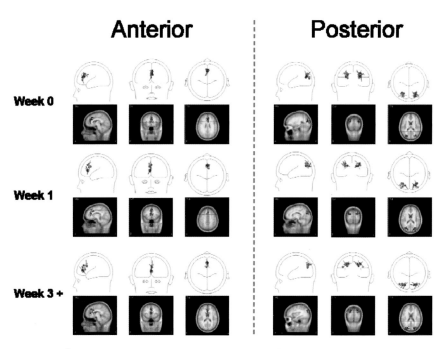

FIGURE 9.16 Within-subject reliability: SOBI recovered the same neuronal sources across different recording sessions for multiple subjects. ECD locations for the SOBI recovered Anterior component (Left) and Posterior component (Right). Session 1: week 0; Session 2: week 1; Session 3: week 4+. Each ECD location is for one subject.

Part Five: Understanding Cognition and Emotion in the Real World: SOBI As an Enabling Technology for Investigating Neuronal Variability

In this chapter, we have argued that to understand cognition and emotion in the real world, it is critical to investigate the phenomena of interest within the rich moment-to-moment context of the real world, that richness of the context as a result of individual history and immediate stimulus environment is encoded in the high-dimensional state of the brain, and that with appropriate signal processing using SOBI, such high dimensional brain states can be observed and characterized with surprisingly high SNR even in moment-to-moment measures.

In contrast to other chapters in this volume that focus on variations at the level of single neurons or at the level of small networks, our analysis is focused on the level of systems. While at the single-neuron level, one speaks of how the firing rate or timing of a single-neuron may vary from one trial to another, at the systems level, we speak of how the final perceptual, cognitive, or emotional outcomes vary from one instance to another, and we speak of how the state of the entire brain as represented in a high dimensional space vary in parallel. Analogous to understanding trial-to-trial variations in single-neuron or small network firing patterns, we seek to understand moment-to-moment variations in psychological outcomes at the systems level in terms of moment-to-moment variations across a set of localizable neuronal sources that characterize the individual's brain state.

Toward this goal, we presented a brief summary of recent advances in high-density EEG signal processing that enables a transition from a sensor-based to source-based language for a dynamic characterization of brain state. We argued for why such a transition is critical for addressing a fundamental question in neuroscience relating specific brain functions to specific brain structures and their dynamic interactions. It is important to accompany these statements with the disclaimer that a relative advantage of a source-based language over a sensor-based language in the context of relating *function to structure* does *not* imply that no valuable information can be gained using a sensor-based language.

It is also important to point out that although SOBI is the algorithm for which we have chosen to provide extensive empirical studies, the use of time correlation (as in the case of SOBI) is only one way of separating sources from mixture of signals (Cardoso, 2001). SOYA (Gorodnitsky and Belouchrani, 2001) and M-COMBI (Tichavsky et al., 2008) are two newer algorithms that have improved upon SOBI. These newer algorithms have desirable properties based on theoretical grounds and simulated data and their success in separating large numbers of neuronal sources from high density EEG data within a wide range of contexts remains to be demonstrated.

Acknowledgments

Supported by grants from the Defense Advanced Research Program Agency (DARPA) and Sandia National Laboratory (SNL) to ACT.

REFERENCES

Belouchrani, A., Abed-Meraim, K., Cardoso, J.F., Moulines, E. (1997) A blind source separation technique using second-order statistics. *IEEE Transactions on Signal Process*, 45, 434–444.

Belouchrani, A., Meraim, K.A., Cardos, J.F., Moulines, E. (1993) Second-order blind separation of temporally correlated sources. In *Proc. Int. Conf. on Digital Sig. Proc.* Nicosia, Cyprus.

Cardoso, J.F. (2001) The three easy routes to independent component analysis: Contrasts and Geometry. Paper read at Proceedings of the 3rd International Conference on Independent Component Analysis and Signal Separation, San Diego, Calif.

Delorme, A., and Makeig, S. (2004) EEGLAB: an open source toolbox for analysis of single-trial EEG dynamics including independent component analysis. *J Neurosci Methods, 134 (1)*, 9–21.

Falk, C. X., Wu, J.Y., Cohen, L.B., Tang, A.C. (1993) Nonuniform expression of habituation in the activity of distinct classes of neurons in the Aplysia abdominal ganglion. *J of Neuroscience, 13 (9)*, 4072–4081.

Fisher, R. (1962) The Arrangement of Field Experiments. *Journal of the Ministry of Agriculture of Great Britain, 33*, 503–513.

Fu, Y. X., Djupsund, K., Gao, H., Hayden, B., Shen, K., Dan, Y. (2002) Temporal specificity in the cortical plasticity of visual space representation. *Science, 296 (5575)*, 1999–2003.

Gorodnitsky, I.F., and Belouchrani, A. (2001) Joint cumulant and correlation based signal separation with application to EEG data analysis. Paper read at Proceedings of the 3rd International Conference on Independent Component Analysis and Signal Separation, San Diego, Calif.

Hamalainen, H., Hari, R., Ilmoniemi, R. J., Knuutila, J., Lounasmaa, O.V. (1993) Magnetoencephalography: Theory instrumentation, and applications to noninvasive studies of the working human brain. *Reviews of Modern Physics, 65*, 413–497.

Holmes, M., Brown, M., Tucker, D. (2005) Dense array EEG and source analysis reveal spatiotemporal dynamics of epileptiform discharges. *Epilepsia, 46 (Suppl 8)*, 136.

Ioannides, A.A., Bolton, J.P.R., Clarke, C.S.J. (1990) Continuous probabilistic solutions to the biomagnetic inverse problem. *Inverse Probl, 6*, 523–542.

Kagan, Jerome. (1996) Three pleasing ideas. *American Psychologist, 51 (9)*, 901–908.

Mainen, Z. F., and Sejnowski, T.J. (1995) Reliability of spike timing in neocortical neurons. *Science, 268 (5216)*, 1503–1506.

Makeig, S., Jung, T.P., Bell, A.J., Ghahremani, D., Sejnowski, T.J. (1997) Blind separation of auditory event-related brain responses into independent components. *Proceedings of the National Academy of Sciences, 94 (20)*, 10979–10984.

Makeig, S., Westerfield, M., Jung, T.P., Enghoff, S., Townsend, J., Courchesne, E., Sejnowski, T.J. (2002) Dynamic brain sources of visual evoked responses. *Science, 295 (5555)*, 690–694.

Markram, H., Lubke, J., Frotscher, M., and Sakmann, B. (1997) Regulation of synaptic efficacy by coincidence of postsynaptic APs and EPSPs. *Science, 275 (5297)*, 213–215.

Mauguiere, F., Merlet, I., Forss, N., Vanni, S., Jousmaki, V., Adeleine, P., and Hari, R. (1997) Activation of a distributed somatosensory cortical network in the human brain. A dipole modelling study of magnetic fields evoked by median nerve stimulation. Part I: Location and activation timing of SEF sources. *Electroencephalography and clinical Neurophysiology, 104 (4)*, 281–9.

McKinney, C. J., Sutherland, M.T., Tang, A.C. (2003) Somatosensory to visual cross-modal interaction: Evidence of visual alpha resetting by median nerve stimulation. In *Annual Cognitive Neuroscience Society Meeting*, New York.

Niedermeyer, Ernst, and Lopes da Silva, F.H. (2004) *Electroencephalography, basic principles, clinical applications, and related fields.* (5th Edition) Hagerstown: Lippincott Williams & Wilkins.

Otten, Leun J., Quayle, A.H., Akram, S., Ditewig, T.A., Rugg, M.D. (2006) Brain activity before an event predicts later recollection. *Nature Neuroscience, 9 (4),* 489–491.

Rosenthal, R. and Rosnow, R.L. (2008) *Essentials of behavioral research: methods and data analysis.* (3rd Edition) New York: McGraw-Hill.

Rosnow, R. L. and Rosenthal, R. (2008) *Beginning Behavioral Research: A conceptual primer.* N.J.: Prentice Hall.

Rugg, M. D. and Coles, M.G.H. (1995) *Electrophysiology of mind:Eevent-related brain potentials and cognition.* Oxford/New York: Oxford University Press.

Sarvas, J. (1987) Basic mathematical and electromagnetic concepts of the biomagnetic inverse problem. *Phys Med Biol, 32 (1),* 11–22.

Scherg, M. (Ed.) (1990) *Fundamentals of dipole source potential analysis. In Advances in Audiology,* Grandori, F., Hoke, M., Romani, G.L. (Eds). Basel: Karger.

Sutherland, M. T., and Tang, A.C. (2006) Reliable detection of bilateral activation in human primary somatosensory cortex by unilateral median nerve stimulation. *Neuroimage, 33 (4),* 1042–1054.

Tang, A. C., Bartels, A.M., Sejnowski, T.J. (1997) Effects of cholinergic modulation on responses of neocortical neurons to fluctuating input. *Cerebral Cortex, 7 (6),* 502–509.

Tang, A. C., Liu, J.Y., Sutherland, M.T. (2005) Recovery of correlated neuronal sources from EEG: The good and bad ways of using SOBI. *Neuroimage, 28 (2),* 507–519.

Tang, A. C., Sutherland, M.T., McKinney, C.J. (2005) Validation of SOBI components from high-density EEG. *Neuroimage, 25 (2),* 539–553.

Tang, A. C., Sutherland, M.T., McKinney, C.J., Liu, J.Y., Wang, Y., Parra, L.C., Gerson, A.D., Sajda, P. (2006) Classifying single-trial ERPs from visual and frontal cortex during free viewing. In *IEEE Proceedings of the 2006 International Joint Conference on Neural Networks,* Vancouver, Canada.

Tang, A. C., Sutherland, M.T., Peng, S., Zhang, Y., Nakazawa, M., Korzekwa, A.M., Yang, Z.,and Ding, M.Z. (2007) Top-down versus bottom-up processing in the human brain: Distinct directional influences revealed by integrating SOBI and Granger causality. In *Proceedings of the 7th International Conference on Independent Component Analysis and Signal Separation.* London, UK.

Tang, A. C., Sutherland, M.T., and Wang, Y. (2006) Contrasting Single-Trial ERPs between Experimental Manipulations: Improving Differntiability by Blind Source Separation. *Neuroimage, 29 (1),* 335–346.

Tichavsky, P., Koldovsky, Z., Yeredor, A., Gomez-Herrero, G., Doron, E. (2008) A hybrid technique for blind separation of non-gaussian and time-correlated sources using a multicomponent approach. *IEEE Trans Neural Netw, 19 (3),* 421–430.

Wu, J. Y., Tsau, Y., Hopp, H.P., Cohen, L.B., Tang, A.C., Falk, C.X. (1994) Consistency in nervous systems: trial-to-trial and animal-to-animal variations in the responses to repeated applications of a sensory stimulus in Aplysia. *J of Neuroscience, 14 (3 Pt 1),* 1366–13684.

10

Linking Neuronal Variability to Perceptual Decision Making via Neuroimaging

Paul Sajda, Marios G. Philiastides, Hauke Heekeren, and Roger Ratcliff

Introduction

One of the fundamental questions posed by systems neuroscience is whether the variability observed in neuronal responses is largely reflective of neurons being noisy processing elements, is a result of unaccounted contextual effects of otherwise identical stimuli (e.g., a memory/hysteresis effect) and/or is reflective of latent processes in the underlying neuronal network. From a behavioral neuroscience perspective, decision making is also confronted with the issue of variability—namely, that even for very simple decisions, accuracy and response time (RT) can vary significantly for nominally identical stimuli. Over the last decade, there has been substantial work focused on linking neuronal variability to this behavioral variability. For the most part, much of the effort has been focused on animal studies, including nonhuman primates. Recent advances in neuroimaging, however, specifically methods for single-trial analysis of noninvasively measured neural activity, has enabled one to address the question with respect to variability and decision making in the human brain.

In this chapter, we review systems, methods, and models we have used to link neuronal variability to perceptual decision making in the human brain. We begin by describing how we identify task-relevant EEG components and use signal detection theory to relate these components to the behavioral data. We then use the well-known diffusion model of two-choice decision making to show that the trial-to-trial variability of these EEG components can be used to improve model fits of the behavioral data, providing evidence that the trial-to-trial variability we see in the EEG contains meaningful information and is not purely noise. We then turn to our work on combining EEG and fMRI to infer the cortical networks underlying perceptual decision making. We briefly discuss how EEG can be used to inform an fMRI analysis to tease apart individual processes underlying perceptual decision making. We then show how the trial-to-trial fluctuations in the EEG can be used to construct regressors that yield fMRI activations that are unobservable, given only behavioral or stimulus derived regressors. These specific results suggest that the trial-to-trial fluctuations we identify in the EEG represent latent processes such as attentional "polling" of the sensory input. In general, our results demonstrate that analysis of trial-to-trial variability of neural activity yields new insights into the constituent brain processes of decision making in the human brain.

Single-Trial Analysis of EEG

Traditionally, the analysis of EEG has relied on averaging event-locked data across hundreds of trials as well as across subjects, to uncover the neural signatures of the neurocognitive process under investigation. The main assumption of this approach is that trial averaging increases signal-to-noise ratio (SNR) by minimizing the background EEG activity relative to the neural activity correlated with experimental events. While this assumption is generally valid, it inevitably conceals inter-trial and inter-subject response variability. This trial-by-trial variability may carry important information regarding the underlying neural processes, which in turn might have important behavioral consequences.

In contrast, single-trial methods are often designed to exploit the large number of sensor arrays by spatially integrating information across channels to generate an aggregate representation (i.e., component) of the data that optimally discriminates between experimental conditions of interest. Spatial integration enhances the signal quality without loss of temporal precision common to trial averaging while the resulting discriminating components are often a better estimator of the underlying neurophysiological activity.

Methods that have been developed to extract components of interest from the EEG include independent component analysis (ICA) (Jung et al., 2001;

Makeig et al., 2002; Onton et al., 2006), common spatial patterns (CSP) (Guger et al., 2000; Ramoser et al., 2000) support vector machines (SVM) (Lal et al., 2004; Thulasidas et al., 2006) and linear discrimination (LD) based on logistic regression (Parra et al., 2002; Parra et al., 2005). LD in particular can be used to compute a set of spatial weights which maximally discriminate between experimental conditions over several different temporal windows, thus allowing the monitoring of the temporal evolution of discriminating activity. Unlike CSP, which tries to identify orientations in sensor space that maximize power, LD tries to maximize discrimination between two classes. Also unlike ICA, which is designed to minimize the correlation between spatial components (i.e., make spatial components as independent as possible (Hyvarinen et al., 2001) LD is used to identify components that maximize the correlation with relevant experimental events. All of these techniques linearly transform the original EEG signal via the following transformation

$$\mathbf{Y} = \mathbf{WX} \tag{1}$$

where $\mathbf{X}$ is the original data matrix, $\mathbf{W}$ is the transformation matrix (or vector) estimated using the different techniques, and $\mathbf{Y}$ is the resulting component/source matrix (or vector). Figure 10.1 summarizes how the LD technique can be used for binary discrimination.

Using the single-trial LD approach highlighted here, we explored the temporal characteristics of perceptual decision making in humans in an attempt to quantify the relationship between neural activity and behavioral output (Philiastides and Sajda, 2006). Motivated from the early work by Newsome and colleagues in primates (Britten et al., 1996; Britten et al., 1992), we reported the first noninvasive neural measurements of perceptual decision making in humans, that lead to neurometric functions predictive of psychophysical performance on a face versus car categorization task (see Figure 10.2A for examples of stimuli that were used). Specifically, we manipulated the difficulty of the task by changing the spatial phase coherence of the stimuli in a range that spanned psychophysical threshold. Carrying out the LD approach at different time windows and coherence levels revealed two EEG components that discriminated maximally between faces and cars as seen in Figure 10.2B for one subject. The early component was consistent with the well-known face-selective N170 (Bentin et al., 1996; Halgren et al., 2000; Jeffreys, 1996; Liu et al., 2000; Rossion et al., 2003) and its temporal onset appeared to be unaffected by task difficulty. The late component, appeared on average around 300 ms after the stimulus at the easiest condition and it systematically shifted later in time and became more persistent as a function of task difficulty. Both of these components showed substantial trial-to-trial variability (see Figure 10.2C) and

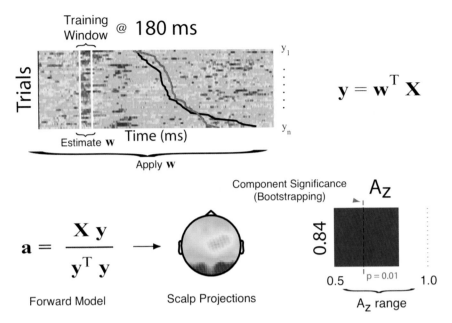

FIGURE IO.I Summary of our linear discriminant (LD) methodology for extracting task-relevant components from single-trial analysis of the EEG. Each row of the discriminant component map represents a single trial across time. Discriminant components are represented by the y vectors. Trials are aligned to the onset of the stimulus (black vertical line) and are sorted by reaction time (sigmoidal curves). To construct this map we choose a training window, indicated by white vertical bars (for this example starting at 180 ms post-stimulus), during which we train the linear discriminator to estimate a weighting vector $\mathbf{w}$ across all sensors in $\mathbf{X}$, such that $\mathbf{y}$ is maximally discriminating between the two experimental conditions (e.g. trial type 1 vs trial type 2). We use the forward model to project the discriminating component back to the sensors. An example scalp projection $\mathbf{a}$ is shown here and is used for interpreting the neuroanatomical significance of the components. To quantify the discriminator's performance we used ROC analysis and computed the area under the ROC curve (Az value).
Reproduced/adapted from Philiastides and Sajda, 2006.

they were both sensitive to decision accuracy in that a high magnitude discriminator output value (i.e. Y) indicated an easy trial, whereas smaller values indicated more difficult decisions. Additional experimental manipulations enabled us to identify a third component, situated between the early and late components, around 220 ms post-stimulus, which systematically increased with increasing task difficulty. To rule out the possibility that this component is an artifact of the bottom-up processing of the stimulus we used a variant of our original paradigm where we colored the same images red or green and asked our subjects to either perform a simple color discrimination or the original face

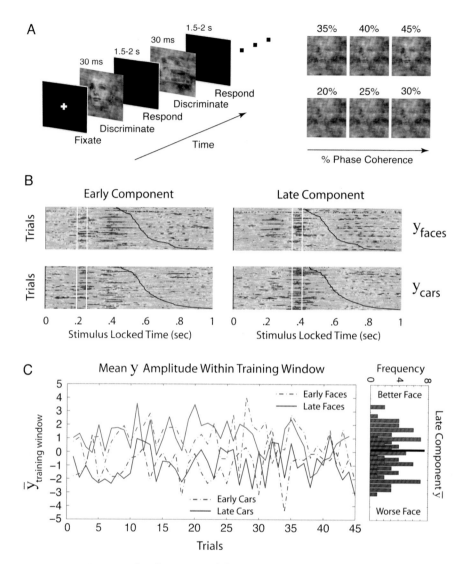

FIGURE 10.2 An example of a perceptual decision-making task and the task-relevant EEG components extracted using linear discrimination, together with their corresponding trial-to-trial variability. A) Behavioral paradigm (left) and sample face stimuli at difference levels of coherence (right). B) Discriminant component maps for one subject at 40% phase coherence. The four panels represent the face-vs-car discriminator output for the two EEG components (one "early" and one "late" relative to stimulus onset). Component maps are shown for both face and car trials using the training windows shown by the vertical white bars. Reaction time profiles are indicated by the black sigmoidal curves. The discriminator was designed to map face trials to positive (red) and car trials to negative values (blue). C) The mean EEG discriminator values within each of the training windows (y bar) for each trial and

FIGURE 10.2 (Continued) for each stimulus class. Shown are trial-by-trial values of the two components for faces and cars at 40% phase coherence only; note that these are not successive trials in the experiment, they are successive presentations of the stimulus condition to illustrate trial-to- trial variability. The amplitudes for the late component are also shown as a histogram (lower panel, right) with a cutoff to separate trials (into "better" face versus "worse" face) denoted by the thick black line. Reproduced from Ratcliff et al., 2009).

categorization task (Philiastides et al., 2006). This manipulation allowed us to keep the stimulus evidence unchanged while comparing the amplitude of the third component between a challenging face/car and a trivial color discrimination. We found that, for the same images, this component was significantly reduced when the subjects were merely discriminating the color of the stimulus confirming that this component is related to task difficulty.

These results taken together suggest that the different EEG components can be thought of as representing distinct cognitive events during perceptual decision making. Specifically, the early component appears to reflect the stimulus quality independent of the task (face/car or color discrimination) and is likely to represent early sensory processing. In contrast, the late component better represents information in the actual face/car decision process as it was shown to be a good predictor of overall behavioral performance during face categorization while its responses to the color discrimination were virtually diminished. Consistent with a top-down attentional control system, the difficulty component appears to be implicated in the recruitment of the relevant attentional and other neuronal resources required to make a difficult decision. Next we consider how the variability in these EEG components can be further interpreted within the context of a well-established and tested model of two-choice decision making.

Linking Trial-to-Trial Variability of EEG Components to Behavior Via the Diffusion Model

Advances in understanding decision processes in both psychology and neuroscience have produced models that require several sources of variability in order to fit experimental data. In psychological applications, the models attempt to fit accuracy and RT distributions for both correct and error responses. The need for assumptions about variability in the various components of processing come about because of the need to fit detailed behavior of error RTs. The major generalizations are that when accuracy is high and speed is stressed,

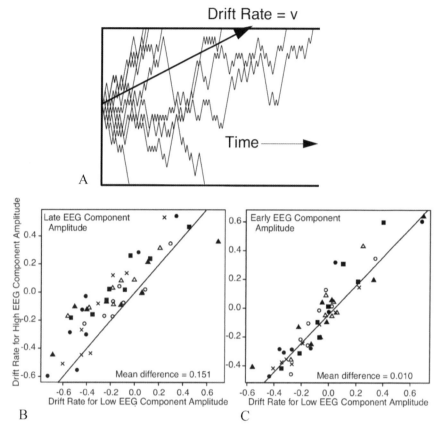

FIGURE 10.3 Linking EEG component variability to the diffusion model for two choice decision making. A) Simulated diffusion processes with the same mean drift rate, demonstrating that behavioral variability can be generated via the model. B) Fits for diffusion model drift rates for data sorted using "late" EEG component values. Drifts rates are systematically higher for EEG components having high values. D) When the "early" EEG component values are used to sort the data, there is no significant difference in the drift rates for high vs low EEG component amplitudes.
Adapted from Ratcliff et al., 2009.

errors are faster than correct responses, but when accuracy is lower and accuracy is stressed, errors are slower than correct responses. This pattern was very difficult to model and error RTs were ignored to a large degree in modeling until the mid 1990s.

In psychology, diffusion models have been shown to be able to successfully account for behavioral data in a range of experimental paradigms. These models assume a gradual accumulation of noisy evidence towards one of two decision criteria as in Figure 10.3A. The parameters of the model include the drift rate, or rate of accumulation of evidence.

In perceptual decision making, this represents the quality of the perceptual signal. The amount of evidence required to make a decision is represented by the distance between the two boundaries, and any bias towards one or other response is represented by any asymmetry between the starting point and either boundary. In addition to these parameters, the other components of processing, such as stimulus encoding and response output are represented by a single parameter which represents the duration of the non-decision components of processing.

The diffusion model, being a dynamic sequential sampling model, can be contrasted with signal detection theory (SDT) which is a static model. In SDT, there is only one source of variability, variability in perceptual strength across trials. This corresponds to variability in drift rate across trials in a diffusion model (see Figure 10.3A). Because there is only one source of variability in SDT, however, all sources of variability are collapsed into the one source. If we believe that there are multiple sources of variability, then SDT is clearly not adequate. We also know that subjects can trade speed for accuracy. A diffusion model analysis shows that to a good approximation, drift rates are invariant under such instructions with differences in accuracy and RT accounted for by a change in the parameter representing boundary separation. In contrast, SDT produces differences in discriminability as a function of speed-accuracy instruction manipulations.

Behavioral models of simple decision making require several sources of variability in order to fit data. Traditionally, behavioral measures (e.g. accuracy and RT) have been the sources of this variability. Neurophysiological measures, however, can also potentially be exploited. For instance, in terms of noninvasive neuroimaging, single-trial EEG offers the ability to track processing in a way that behavioral measures do not. EEG provides a millisecond by millisecond measure of the brain's electrical activity and therefore it is possible to link this activity to different parameters resulting from the psychological models of processing. (Philiastides et al., 2006) showed that the late component of processing correlated highly with drift rate from diffusion model fits to the experimental data. Because this late component provides an estimate of the quality of evidence on single trials we examined whether it could be used to index drift rate in a diffusion model analysis.

In our analysis, the data was divided in half as a function of the size of the late EEG component value. So for each trial, we decided whether the component values was greater or less than the mean for that condition (e.g., the histograms in Figure 10.2C) and then sorted the data into two groups for each condition for each subject. In the diffusion model, this would be equivalent to dividing the drift rates in each condition into two halves if the component value was an estimate of drift rate for each trial. The diffusion model was fit to the two groups of data for each subject, and results showed that for the more face-like group of data, drift rates were more face-like than for the less face-like group of data (see Figure 10.3B). A similar analysis based on the early component of processing showed no difference (Figure 10.3C). In addition, the estimate of variability across trials in drift rate averaged over subjects was significantly lower than the value obtained by fitting all the data for each subject.

These results show a close connection between the variability of the late single trial EEG component value and drift rate in the diffusion model produced by fitting the behavioral data. This provides additional support for both the psychological reality of sequential sampling models. To better understand the neuronal origins of this variability however, one needs to use the single-trial information obtained from the EEG to inform the analysis of fMRI data collected for the same task. The next section describes our efforts of combining EEG and fMRI to describe decision making with high temporal as well as high spatial precision.

Coupling EEG to fMRI for Inferring Cortical Networks Underlying Perceptual Decision-Making

Despite significant progress made in understanding perceptual decision making in humans using EEG and fMRI in isolation, the spatial localization restrictions of EEG and the temporal resolution constraints of fMRI suggest that only a fusion of these modalities can provide a full spatiotemporal characterization of this process. Animal experiments have already demonstrated that hemodynamic signals are more closely coupled to synaptic than spiking activity and that changes in the fMRI BOLD signal can correlate tightly with synchronized oscillatory activity recorded from local field potentials (LFPs) (Logothetis, 2008; Logothetis and et al., 2001; Niessing et al., 2005; Viswanathan and Freeman, 2007). Under these premises, it is reasonable to assume that neural activity reflected in the EEG could also correlate well with the underlying BOLD hemodynamic response.

We have used two methods for coupling EEG and fMRI activity. One is to record EEG and fMRI simultaneously, and explicitly utilize the trial-to-trial fluctuations in the EEG components to construct regressors for use in the analysis of the fMRI activity. In a second approach, we use each modality separately and, given an appropriate experimental design, derive MRI regressors that are modulated by average amplitudes of EEG components associated with different experimental conditions. Specifically, we first perform single-trial LD to identify EEG components of interest (e.g. early, late and difficulty components). Assuming the discriminator is trained with T samples within each window (τ) of interest, the output ($\mathbf{y}_\tau$) has dimensions $T{\times}N$, where N is the total number of trials. To achieve more robust single-trial estimates for $\mathbf{y}_\tau$, averaging across all training samples is performed:

$$\bar{\mathbf{y}}_{\tau,i} = \frac{1}{T} \sum_{j=1}^{T} \mathbf{y}_{\tau,i,j}$$

(2)

Where i is used to index trials and j training samples. For the first approach, $\bar{\mathbf{y}}_{\tau,i}$ is then used to modulate the amplitude of the different fMRI regressor events. Finally, the parametric regressor is convolved with a prototypical hemodynamic response function, which is used to model the fMRI data in the context of a general linear model (GLM). This process can be repeated for multiple windows/components (τ) each resulting in a separate regressor (see Figure 10.5 for a summary of this approach). Identifying the brain regions that correlate with each of these regressors will enable a comprehensive characterization of the cortical network involved in perceptual decision making.

In the absence of simultaneous EEG/fMRI measurements, the second method, namely using average values of EEG components to modulate regressors which are a function of the experiment condition (e.g. trial type). can be used instead. In this case the discriminator output associated with each component and each experimental condition is averaged across trials:

$$\bar{\mathbf{y}}_{\tau,i}^{c} = \frac{1}{N} \frac{1}{T} \sum_{i=1}^{N} \sum_{j=1}^{T} \mathbf{y}_{\tau,i,j}^{c}$$

(3)

where c is used to index the different experimental conditions. The average discriminator output per component and experimental condition obtained from equation 4 can be used to model the fMRI data. Importantly, $\bar{\mathbf{y}}_{\tau,i}^{c}$ is now a scalar - that is, in the absence of single-trial information during the fMRI session, all like trials will be modeled in the same way. Though inter-trial variability is ultimately concealed in this formulation, important information regarding the localization of each of the EEG components, that would otherwise be unattainable using EEG or fMRI alone, can now be obtained.

We first considered the latter approach for the perceptual decision making work presented above (Philiastides et al., 2006; Philiastides and Sajda, 2006). As highlighted earlier, the strength of our early EEG component was proportional to the stimulus evidence (i.e., stronger for easy than hard trials) and it remained unchanged during the face/car and color discriminations. The late EEG component also responded proportionally to the stimulus evidence during the face/car discrimination, but it was stronger across all difficulty levels relative to the early one. Unlike the early component, however, the strength of the late component was significantly reduced during the color discrimination.

In contrast to both the early and late components, the strength of the difficulty component was inversely proportional to the amount of stimulus evidence (i.e., stronger for hard rather than easy trials).

As a result of these observations, we constructed three parametric fMRI regressors, one for each of the early, difficulty, and late components in order to analyze the fMRI data collected for the same task. To modulate the heights of the corresponding regressor events we estimated the relative strengths of our components with respect to the difficulty (i.e., low [L] vs high [H] coherence) and the type of task (i.e., face vs car [FC] or red vs green [RG]) (i.e. $\bar{y}_{\tau,i}^{FC,L}$, $\bar{y}_{\tau,i}^{FC,H}$, $\bar{y}_{\tau,i}^{RG,L}$, $\bar{y}_{\tau,i}^{RG,H}$ where $\tau = (early, difficulty, late)$).

Figure 10.4 summarizes our findings in a form of a spatiotemporal diagram and demonstrates that a cascade of events associated with perceptual decision making takes place in a highly distributed neural network. These include early visual perception (early component), task/decision difficulty (difficulty component) and postsensory/decision-related events (late component). Clear is that by exploiting the variability across EEG component and trial types (i.e. the variability in the $\bar{y}_{\tau,i}^{FC,L}$, $\bar{y}_{\tau,i}^{FC,H}$, $\bar{y}_{\tau,i}^{RG,L}$, $\bar{y}_{\tau,i}^{RG,H}$) we were able to infer a more detailed picture of the cortical networks underlying perceptual decision making.

Next, we wanted to demonstrate the efficacy of the first method of exploiting the trial-to-trial variability measured during simultaneous acquisition of EEG and fMRI. Simultaneous EEG/fMRI is a relatively new neuroimaging modality that enables the simultaneous measurement of electrical and blood oxygenation level dependent (BOLD) activity. The electrical activity measured via EEG is temporally precise (millisecond resolution) and is a direct measure of neural activity whereas the BOLD activity measured via fMRI is more spatially localized (millimeter resolution) and represents an indirect measure of neural activity. We have conducted experiments that use such multimodal neuroimaging to correlate the trial-to-trial variability of temporally precise EEG components with simultaneously measured BOLD activity. The underlying hypothesis is that the trial-to-trial variability in the EEG components has information content that is meaningful, for example representing the dynamics of latent brain states that are unobservable via stimulus or behaviorally derived measures.

Given the technical challenges in acquiring EEG and fMRI simultaneously, we first focused on a very simple and classic perceptual detection paradigm, the auditory oddball task (Donchin and Coles, 1988; Picton, 1992; Polich, 2007). A detailed description of the paradigm and data acquisition can be found in (Goldman et al., 2009). Here we focus on the method for coupling the single-trial variability of the EEG components with the fMRI measured BOLD activity.

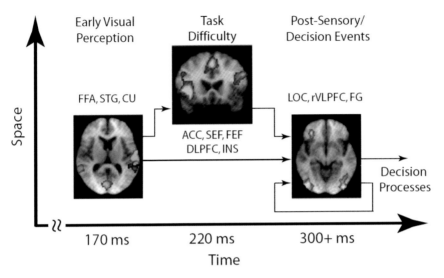

FIGURE IO.4 Spatio-temporal processing timing diagram resulting from an EEG-informed fMRI analysis For the early component, we see significant correlations with activity in areas implicated in early visual processing of objects/faces such as the fusiform face area (FFA) and the superior temporal sulcus (STS), (Allison et al., 1999; Haxby et al., 2000; Hoffman and Haxby, 2000; Kanwisher et al., 1997; Puce et al., 1998). The difficulty component is correlated with activity in the supplementary and frontal eye fields (SEF/FEF), the anterior cingulate cortex (ACC), the dorsolateral prefrontal cortex (DLPFC) and the anterior insula (INS). These observations are consistent with the interpretation that there exist an attentional control system that exerts top-down influence on decision making (Heekeren et al., 2004; Heekeren et al., 2008). Finally, the late component is correlated with activity in the lateral occipital complex (LOC) and in the right ventrolateral prefrontal cortex (rVLPFC). Aside from its involvement in object categorization (Grill-Spector et al., 2004; Grill-Spector et al., 2001; Grill-Spector et al., 1999; James et al., 2000, 2002), the LOC has been implicated in "perceptual persistence" (Ferber et al., 2002; Large et al., 2005), a process in which a percept assembled by lower-visual areas is allowed to remain in the visual system, via feedback pathways, as a form of iconic memory (Coltheart, 1980; DiLollo, 1977; VanRullen and Koch, 2003).

Adapted from Philiastides and Sajda, 2007.

Figure 10.5 shows specifically how we utilize the trial-to-trial variability in the EEG components to construct novel regressors for correlating with the BOLD activity. In this example two EEG components are identified after stimulus onset, one at 250ms and the other at 400ms. Both of these components discriminate target from nontarget stimulus and both are stimulus locked. Note that though both components have discriminative power in terms of

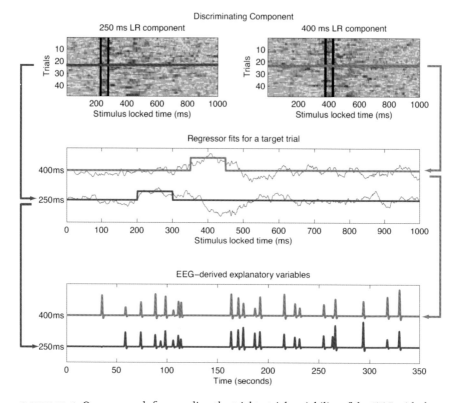

FIGURE 10.5 Our approach for coupling the trial-to-trial variability of the EEG with the BOLD signal, given simultaneous EEG/fMRI acquisition. (top) Output for all trials of the single-trial EEG discriminator for two stimulus-locked 50 ms windows (data between black vertical bars) centered at 250 ms and 400 ms post stimulus-onset. Hot to cold color scale indicates positive to negative values of the discriminator output (i.e. positive and negative correlations). (middle) EEG discriminator output for a single target trial for each of the two components (black curves), showing the fMRI event model amplitude as the average of the discriminator output for each window, 250 ms (blue) and 400 ms (red), for the trial. (bottom) Single-trial fMRI model for target trials across the entire session for the 250 ms and 400 ms windows. Note that the event timing for each of the two windows is the same, but the event amplitudes are different. Reproduced from Goldman et al. (2009).

target from non-target trials, their trial-to-trial variability is not 100% correlated, and therefore their individual trial-to-trial variability in principal could capture different aspects of the decision making process. For each of these components, we construct regressors by using the amplitude of the component on each trial to modulate the amplitude of a boxcar regressor. A regressor is constructed for each EEG component and then convolved with the hemodynamic response function. This leads to two explanatory variables that capture the trial-to-trial variability of the EEG components and can be used in a general linear model (GLM) analysis to correlate with the BOLD activity. Finally we orthogonalize these EEG-derived explanatory variables with respect to traditional stimulus and behaviorally derived regressors, thus ensuring the activity they capture is purely correlation with the EEG component trial-to-trial variability.

Figure 10.6 shows results for statistically significant fMRI activations resulting from trial-to-trial variability in the EEG during an auditory oddball paradigm. (Additional details can be found in (Goldman et al., 2009). Several interesting observations can be made. The first is that the locations of the fMRI

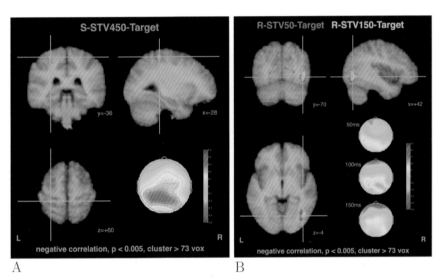

FIGURE 10.6 (A) fMRI activations for the stimulus-locked single-trial analysis showing regions with significant BOLD signal correlation (p<0.005, cluster>73 voxels, negative correlation) with single-trial variability to targets for the 450ms window, S-STV450-Targ. For target tones, only the stimulus-locked 450ms window passed both the EEG and fMRI thresholds. Shown also is the scalp topography of the corresponding 450ms window stimulus-locked EEG discriminating component (arbitrary units). (B) fMRI activations for the response-locked single-trial analysis showing regions with significant BOLD signal correlation (p<0.005, cluster>73 voxels, negative correlation) to response-locked single-trial variability to target tones. The response-locked 50ms window, R-STV50-Targ (blue), and 150ms window, R-STV150-Targ (green), passed both the EEG and fMRI thresholds. The scalp maps of the output of the EEG discriminator for the 3 windows from 50-150ms response-locked are also shown (arbitrary units). Reproduced from Goldman et al. (2009).

activations that arise from the trial-to-trial variability are remarkably consistent with the scalp projections of the corresponding EEG components. Since only the trial-to-trial variability of the EEG components is used in the GLM analysis, no information about the locations of the EEG components (i.e., scalp projections) is used to constrain the spatial location of the fMRI activations. Thus, the fact that that EEG trial-to-trial variability leads to consistent localizations in both modalities supports the interpretation that that this variability is neurophysiologically meaningful. A second observation pertains to the specific locations of the activated regions. Figure 10.6A shows activations localized to somatosensory cortex with Figure 10.6B showing activations in lateral occipital complex. Given that the paradigm is an auditory oddball task, why would two cortical areas selective to other modes of sensory input (somatosensation and vision) be activated? The third observation provides a clue, namely that these activation are negatively correlated with the EEG component trial-to-trial variability. In other words, on a trial, when the EEG component increases the fMRI BOLD signal decreases, and vice versa. A possible interpretation of these three observations is that the trial-to-trial variability represents an attentional "polling" of the sensory inputs, with attention allocated in a "push-pull" fashion—i.e. when attention is directed to one modality it is pulled from the other sensory modalities. We are further investigating this hypothesis with additional experiments that consider activations elicited when the oddball paradigm is performed via a different sensory modality (e.g., visual or somatosensory). In general, these findings suggest that the trial-to-trial variability in EEG components may reflect latent brain states that, when combined with fMRI, can yield novel insight into perceptual decision making. Currently, we are conducting experiments for the face/car paradigm, within the context of this type of simultaneous EEG/fMRI analysis. We believe that this will enable us better elucidate additional details of the underlying cortical networks (i.e. improve upon the accuracy of the spatio-temporal diagram of Figure 10.6).

Conclusions

Our efforts using spatially and temporally precise neuroimaging, machine learning and signal processing, and cognitive modeling to measure and analyze neuronal variability have so far been aimed at understanding how we make very simple decisions. The ultimate challenge is to understand the cortical circuits involved in making typical, everyday decisions such as "Should I take the subway or walk to work today?" or "Should I read this chapter given how busy I am?" The neuronal variability underlying these everyday decisions may in fact be the key to understanding what makes each of us unique—i.e,. what differentiates individuals from one another. In addition, analysis of such neuronal variability may be critical for identifying precursors to behavioral changes, including pathological changes that are associated with cognitive deficits and disease. Thus the imaging, analysis and modeling methods we have described can be seen as a suite of tools, to be used in concert, for measuring and analyzing neuronal variability associated with both normal and abnormal decision making in the human brain.

Acknowledgments

This research was supported by funding from the NIH (grants R33-EB004730 and R01-MH085092) and DARPA (contract NBCHC080029).

REFERENCES

Allison, T., Puce, A., Spencer, D.D., McCarthy, G. (1999) Electrophysiological studies of human face perception: potentials generated in occipitotemporal cortex by face and nonface stimuli. *Cereb Cortex, 9,* 415–430.

Bentin, S., Allison, T., Puce, A., Perez, A., McCarthy, G. (1996) Electrophysiological studies of face perception in humans. *Journal of Cognitive Neuroscience, 8,* 551–565.

Britten, K.H., Newsome, W.T., Shadlen, M.N., Celebrini, S., Movshon, J.A. (1996) A relationship between behavioral choice and visual responses of neurons in macaque MT. *Vis Neurosci, 14,* 87–100.

Britten, K.H., Shadlen, M.N., Newsome, W.T., Movshon, J.A. (1992) The analysis of visual motion: A comparison of neuronal and psychophysical performance. *J of Neuroscience, 12,* 4745–4765.

Coltheart, M. (1980) The persistences of vision. *Philos T Roy Soc B, 290,* 57–69.

DiLollo, V. (1977) Temporal characteristics of iconic memory. *Nature, 267,* 241–243.

Donchin, E., Coles, M.G. (1988) Is the P300 component a manifestation of context updating? *Behavioral and Brain Sciences, 11,* 357–374.

Ferber, S., Humphrey, G.K., Vilis, T. (2002) The lateral occipital complex subserves the perceptual persistence of motion-defined groupings. *Cereb Cortex, 35,* 793–801.

Goldman, R.I., Wei, C.-Y., Philiastides, M.G., Gerson, A.D., Friedman, D., Brown, T.R., Sajda, P. (2009) Single-trial discrimination for integrating simultaneous EEG and fMRI: Identifying cortical areas contributing to trial-to-trial variability in the auditory oddball task. *Neuroimage, 47,* 136–147.

Grill-Spector, K., Knouf, N., Kanwisher, N. (2004) The fusiform face area subserves face perception, not generic within-category identification. *Nat Neurosci, 7,* 555–562.

Grill-Spector, K., Kourtzi, Z., Kanwisher, N. (2001) The lateral occipital complex and its role in object recognition. *Vision Res, 41,* 1409–1422.

Grill-Spector, K., Kushnir, T., Edelman, S., Avidan, G., Itzchak, Y., Malach, R. (1999) Differential processing of objects under various viewing conditions in the human lateral occipital complex. *Neuron, 24,* 187–203.

Guger, C., Ramoser, H., Pfurtscheller, G. (2000) Real-time EEG analysis with subject-specific spatial patterns for a brain computer interface BCI. *IEEE Trans Rehabil Eng, 8,* 441–446.

Halgren, E., Raij, T., Marinkovic, K., Jousmaki, V., Hari, R. (2000) Cognitive response profile of the human fusiform face area as determined by MEG. *Cereb Cortex, 10,* 69–81.

Haxby, J.V., Hoffman, E.A., Gobbini, M.I. (2000) The distributed human neural system for face perception. *Trends Cogn Sci, 4,* 223–233.

Heekeren, H.R., Marrett, S., Bandettini, P.A., Ungerleider, L.G. (2004) A general mechanism for perceptual decision-making in the human brain. *Nature, 431,* 859–862.

Heekeren, H.R., Marrett, S., Ungerleider, L. (2008) The neural systems that mediate human perceptual decision making. *Nat Rev Neurosci, 9,* 467–479.

Hoffman, E., Haxby, J.V. (2000) Distinct representation of eye gaze and identity in the distributed human neural system for face perception. *Nat Neurosci, 3,* 80–84.

Hyvarinen, A., Karhunen, J., Oja, E. (2001) *Independent component analysis.* New York: John Wiley and Sons.

James, T.W., Humphrey, G.K., Gati, J.S., Menon, R.S., Goodale, M.A. (2000) The effects of visual object priming on brain activation before and after recognition. *Curr Biol, 10,* 1017–1024.

James, T.W., Humphrey, G.K., Gati, J.S., Menon, R.S., Goodale, M.A. (2002) Differential effects of viewpoint on object-driven activation in dorsal and ventral streams. *Neuron, 35,* 793–801.

Jeffreys, D.A. (1996) Evoked studies of face and object processing. *Visual Cognition, 3,* 1–38.

Jung, T.P., Makeig, S., McKeown, M.J., Bell, A.J., Lee, T.W., Sejnowski, T.J. (2001) Imaging brain dynamics using independent component analysis. *Proc IEEE, 89,* 1107–1122.

Kanwisher, N., McDermott, J., Chun, M.M. (1997) The fusiform face area: A module in human extrastriate cortex specialized for face perception. *Jl of Neurocience, 17,* 4302–4311.

Lal, T.N., Schroder, M., Hinterberger, T., Weston, J., Bogdan, M., Birbaumer, N., Scholkopf, B. (2004) Support vector channel selection in BCI. *IEEE Trans Biomed Eng, 51,* 1003–1010.

Large, M.E., Aldcroft, A., Vilis, T. (2005) Perceptual continuity and the emergence of perceptual persistence in the ventral visual pathway. *J of Neurophysiology, 93,* 3453–3462.

Liu, J., Higuchi, M., Marantz, A., Kanwisher, N. (2000) The selectivity of the occipitotemporal M170 for faces. *Neuroreport, 11*, 337–341.

Logothetis, N.K. (2008) What we can do and what we cannot do woth fMRI. *Nature, 453*, 869–878.

Logothetis, N.K., et al., J.P. (2001) Neurophysiological investigation of the basis of the fMRI signal. *Nature, 412*, 150–157.

Makeig, S., Westerfield, M., Jung, T.P., Enghoff, S., Townsend, J., Courchesne, E., Sejnowski, T.J. (2002) Dynamic brain sources of visual evoked responses. *Science, 295*, 690–694.

Niessing, J., Ebisch, B., Schmidt, K.E., Niessing, M., Singer, W., Galuske, R.A.W. (2005) Hemodynamic signals correlate tightly with synchronized gamma oscillations. *Science, 309*, 948–951.

Onton, J., Westerfield, M., Townsend, J., Makeig, S. (2006) Imaging human EEG dynamics using independent component analysis. *Neurosci Biobehav Rev, 30*, 802–822.

Parra, L., Alvino, C., Tang, A., Pearlmutter, B., Young, N., Osman, A., Sajda, P. (2002) Linear spatial integration for single-trial detection in encephalography. *Neuroimage, 17*, 223–230.

Parra, L.C., Spence, C.D., Gerson, A.D., Sajda, P. (2005) Recipes for the linear analysis of EEG. *Neuroimage, 28*, 326–341.

Philiastides, M.G., Ratcliff, R., Sajda, P. (2006) Neural representation of task difficulty and decision-making during perceptual categorization: a timing diagram. *J of Neuroscience, 26*, 8965–8975.

Philiastides, M.G., and Sajda, P. (2006) Temporal characterization of the neural correlates of perceptual decision making in the human brain. *Cereb Cortex, 16*, 509–518.

Philiastides, M.G., and Sajda, P. (2007) EEG-informed fMRI reveals spatiotemporal characteristics of perceptual decision making. *J of Neuroscience, 27*, 13082–13091.

Picton, T.W. (1992) The P300 wave of the human event-related potential. *J Clin Neurophysiol, 9*, 456–479.

Polich, J. (2007) Updating P300: an integrative theory of P3a and P3b. *Clin Neurophysiol, 118*, 2128–2148.

Puce, A., Allison, T., Bentin, S., Gore, J.C., McCarthy, G. (1998) Temporal cortex activation in humans viewing eye and mouth movements. *J of Neuroscience, 18*, 2188–2199.

Ramoser, H., Müller-Gerking, J., Pfurtscheller, G. (2000) Optimal Spatial Filtering of Single Trial EEG During Imagined Hand Movement. *IEEE Trans. Rehab. Eng, 8*, 441–446.

Ratcliff, R., Philiastides, M.G., Sajda, P. (2009) Quality of evidence for perceptual decision making is indexed by trial-to-trial variability of the EEG. *Proceedings of the National Academy of Science, 106*, 6539–6544.

Rossion, B., Joyce, C., Cottrell, G.W., Tarr, M.J. (2003) Early laterization and orientation tuning for face, word, object processing in the visual cortex. *Neuroimage, 20*, 1609–1624.

Thulasidas, M., Guan, C., Wu, J. (2006) Robust classification of EEG signals for brain-computer interface. *IEEE Trans Neural Syst Rehabil Eng, 14,* 24–29.

VanRullen, R., Koch, C. (2003) Visual selective behavior can be triggered by a feed-forward process. *Journal of Cognitive Neuroscience, 15,* 209–217.

Viswanathan, A., Freeman, R.D. (2007) Neurometabolic coupling in cerebral cortex reflects synaptic more than spiking activity. Neurometabolic coupling in cerebral cortex reflects synaptic more than spiking activity. *Nat Neurosci, 10,* 1308–1312.

II

Spatiotemporal Dynamics of Synchronous Activity across Multiple Areas of the Visual Cortex in the Alert Monkey

Charles M. Gray and Baldwin Goodell

Introduction

The variability of neuronal activity in the brain is enigmatic. In mammals, complex neural interactions, occurring in parallel across widely distributed networks, enable an astounding repertoire of flexible behavior. One might assume that such analytical and computational power, to borrow a phrase from information technology, would be associated with highly reliable and robust neural activity patterns that are tightly correlated with behavior. Yet, when measured from just about any location in the Telencephalon, neuronal activity appears noisy, unreliable and often weakly linked to behavior and events in the external world. Detecting the relationships that do exist typically requires extensive behavioral training of the subject and repeated measurements to "average out the noise.". Perhaps this situation is to be expected, given that neurons are intrinsically nonlinear and much of their activity depends on patterns of input from tens of thousands of weak, probabilistic and plastic synapses. It does, however, beg the question of how such variable and dynamic neuronal activity can underlie the impressive perceptual, motor and cognitive capabilities of mammals. Perhaps we are simply unable to measure the activity of enough neurons simultaneously to identify the networks that are engaged in particular cognitive processes. Or, perhaps more likely, we have yet to identify the neural dynamics that underlie specific cognitive functions. One can't help but be impressed with how much we don't understand.

The realization that the brain is a nonlinear dynamical system (Freeman and Skarda, 1985; Kelso, 1995; Friston, 2000; Izhikevich, 2007; Izhikevich and Edelman, 2008) may account for some of the difficulty. The brain, and the cortex in particular, is generally regarded as a parallel distributed system, composed of enormous numbers of highly nonlinear and adaptable neurons, that are organized into hierarchical networks with multiple, nested levels of feedback. Even simple systems having these properties are notorious for their emergent and unpredictable behavior, and the brain is certainly the epitome of such a system. Thus, it should come as no surprise that the activity of individual neurons, embedded within distributed neural networks, often shows little or no relation to experimental manipulations and displays inexplicable variability. Unlike explanatory theories in physics and chemistry, however, the development of a systems level theory of distributed neural processing is still at an early stage (Buzsáki, 2006). We therefore lack a clear search image for identifying large-scale, emergent patterns of neural activity that are robustly linked to behavior. This often leads to a heuristic approach and a focus on problems that are technically feasible. This problem is analogous to that faced by the drunk who is looking for his lost keys under the streetlight because that's where the light is.

This is not to discount or ignore the many impressive advances in systems neuroscience, but rather highlight the unique challenges posed by understanding distributed neural processing. Perhaps the field is at a developmental stage similar to what Kuhn (1962) referred to as a 'pre-paradigm period,'" in which competing schools of thought use different methods and are guided by differing theories and presuppositions. If one accepts this premise, it implies that cognitive/systems neuroscience is largely an empirical enterprise, which raises the question of what aspects of neural activity should be measured and analyzed to gain the greatest insights. A case can be made that a useful approach is to cast a broad net, ground one's observations in sound physiological principles, and characterize phenomena closely related to behavior.

In this chapter, we present preliminary results from experiments that have attempted to take this approach at face value. Our broad net has been to initiate the design and development of instruments that enable the recording of unit activity and local field potentials from large numbers of chronically implanted, and independently movable, microelectrodes. We have borrowed design concepts from other successful efforts (Wilson and McNaughton, 1993; deCharms et al., 1999; Hoffman and McNaughton, 2002; Csicsvari et al., 2003; Miller and Wilson, 2008) and developed new devices for long-term recordings of distributed neural activity in awake/behaving monkeys. Our grounding in neurophysiology, and the behavioral correlates of mesoscopic brain states, stems from our own work (Gray et al., 1986, 1989; Gray and McCormick, 1996; Azouz and Gray, 2000; Maldonado et al., 2000), and that of many others (Freeman and Skarda, 1985; Bressler 1995; Singer, 1999; Usrey and Reid, 1999; Freeman, 2000; Varela et al., 2001; Buzsáki and Draguhn, 2004; Fries 2005; Buzsáki, 2006), and focuses on the properties, underlying neural mechanisms, and behavioral correlates of distributed patterns of synchronous neuronal activity.

We infer, on the basis of a large body of existing evidence, that spatially distributed patterns of synchronous activity play a fundamental role in cognitive brain function and that extensive characterization of these phenomena is needed. Our justification follows two lines of reasoning. At the cellular level, synchronous synaptic activity is known to be highly effective at driving postsynaptic responses (Alonso et al., 1996; Azouz and Gray, 2000, 2003) and plays a key role in regulating activity dependent synaptic plasticity (Markram et al., 1997; Bi and Poo, 1998). At the network level, distributed patterns of synchronous activity are robust, prevalent, and well correlated with sensory stimulation and cognitive aspects of behavior (for reviews see Gray, 1994; Singer and Gray, 1995; Bressler, 1995; Singer, 1999, 2009; Usrey and Reid, 1999; Buzsáki and Draguhn, 2004; Buzsáki, 2006; Fries, 2009, and more recent studies by Langheim et al., 2006; Buschman and Miller, 2007; Saalmann et al., 2007; Zhang et al., 2008; Pesaran et al., 2008; Lubenov and Siapas, 2009; Gregoriou et al., 2009). In spite of this extensive work, however, we believe that the characterization of distributed activity patterns and their relationships to cognition and behavior, and the development of new theory, is still in its infancy. This situation is somewhat analogous to the state of astronomy, circa 1920, before the discovery of galaxies lying beyond the Milky Way (Ferris, 1997). New instruments, in the form of large telescopes utilizing spectral analysis, confirmed the existence of distant galaxies and an expanding universe. This led to a wave of experimentation and theory development that continues unabated to this day.

With this context, we describe the results of our initial measurement and characterization of the spatiotemporal dynamics of the local field potential recorded from several areas of the visual cortex in an alert macaque monkey that is freely viewing a dynamic natural scene. Our findings indicate that perceptual and cognitive processes involve large-scale, distributed patterns of synchronization that occur within and between multiple cortical areas. These patterns of correlated activity are transient, non-stationary, occur in multiple frequency bands, and reflect the time course of sensory and behavioral events.

Methods

We performed unit and local field potential recordings in a female macaque monkey, using a semi-chronically implanted array of sixty independently movable microelectrodes. Prior to recording, the animal was implanted with a post for fixation of the head, a scleral search coil for monitoring eye position, and a custom, hermetically-sealed recording chamber to enable mounting of the microdrive (Gray et al., 2007). The chamber was centered over area V4 in the left hemisphere. The monkey was trained to visually fixate a central target, to permit the mapping of cellular receptive fields, and to freely scan brief presentations of static natural scenes and movies.

The Chamber and Microdrive

The recording chamber system incorporates a replaceable Silastic membrane that provides a water-tight seal and an effective barrier to infection (see Gray et al., 2007, for details). The microdrive houses sixty linear actuators and contact with the microelectrodes (Tungsten-in-glass, Alpha Omega, Inc.) is established through a printed circuit board. The inter-electrode spacing is 1.2 mm and each actuator enables 6 mm of bi-directional electrode travel. The microdrive is 15 mm in diameter, 32 mm in height and, when mounted within the chamber, the bottom surface of the drive lies flush against the Silastic membrane.

Figure 11.1 shows the fully loaded microdrive with fifty-seven of the sixty electrodes advanced for testing impedance and the mechanical integrity of each actuator. (Three of the actuators failed during the loading process.) Prior to mounting the microdrive in the chamber, the guide holes in the bottom of the drive were back-filled with ophthalmic antibiotic ointment, and the bottom surface of the drive was covered with a thin layer of sterile, molten bone wax (Swadlow et al., 2004). These steps insure sterility and minimize the back flow of fluid into the actuators. Once these steps were completed, the microdrive was mounted within the chamber, fixed in place with a retaining cap, and the assembly reinforced with a supplemental layer of acrylic cement that extended up to the lower flange on the retaining cap.

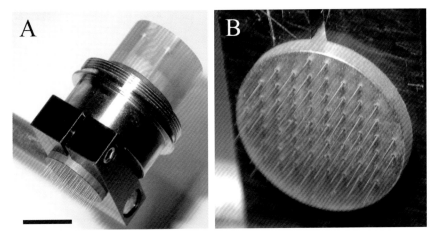

FIGURE 11.1 Photographs of the semichronic microdrive prior to its implantation.
A) Tilted view of the microdrive mounted in a holder. All 57 electrodes are advanced.
B) Close up view of the electrode tips. Scale bar in A is 6 mm.

Electrophysiological Recording

Once the microdrive was mounted within the chamber, the microelectrodes
were gradually advanced into the cortex over a period of five to seven days, and
recordings of unit activity and local field potentials were performed five days a
week for a total of twenty-five days. Each day the monkey viewed a color movie
on a computer monitor placed at a distance of 57 cm. Data sets were collected
during periods of one to three minutes of continuous viewing at the beginning
of each session and after a set of electrodes (typically five to ten) had been incre-
mentally advanced to isolate activity at new sites.

At the end of this first experiment, a second microdrive, containing
thirty-two independently movable microelectrodes (20 mm travel, 2 mm inter-
electrode spacing), was implanted at the same location in the right hemisphere.
A similar series of measurements were made using this drive. These data are
still being analyzed. Following the second experiment, the animal was eutha-
nized, perfused transcardially with fixative and the brain removed and photographed with the overlying skull and implant intact. This enabled us to
accurately identify the recording locations of each of the electrodes in both
hemispheres relative to the sulcul landmarks. The reconstructed recording
locations in the left hemisphere are shown in Figure 11.2. The recording array
spanned at least four separate areas of the visual cortex, including areas V1, V2,
V4 and 7a.

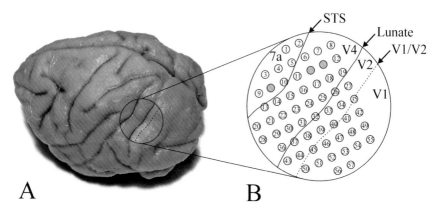

FIGURE 11.2 Reconstruction of the recording locations from the 60-channel array
A) Photograph of the left hemisphere of the monkey's brain. The boundary of the
recording chamber is shown by the circle. B) Expanded schematic of the recording
locations of each of the 57 electrodes. The sulci and visual cortical areas are labeled.
An estimate of the V1/V2 boundary is shown by the dashed line. Bad channels are
shown by the gray filled circles. STS – Superior Temporal Sulcus.

Data Analysis

The aim of the data analysis was to measure and characterize the spatiotemporal patterns of correlated local field potential (LFP) fluctuations measured
across the array. For this, we employed a sliding window cross-correlation analysis, previously developed by us to characterize synchronous activity in area 17
of the cat (Gray et al., 1992). Each signal from the electrode array was bandpass
filtered (10-100 Hz) and down-sampled to a rate of 1 kHz. A 2 sec segment of
the filtered signals from fifty-seven electrodes is shown in Figure 11.3. This
example, taken from ~1 minute of data while the monkey was visually scanning
a movie, illustrates the highly dynamic nature of the spatial and temporal properties of the LFP. Higher numbered channels, located within V1, and possibly
V2 (see Figure 11.2B), exhibit pronounced episodes of synchronized gamma-
band (30–60 Hz) activity. Lower and intermediate numbered channels exhibit
signals in the beta-band (12–30 Hz) having varying degrees of correlation, and
also appear to be independent of the activity occurring in areas V1 and V2.

To evaluate these spatiotemporal interactions with high resolution, we calculated a time-lagged cross-correlogram (1 ms resolution) within a sliding
window (110 ms duration, 20 ms step size) spanning a range of ±20 ms time
lags for all possible channel combinations (n=1596 chn pairs) in the array.
Figure 11.4 illustrates the analysis method. A short segment of the LFP data
taken from two channels in the array (blue and green) is shown in A. Part B shows

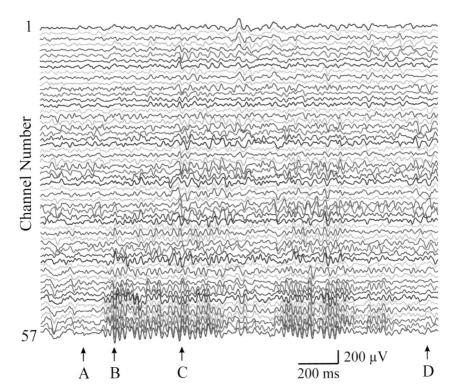

FIGURE 11.3 LFP signals from 57 channels of the array during a 2 second period while the monkey freely viewed a movie. The signals were band pass filtered (10-100 Hz). The arrows labeled A-D mark time points that correspond to the correlation maps in Figure 7.

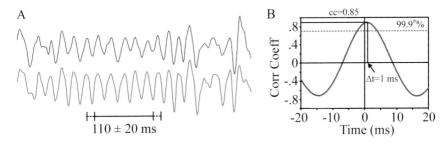

FIGURE 11.4 Sliding window correlation analysis A) Short segment of LFP signals (bandpass filtered 10-100 Hz) from two adjacent channels. The scale bar indicates the duration of the sampling window and the dashed lines indicate the range of time lags and the magnitude of the time step of the windowed analysis. B) Cross correlogram computed from the data segment shown by the scale bar in A. The red dashed line indicates the 99.9% confidence limit. The magnitude and time lag of the correlogram peak are indicated by the horizontal and vertical lines, respectively.

the cross-correlogram computed from the segment shown below the traces in A. For each step in the windowed analysis, we determined the magnitude and time-lag (i.e. phase) of the positive correlation peak closest to time 0. In this example, the positive peak had a value of 0.85 at a delay (Δt) of +1 ms. To test for the significance of this value, we computed a set of 1,000 surrogate correlation coefficients at 0 ms time-lag by independent and random sampling of the window locations in the two channels across the entire recording session. This yielded a Gaussian distribution of correlation coefficients with a maximum centered near 0. The positive value in this distribution, at which 99.9% of the data fell below, served as the threshold for statistical significance. This value, indicated by the dashed red line in B, served as the significance threshold for all time steps of the windowed analysis across the data set for this channel pair. An identical calculation was performed for each channel pair across the array, thereby providing a separate significance threshold for each pair of LFP signals. (The resulting threshold values fell within a narrow range across channels.)

An example of the results of this analysis for two different channel pairs (electrodes 29–55, 55–57), is shown in Figure 11.5. Channel 29 sampled activity from area V4 and channels 55 and 57 were located within area V1 and separated by approximately 2.2 mm (see Figure 11.2). The traces in A (chns 55, 57) and B (chns 29, 55) show the LFP signals (red, blue) and the peak correlation coefficient (black) as a function of time for a 2 sec epoch of the recording. The scale for the correlation coefficients is shown at left, and the threshold for significance (P<.001) is indicated by the black dashed line. The two signals in V1 (A) were highly correlated, with correlation coefficients often rising above the significance threshold. In contrast, the signals on channels 29 and 55 (B) appeared to be largely independent of one another, having only one time step where the correlation coefficient exceeded the significance threshold. The phase differences between the two pairs of signals (i.e. time-lag in ms) are shown in part C. The blue and green traces correspond to the channel pairs in A (55–57) and B (29–55), respectively. The signals recorded in V1 (55-57) tend to remain close to 0 ms time-lag, particularly during the periods where the correlation coefficients exceed the significance threshold. The second pair of signals (29–55), recorded in V4 and V1, display a broad range of time-lags indicative of two independent signals.

We applied this analysis to the same channel pairs for the entire 1-minute duration of the session. Figure 11.6 shows the distributions of significant correlation coefficients (A,D), their corresponding time-lags (B,E), and the durations of temporally continuous periods of significant correlation (C,F). The data from the V1 channel pair (55–57) and the V4/V1 channel pair (29–55) are shown in the top and bottom rows, respectively. For the V1 pair, significant

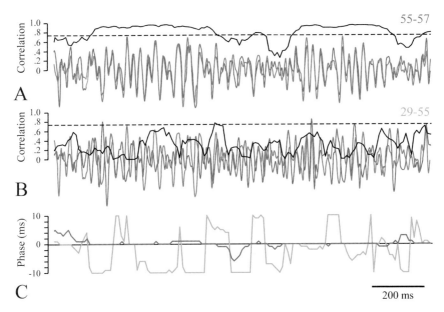

FIGURE II.5 Sliding window correlation analysis The plots in A and B show pairs of
LFP signals (red, blue) and their corresponding time-dependent correlation
coefficients (black) for a 2 sec segment of data taken from channels 55–57 (A) and
29–55 (B). The 99.9% confidence limit is marked by the dashed lines in each plot. The
plot in C shows the corresponding time-lags of the correlation peaks as a function of
time. The blue and green traces were computed from the signal pairs in A and B,
respectively.

correlations were robust and prevalent. The mean value of the correlation coefficients that exceeded the significance threshold was 0.85, and the two signals
were significantly correlated 58% of the time. The distribution of time-lags for
these coefficients was centered at 0 (mean=0.1 ms) and displayed very little
variation (stdev=1.06 ms). In addition, when the two signals became correlated, the duration of these events had a median value of 160 ms and a maximum of ~1 sec.

In contrast, the correlations between the V4/V1 pair were much weaker
and very sparse. The mean significant correlation coefficient was 0.76, and
the signals were significantly correlated only 1% of the time. The distribution
of time-lags was essentially random. There was no clear peak in the distribution and the standard deviation was 14.6 ms. Moreover, the distribution of
correlation durations had a median value of 20 ms, suggesting that nearly all
the significant correlation events were due to chance crossings of the significance threshold at some random phase. These data showed no indication of

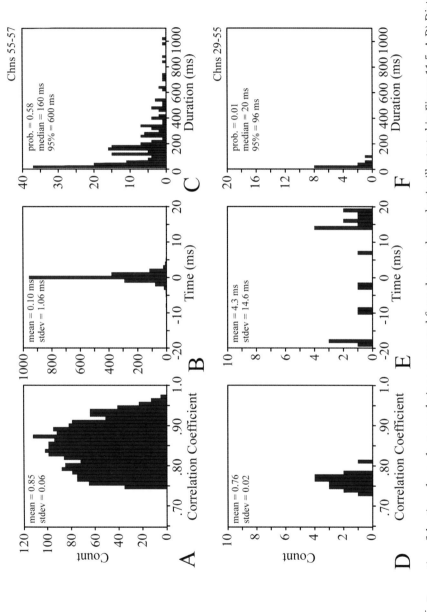

FIGURE 11.6 Properties of the time-dependent correlations computed from the two channel pairs illustrated in Figure 11.5. A,D) Distribution of significant correlation coefficients (p<.001). B,E) Distribution of the corresponding time-lags. C,F) Distribution of the duration of continuous periods of significant correlation.

systematic temporal correlation and suggest that this pair of V4 and V1 signals are independent.

In order to characterize the spatiotemporal patterns of synchronization, we considered it important to identify, and then exclude, correlations in the data that were likely to have occurred by chance, and thus not reflect true corti-co-cortical interactions. Evidence for these types of spurious correlations was apparent in the V4/V1 signal pair shown in Figure 11.6. We therefore applied the same analysis to all channel pairs in the data set (n=1596) and plotted the results as a function of the spatial separation between the electrode pairs (data not shown). *(Note that the separations were calculated from the electrode spacing in the array and did not take into account the depths of the electrodes or the cortical separation distance based on the curvature and sulcal patterns in the cortex.)* These data revealed that the magnitude, duration and probability of significant correlation decreased with distance, while the variance in the time-lag of the correlations increased with distance. We used these data, along with inspection of the individual time-lag histograms, to select thresholds for exclusion of channel pairs and individual correlation coefficients, whose values were indicative of chance correlations. A channel pair was excluded from the analysis when at least one of the following conditions was met: (1) the mean significant correlation coefficient was < 0.7 *(this led to the exclusion of only one channel pair)*, (2) the standard deviation of the time lag distribution was > 9 ms, (3) the median duration of the correlation events was < 60 ms, and (4) the percentage of time the signals were significantly correlated was < 1%. Even when these criteria were applied, we continued to find correlations in the remaining signal pairs in which the distribution of time-lags was centered at, or near, 0 ms, but had some large values lying outside the central distribution. We suspected that these events also represented spurious correlations and applied the additional threshold to exclude correlation coefficients in which the absolute value of the time lag was > 6 ms.

Results

Having applied these thresholds, we were able to characterize the spatiotempo-ral properties of synchronous activity across the array. An example of this is shown in Figure 11.7. The four panels show separate snapshots of the spatial distribution of significant correlation coefficients for the four corresponding epochs labeled A–D in Figure 11.3. There are at least three distinct correlated networks that are apparent in these examples. During the period marked by A, the distribution of correlations is sparse, comparatively weak and relatively

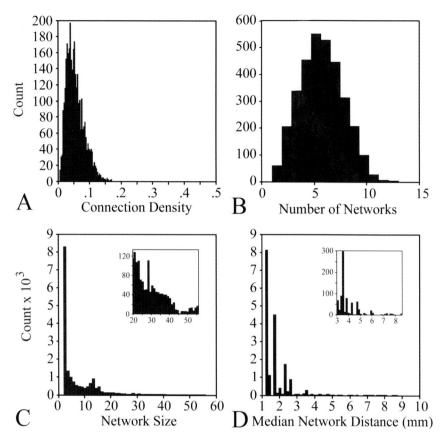

FIGURE 11.8 Histograms of connection density (A), number of networks (B), network size (C) and median network distance (D) computed from the entire 1-minute of data sampled from the 60-channel array while the monkey freely viewed a movie.

observed networks is 4, indicating that networks of only a few connections are by far the most common (C), but larger networks are also prevalent (see inset in C). We also characterized the spatial dimensions of the synchronous networks by calculating the median length (in millimeters) among the connections in all observed networks (D). As expected, these data demonstrate that most networks are composed of connected nodes that are adjacent or nearby to one another. Occasionally, however, networks of larger spatial scale are present (see inset in D). Finally, scatter plots of these variables revealed that as connection density across the array increased the number of networks decreased, and the maximum network size increased (data not shown). Thus increases in connectivity across the array were associated with fewer numbers of networks having larger sizes.

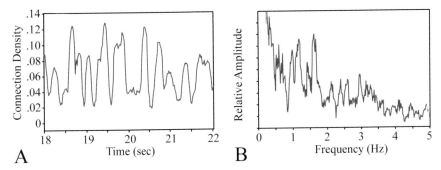

FIGURE II.9 Time dependent properties of the synchronous networks A. Connection density as a function of time for a 2-second segment of data. B. Power spectrum of the connection density versus time for the entire 1-minute period of data collection.

In order to gain some additional insight into the temporal organization of these networks, we performed some additional analyses of the time-dependent changes in these network parameters. Because both network size and the number of networks were closely correlated with connection density, we restricted our analysis to the latter variable. Figure 11.9 shows the time-dependent changes in connection density across the array. The plot in A shows a 2-second segment of connection density as a function of time. Large, semi-periodic fluctuations are apparent with time scales on the order of ~200-500 ms. The power spectrum of connection density for the entire 1-minute recording session (B) supports this observation. Multiple frequency components are present in the data and prominent peaks occur at approximately 1, 1.5, 2.5 and 3 Hz. Thus, there is a striking dynamic organization to the time-dependent changes in synchronous cortical networks. Large changes in the number of visual cortical networks, their connection density, and their size occur rapidly, on the order of hundreds of milliseconds, as the monkey freely scans a dynamic natural scene.

These findings of course raise the question of how the network organization varies with respect to the properties of the visual scene and the animal's saccadic eye movements. These questions are unfortunately beyond the scope of our initial investigation. In these early recordings, our ability to acquire the eye position signals during the free-viewing task was constrained by some technical factors. We were thus unable to evaluate the network dynamics with respect to eye movements and the image properties in the movie. In the second series of experiments, utilizing a thirty-two-channel array in the opposite hemisphere (see Methods), we solved the former problem and are thus able to provide some limited insight into the relation between network organization and eye movements. The placement of this second array was very similar to that of the first. The electrodes sampled activity from areas V1, V2, V4 and 7a. We collected data from the monkey over a period of eight weeks, and on each recording day the animal freely viewed a movie for several sessions, each lasting several minutes.

The analysis of these data is still in progress, but visual inspection of the raw data has revealed some interesting relationships between saccadic eye movements and the occurrence and properties of synchronous networks. A typical example of these data is shown in Figure 11.10. This plot shows the vertical and horizontal components of the monkey's eye movements (V,H) along with the broadband (0.5 Hz – 10 kHz) signal recorded from electrodes in V1, near the V1/V2 border, for a 2-second period. The onset of visual fixation, at each new target chosen by the animal, is marked by a vertical line. A striking property of these signals is the occurrence of brief synchronous gamma-band oscillations that follow the onset of some visual fixations and

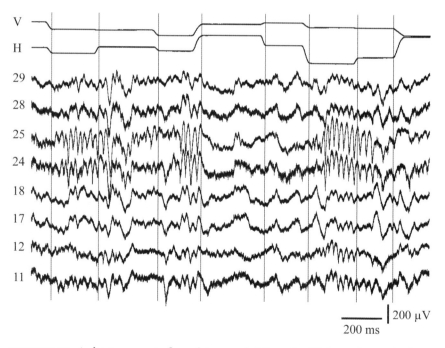

FIGURE 11.10 A short segment of raw data sampled from the 32-channel array in the right hemisphere while the monkey freely viewed a movie. The upper two traces show the vertical and horizontal components of the eye movements. The remaining traces show the broadband signal (1 Hz – 10 kHz) sampled from 8 of the electrodes located in area V1 near the V1/V2 border.

not others. The latency, duration, amplitude and spatial distribution of these bursts also vary across fixations. In some instances the synchronous activity spans multiple fixations or can be truncated by the evoked response following the onset of a new fixation. While these data are preliminary, and we have not characterized the image properties in relation to the animal's eye movements, we can be certain that the image projected on the retina changes markedly from one visual fixation to the next. Thus, it is reasonable to assume that the fluctuations in network organization described above are strongly dependent on the properties of the visual images.

Discussion

Using a newly developed instrument, and time-dependent correlation analysis, to measure correlated local field potential fluctuations from multiple visual cortical areas simultaneously, we find striking stimulus-dependent, dynamic patterns of synchrony that occur within and between several areas of the visual cortex. These findings are consistent with a number of theoretical predictions concerning the dynamics of cortico-cortical interactions (Gray, 1999; Singer, 1999, 2009; Friston, 2000; Fries, 2005; Buzsáki, 2006). They demonstrate that multiple, independent synchronous assemblies can form and dissipate rapidly, follow complex spatiotemporal trajectories, and vary in their spatial distribution and spectral composition over a wide range of frequencies. The synchronous networks tend to remain confined to cortical area boundaries, but also encompass multiple areas in many instances. These initial data suggest that gamma-band networks are formed largely in V1, possibly V2, and that they follow the onset of fixation at a latency ranging from 50-100ms, a result supported by a recent study in V1 of free-viewing monkeys (Maldonado et al., 2008).

These results are also cause for optimism. While not reported here, we have found from ongoing measurements in V1, as well as prefrontal and posterior parietal cortex (Salazar et al., 2008), that it is possible to measure multi- and single-unit activity from fixed recording locations for periods lasting one to two weeks or longer. These data suggest that the chronic recordings are not damaging the cortical tissue, as might be expected if the brain were moving relative to the recording array that is rigidly mounted on the skull. Moreover, an advantage of the method is that once adequate data has been sampled, or if activity has deteriorated over time, new signals (units and field potentials) can be sampled by advancing one or all of the electrodes. In this way it is possible to collect extensive data sets that not only span multiple cortical areas, but also sample activity across cortical layers, into the depths of sulci, and from subcortical nuclei.

The data presented here are clearly preliminary, however, and many questions remain to be addressed. Detailed analysis needs to be performed to establish the relationship between saccadic eye movements, the properties of the visual image during each period of fixation, and the spatiotemporal organization of the synchronous networks. In our second set of recordings, described in Figure 11.10, we have found many instances in which evoked responses follow saccades at short latency. These common events are readily detected by our method and are likely to account for some fraction of the synchronous networks we have measured. Other robust networks, such as those detected in V1, follow the onset of fixation and occasionally span saccadic eye movements suggesting a potential mechanism for temporal integration across successive visual fixations. In retinotopically organized areas we should expect to find transient synchronous networks that reflect the features in the retinal image or the salience of objects (Gray, 1999). Whereas in nonretinotopic areas the patterns may be indicative of the behavioral significance of the images, the intention to make an eye movement to a particular location or target, or the attention directed to some aspect of the visual scene.

Analytically, there is much room for improvement as well. We chose to measure correlations in the time domain because this enabled us to use smaller temporal windows than conventional time-frequency analysis (Mitra and Pesaran, 1999; Grinsted et al., 2004) and avoid the need for repeated observations or signal averaging (Ding et al., 2000) which would have eliminated the real-time nature of the measurements. This prevented us from characterizing the frequency distribution of the interactions and forced us to express phase in units of milliseconds. Perhaps other more powerful methods, such as Empirical Mode Decomposition (Liang et al., 2005) or Frequency Flows Analysis (Rudrauf et al., 2006) could provide a more effective basis for analysis of these data.

Finally, our findings, and the feasibility of the recording methods, may open up a broad new area of investigation of distributed processing in the mammalian brain. The chamber system and microdrive array can easily be expanded to sample activity from much larger areas of the brain. New devices can extend the travel of the electrodes, decrease the inter-electrode spacing to enable higher sampling density, and incorporate additional instruments for electrical stimulation, drug delivery or the use of an optical neural interface (Aravanis et al., 2007; Han et al., 2009). Currently, we are developing a system to enable high-density microelectrode recording from an entire hemisphere in macaque monkeys (Goodell and Gray, 2008). Implementation of such a device will no doubt present many challenges. It will also provide unprecedented access to the brain to permit the analysis of distributed processes on a scale comparable to functional imaging methods, but with much higher spatial and temporal resolution. Data from these and related instruments will likely lead to the development of new analytical methods to observe and characterize distributed patterns of neural activity that have been beyond the scope of our current methods. Perhaps then we will metaphorically see beyond our own galaxy and observe the large scale dynamics of the brain.

REFERENCES

Alonso, J.M., Usrey, W.M., Reid, R.C. (1996) Precisely correlated firing in cells of the lateral geniculate nucleus. *Nature, 383,* 815–819.
Aravanis, A., Wang, L.P., Zhang, F., Meltzer, L., Mogri, M., Schneider, M.B., Deisseroth, K. (2007) An optical neural interface: *in vivo* control of rodent motor cortex with integrated fiberoptic and optogenetic technology. *Journal of Neural Engineering, 4,* S143–S156.
Azouz, R., Gray, C.M. (2000) Dynamic spike threshold reveals a mechanism for synaptic coincidence detection in cortical neurons *invVivo.* Proceedings of the Nationall Academy of Science, 97(14), 8110–8115.
Azouz, R., Gray, C.M. (2003) Adaptive coincidence detection and dynamic gain control in visual cortical neurons *in vivo. Neuron, 37,* 513–523.
Bassett, D.S., Bullmore, E. (2006) Small-world brain networks. *Neuroscientist, 12(6),* 512–523.
Bi, G.Q., Poo, M.M. (1998) Synaptic modifications in cultured hippocampal neurons: dependence on spike timing, synaptic strength, and postsynaptic cell type. *J of Neuroscience, 18,* 10464–10472.
Bressler, S.L. (1995) Large-scale cortical networks and cognition. *Brain Res Rev, 20,* 288–304.
Buschman, T.J. and Miller, E.K. (2007) Top-down versus bottom-up control of attention in the prefrontal and posterior parietal cortices. *Science, 315,* 1860-1862.
Buzsáki G. (2006) Rhythms of the Brain. Oxford University Press.
Buzsáki, G. and Draguhn, A. (2004) Neuronal oscillations in cortical networks. *Science, 304,* 1926–1929.
Csicsvari, J., Henze, D.A., Jamieson, B., Harris, K.D., Sirota, A., Wise, K.D., Buzsáki, G. (2003) Massively parallel recording of unit and local field potentials with silicon-based electrodes. *J of Neurophysiology, 90,* 1314–1323.
DeCharms, R.C., Blake, D.T., Merzenich, M.M. (1999) A multielectrode implant device for the cerebral cortex. *J. Neurosci Meth., 93,* :27–35.
Ding, M., Bressler, S.L., Yang, W., Liang, H. (2000) Spectral analysis of cortical event-related potentials by adaptive multivariate autoregressive modeling: Model order, stability and consistency. *Biol Cybern, 83,* 35–45.
Ferris T. (1997) The whole shebang. New York: Touchstone.

Freeman, W.J. (2000) Mesoscopic neurodynamics: from neuron to brain. *J Physiol Paris, 94,* 303–322.

Freeman, W.J. and Skarda, C.A. (1985) Spatial EEG patterns, non-linear dynamics and perception: the neo-Sherringtonian view. *Brain Res, 357,* 147–175.

Fries, P. (2005) A mechanism for cognitive dynamics: neuronal communication through neuronal coherence. *Trends Cogn Sci, 9,* 474–480.

Fries, P. (2009) Neuronal gamma-band synchronization as a fundamental process in cortical computation. *Annu Rev Neurosci, 32,* 209–224.

Friston, K.J. (2000) The labile brain. I. Neuronal transients and nonlinear coupling. *Philos Trans R Soc Lond B Biol Sci, 355,* 215–236.

Goodell, A.B. and Gray, C.M. (2008) A large-scale, distributed recording system for semi-chronic monitoring of cortical and sub-cortical neuronal activity in alert monkeys. *Soc Neurosci Abs,* 101.7.

Gray, C.M. (1994) *Synchronous oscillations in neuronal systems: mechanisms and functions. J. of Computational Neuroscience, 1,* 11–38.

Gray, C.M. (1999) The temporal correlation hypothesis of visual feature integration: Still alive and well. Neuron, 24, 31–47.

Gray, C.M., Engel, A.K, Koenig, P., Singer, W. (1992) Synchronization of oscillatory neuronal responses in cat striate cortex: Temporal properties. *Visual Neuroscience, 8,* 337–347.

Gray, C.M., Freeman, W.J., Skinner, J.E. (1986) Chemical dependencies of learning in the olfactory bulb: acquisition of the transient spatial pattern change depends on norepinephrine. *Behavioral Neuroscience, 100(4),* 585–596.

Gray CM, Goodell AB, Lear AT. (2007) A Multi-Channel Micromanipulator and Chamber System for Recording Multi-Neuronal Activity in Alert, Non-Human Primates. *J. Neurophysiol., 98,* 527–536.

Gray. C.M., Koenig, P., Engel, A.K., Singer, W. (1989) Stimulus-specific neuronal oscillations in cat visual cortex exhibit inter-columnar synchronization which reflects global stimulus properties. *Nature, 338,* 334–337.

Gray, C.M., McCormick, D.A. (1996) Chattering cells: Superficial pyramidal neurons contributing to the generation of synchronous oscillations in visual ortex. *Science, 274,* 109–113.

Gregoriou, G.G., Gotts, S.J., Zhou, H., Desimone, R. (2009) High-frequency, long-range coupling between prefrontal and visual cortex during attention. *Science, 324,* 1207–1210.

Grinsted, A., Moore, J.C., Jevrejeva, S. (2004) Application of the cross wavelet transform and wavelet coherence to geophysical time series. *Nonlinear Processes in Geophysics, 11,* 561–566.

Han, X., Qian, X., Bernstein, J.G., Zhou, H.H., Franzesi, G.T., Stern, P., Bronson, R.T., Graybiel, A.M., Desimone, R., Boyden, E.S. (2009) Millisecond-timescale optical control of neural dynamics in the nonhuman primate brain. *Neuron, 62,* 191–198.

Hoffman, K.L. and McNaughton, B.L. (2002) Coordinated reactivation of distributed memory traces in primate neocortex. *Science, 297,* 2070–2073.

Izhikevich, E.M. (2007) *Dynamical systems in neuroscience: The geometry of excitability and bursting*. Cambridge: MIT Press.

Izhikevich, E.M. and Edelman, G.M. (2008) Large-scale model of mammalian thalamo-cortical systems. *Proceedings of the National Academy of Science*, 105, 3593–3598.

Kelso, J. (1995) *Dynamic patterns: The self-organization of brain and behavior*. Cambridge: MIT Press.

Kuhn, T.S. (1962) *The structure of scientific revolutions*. Chicago: University of Chicago Press.

Langheim, F.J., Leuthold, A.C., Georgopoulos, A.P. (2006) Synchronous dynamic brain networks revealed by magnetoencephalography. *ProcEedings of the National Academy of Science, 103*, 455–459.

Liang, H., Bressler, S.L., Buffalo, E.A., Desimone, R., Fries, P. (2005) Empirical mode decomposition of field potentials from macaque V4 in visual spatial attention. *Biol Cybern., 92*, 380–392.

Lubenov, E.V. and Siapas, A.G. (2009) Hippocampal theta oscillations are travelling waves. *Nature, 459*, :534–539.

Maldonado, P., Babul, C., Singer, W., Rodriguez, E., Berger, D., Gruen, S. (2008) Synchronization of neuronal responses in primary visual cortex of monkeys viewing natural images. *J of Neurophysiology 100*, 1523–1532.

Maldonado, P.E., Friedman-Hill. S.R., Gray, C.M. (2000) Dynamics of striate cortical activity in the alert macaque: II. Fast time scale synchronization. *Cerebral Cortex, 10*, 1117–1131.

Markram, H., Lubke, J., Frotscher, M., Sakmann, B. (1997) Regulation of synaptic efficacy by coincidence of postsynaptic APs and EPSPs. *Science, 275*, 213–215.

Miller, E.K. and Wilson, M.A. (2008) All my circuits: using multiple electrodes to understand functioning neural networks. Neuron, 60, 483–488.

Mitra, P.P. and Pesaran, B. (1999) Analysis of dynamics brain imaging data. *Biophys J, 76*, 691–708.

Pesaran, B., Nelson, M.J., Andersen, R.A. (2008) Free choice activates a decision circuit between frontal and parietal cortex. *Nature, 453*, 406–409.

Rudrauf, D., Douiri, A., Kovach, C., Lachaux, J.P., Cosmelli, D., Chavez, M., Adam, C., Renault. B., Martinerie, J., Le Van Quyen. M. (2006) Frequency flows and the time-frequency dynamics of multivariate phase synchronization in brain signals. *Neuroimage, 31*, 209–227.

Sakkalis, V., Oikonomou, T., Pachou, E., Tollis. I., Micheloyannis. S., Zervakis M. (2006) Time-significant wavelet coherence for the evaluation of schizophrenic brain activity using a graph theory approach. *Conf Proc IEEE Eng Med Biol Soc, 1*, 4265–4268.

Saalmann, Y.B., Pigarev, I.N., Vidyasagar, T.R. (2007) Neural mechanisms of visual attention: how top-down feedback highlights relevant locations. *Science, 316*, 1612–1615.

Salazar, R.F., Bressler, S, Richter, C., Gray, C.M. (2008) Fronto-parietal coherence is task and rule specific. *Soc Neurosci Abs*, 418, 9.

Singer, W. (1999) Neuronal synchrony: a versatile code for the definition of relations? *Neuron, 24*, 49–65.

Singer, W. (2009) Distributed processing and temporal codes in neuronal networks. *Cogn Neurodyn., Jun 28*. [Epub ahead of print]

Singer, W. and Gray, C.M. (1995) Visual feature integration and the temporal correlation hypothesis. *Ann. Rev. Neurosci, 18*, 555–586.

Sporns, O. (2002) Graph theory methods for the analysis of neural connectivity patterns. In Kotter, R. (Ed.), *Neuroscience Databases. A Practical Guide.* Boston: Kluwer; 171–186.

Swadlow, H.A., Bereshpolova, Y., Bezdudnaya, T., Cano, M., Stoelzel, C.R. (2004) A multi-channel, implantable microdrive system for use with sharp, ultra-fine "Reitboeck" microelectrodes. *J. of Neurophysiology, 93*, 2959–2965.

Usrey, W.M., and Reid, R.C. (1999) *Synchronous activity in the visual system. Annual Review of Physiology, 61*, 435-56.

Varela, F., Lachaux, J.P., Rodriguez, E., Martinerie. J. (2001) The brainweb: phase synchronization and large-scale integration. *Nat. Rev. Neurosci, 2*, 229–239.

Watts, D.J. and Strogatz, S.H. (1998) Collective dynamics of "small-world" networks. *Nature, 393*, 440–442.

Wilson, M.A. and McNaughton, B.L. (1993) Dynamics of the hippocampal ensemble code for space. *Science, 261*, 1055–1058.

Zhang, Y., Wang, X., Bressler, S.L., Chen, Y., Ding, M. (2008) Prestimulus cortical activity is correlated with speed of visuomotor processing. *J Cogn Neurosci, 20*, 1915–1925.

12

Behavioral and Neural Variability Related to Stochastic Choices during a Mixed-Strategy Game

Daeyeol Lee and Hyojung Seo

Introduction

Behavioral responses of humans and animals frequently display a substantial amount of variability, even when they are tested repeatedly under the same physical conditions. For example, the time it takes a subject to produce a particular motor response after the onset of a sensory stimulus, often referred to as reaction time, varies from trial to trial (Luce, 1986). Similarly, the spatial trajectory of the resulting movement is not fixed when the same movement is produced repeatedly (Todorov and Jordan, 2002). In addition to this motoric variability, decisions are often made stochastically. For example, we might often switch between different restaurants or between different types of food. In some cases, this might be due to changes in our underlying preferences and sensory habituation. Humans and animals, however, would often change their choices, even when the reward expected from their actions is constant and homogeneous. Indeed, in the majority of the laboratory experiments on decision making, the type of reward received by the subject is fixed. Most human studies employ money as the potential reward, whereas animal studies frequently use a particular type of food or water. Nevertheless, stochastic choices are observed commonly in many studies.

For many problems in decision making, an optimal strategy is to choose a particular option exclusively, and hence deterministically. For example, if the two alternative options deliver the same amount of reward with different probabilities, it would be optimal to choose the option with the higher reward probability exclusively. Nevertheless, the probability of choosing the high-probability reward is often matched to the probability of reward (Estes, 1962), even though the optimal choice would be to choose the high-probability reward exclusively. In other cases, stochastic behavior might be desirable and even optimal. First, when the outcomes expected from alternative actions and their probabilities are not fully known, decision makers need to explore and improve the accuracy of their estimates of reward probabilities for different actions (Sutton and Barto, 1998). Second, choosing actions stochastically might be beneficial in some competitive social contexts, because it allows the decision makers to avoid getting exploited by their opponents (Lee et al., 2004, 2005; Seo and Lee, 2008).

An important question in systems neuroscience is to understand the nature of underlying neural processes responsible for this behavioral variability. For example, it is well known that the pattern of discharges in individual cortical neurons is highly variable, even when they are driven by the identical sensory stimuli in multiple trials (Softky and Koch, 1993). In fact, many studies have found that the variance of spike count is approximately proportional to the mean spike count (Henry et al., 1973; Tomko and Crapper, 1974; Rose, 1979; Dean, 1981; Tolhurst et al., 1983; Lee et al., 1998), which is expected if the spike trains of cortical neurons are Poisson processes (Rieke et al., 1997). In addition, for saccadic eye movements, variability in their reaction times has been linked to the variability in the rate of rise in the activity of individual neurons in the frontal eye field (Hanes and Schall, 1996). Nevertheless, little is known about how the variability in the neural activity leads to stochastic choice behavior that is useful for exploration and competitive social interactions. In this article, we first review the choice behaviors of rhesus monkeys performing a computer-simulated matching pennies task, which is a binary competitive game for two players. This game requires the players to choose stochastically between the two alternative choices in order to maximize their payoffs, and therefore it is particularly well-suited for studying the relationship between neural and behavioral variabilities. We found that the animals tend to approximate the optimal strategy during the matching pennies game, using a relatively simple reinforcement learning algorithm. We then describe the various types of neural signals identified in the frontal cortex and parietal cortex during the same task that might be used to implement the reinforcement learning algorithm. Finally, we describe the time course of the variability in neural activity during the matching pennies task.

Stochastic Behavior during Competitive Games

People and animals can make decisions individually or as a group. For individual decision making, choices are considered rational when a set of numbers, called utilities, can be assigned to alternative actions so that decision makers always choose the actions with maximum utilities. Of course, human choice behavior often deviates from the predictions of such rational choice theory, and many alternative theories, including the prospect theory, have been proposed to account for the violations of rational choice theory. Understanding the process of decision making in a social context is more difficult. For example, although the same principle of utility maximization can be applied to decision making in a social context, the expected outcomes of choosing a particular action can vary depending on the actions of other decision makers during social interactions. In game theory, this is summarized in a payoff matrix, which defines the payoffs for all the individuals in a group according to their choices.

To illustrate how the payoff matrix can be used to describe a specific game, the payoff matrix for the prisoner's dilemma is illustrated in Figure 12.1A. During the prisoner's dilemma game, each of the two players chooses between cooperation and defection. The maximum payoff is given to the player who defects while the other player cooperates, and the minimum payoff is given to the player who cooperates while the other player defects. For the payoff matrix shown in Figure 12.1A, the maximum and minimum payoffs correspond to 5 and 0, respectively. In addition, the payoff for defection is higher than that for cooperation regardless of whether the other player cooperates or defects. The payoff for mutual defection, however, which is "1" in this example, is lower than the payoff for mutual cooperation. In game theory, a set of choices defined for all players is referred to as a Nash equilibrium, in which none of the players can increase their payoffs any more by changing their strategies individually (Nash, 1950). This implies that a set of rational players trying to maximize their individual payoffs should adopt the Nash-equilibrium strategies. In the prisoner's dilemma's game, mutual defection is the only Nash equilibrium. Interestingly, people do not always choose the Nash-equilibrium strategies during the prisoner's dilemma game, indicating that the assumptions of rationality might be often violated (Sally, 1995; Lee, 2008).

A. Prisoner's dilemma game

Player II

		Cooperate	Defect
Player I	Cooperate	(3, 3)	(0, 5)
	Defect	(5, 0)	(1, 1)

B. Matching pennies game

Player II

		Left	Right
Player I	Left	(1, −1)	(−1, 1)
	Right	(−1, 1)	(1, −1)

FIGURE 12.1 Payoff matrix for the prisoner's dilemma game (A) and matching pennies game (B). Two numbers in each parenthesis indicate the payoffs to the players I and II determined by their choices.

For some games, such as the prisoner's dilemma's game, its Nash-equilibrium strategy is fixed and corresponds to choosing a particular action exclusively, which is referred to as a pure strategy in game theory. In contrast, a mixed strategy refers to choosing multiple actions stochastically. In some cases, a Nash equilibrium might consist of mixed strategies. For example, the matching pennies is a simple two-player zero-sum games in which one of the player ("matcher") wins if the two players choose the same target, and the other player ("nonmatcher") wins otherwise. For the matching pennies with a symmetrical payoff, such as the one shown in Figure 12.1B, the Nash-equilibrium is reached when both players choose the two targets randomly with equal probabilities.

A number of studies have tested whether humans can follow a mixed Nash-equilibrium strategy and make their choices randomly. Almost all of these studies have found that people can play a mixed Nash-equilibrium strategy only approximately (Rapoport and Budescu, 1992; Budescu and Rapoport, 1994; Mookherjee and Sopher, 1994, 1997; Erev and Roth, 1998; Camerer, 2003). This is not surprising, given that a perfect mixed Nash-equilibrium strategy requires the decision makers to make their choices randomly and independently of their previous choices and their outcomes. Instead, actual choice behaviors of subjects during mixed-strategy competitive games, such as the matching pennies game, were better accounted for by various reinforcement learning algorithms. Namely, people tend to choose the actions that were previously successful more frequently than demanded by the Nash-equilibrium strategy.

Reinforcement Learning During the Matching Pennies Game

Previous studies in our laboratory have tested whether rhesus monkeys can learn to play a mixed Nash-equilibrium strategy during simple zero-sum games, such as the matching pennies (Lee et al., 2004, 2005). These experiments were conducted while the animal's head was fixed and the animal indicated its choice between the two alternative targets by shifting its gaze towards its chosen target. The animal began each trial by fixating the central target in a computer screen (Figure 12.2A). Following a 0.5-s fore-period, two identical peripheral targets were presented along the horizontal meridian. The central target was then extinguished after a 0.5-s delay period, and the animal was required to shift its gaze towards one of the two peripheral targets within 1 s. After a 0.5-s fixation period during which the animal was required to maintain its fixation on the chosen target, a red feedback ring was displayed around the target chosen by the computer opponent, and the animal was rewarded only when it chose the same target as the computer opponent. For three animals, we have manipulated the complexity of the algorithm utilized by the computer opponent to test whether the animal's choice behavior changed according to the strategy of its opponent (Lee et al., 2004). As predicted, we found that when the computer opponent unilaterally played the Nash-equilibrium strategy and chose between the two targets randomly with equal probabilities, the animals tended to show idiosyncratic biases to choose one of the targets more frequently. This is not surprising, because during the matching pennies, the expected payoffs from the two targets are equal and constant for any strategies, when the opponent plays the Nash-equilibrium strategies. We then tested the animal's behavior when the computer opponent exploited the statistical biases in the animal's choice sequences. In all three monkeys tested with this algorithm (referred to as algorithm 1 in Lee et al., 2004), this had a dramatic effect and quickly equalized the probabilities for choosing the two different targets. Interestingly, all animals also showed a substantial bias to choose more frequently the targets that were chosen by the computer and therefore rewarded in recent trials. In other words, they tended to make their choices according to

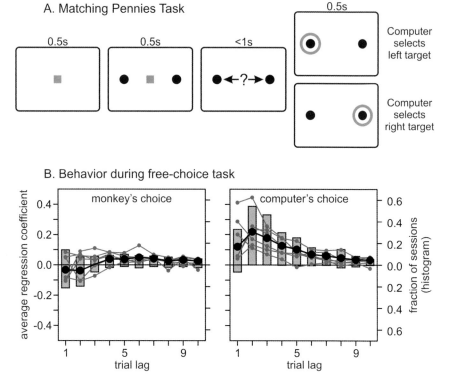

FIGURE 12.2 Task sequence for the computer-simulated matching pennies game (A) and the behavioral performance of six rhesus monkeys during the same task (B). The line plots in B show the average regression coefficients related to the animal's previous choices (left) and the choices of the computer opponent (right). Small gray dots indicate the results from individual animals, whereas black dots are the values averaged across all animals (n=6). Large black disks indicate that the average values were significantly different from zero (t-test, p<0.05). The gray histograms in (B) show the proportion of daily sessions in which the corresponding regression coefficient was significantly positive (upper half) or negative (lower half).

the so-called win-stay-lose-stay strategy, which is also consistent with the use of reinforcement learning algorithm. We also tested whether this bias to use the win-stay-lose-switch strategy could be eliminated by introducing the computer opponent that not only monitored the animal's choice sequences but also exploited any tendency to choose its targets according to its previous choices and their outcomes (referred to as algorithm 2 in Lee et al., 2004). Although a frequent use of win-stay-lose-switch strategy was penalized under this condition, the animals did not completely remove the bias to choose the same targets that were rewarded in previous trials.

To analyze how the animal's choice in a given trial was influenced by its previous choices and their outcomes, we applied the following logistic regression analysis to the behavioral data collected from 6 rhesus monkeys using the more exploitative algorithm (i.e., algorithm 2; Lee et al., 2004; Seo and Lee, 2007, 2008; Seo et al., 2009; Kim et al., 2009). These data were collected in a total of 319 sessions and included 200,228 trials, and the logistic regression model was given by the following:

$$\text{logit} P_t(R) \equiv \log P_t(R)/\{1 - P_t(R)\} = a_0 + A_c \left[c_{t-1} \, c_{t-2} \cdots c_{t-10} \right]$$
$$+ A_o \left[o_{t-1} \, o_{t-2} \cdots o_{t-10} \right],$$

where $P_t(R)$ denotes the probability that the animal would choose the right-hand target in trial t, c_t and o_t the choice of the animal and that of the computer opponent in trial t, respectively (1 and −1 for right-hand and left-hand targets). A_C and A_O are the vectors of regression coefficients, and their individual elements indicate whether the animal had the tendency to choose the same target that it or the computer opponent chose in ten previous trials. The positive values for the elements in A_C would indicate that the animal tended to choose the same target as in the previous trials, whereas the positive values for the elements in A_O would indicate that the animal tended to choose the same target that was chosen by the computer opponent in the previous trials. During this matching pennies task, the animal was rewarded only when it chose the same target as the computer opponent. Therefore, the positive elements in A_O also indicate that the animal was more likely to choose the same target when it was rewarded previously. The results from this logistic regression model showed that there was not a strong tendency for the animals to choose the same target repeatedly (Figure 12.2B, left). In contrast, all animals tested in this experiment showed strong tendencies to choose the same target chosen by the computer opponent in the last several trials (Figure 12.2B, right). This implies that the animals were more likely to choose the target rewarded in previous trials, and suggests that they might have used a reinforcement learning algorithm (Sutton and Barto, 1998; Lee et al., 2004; Seo and Lee, 2007, 2008).

As described above, choices of human subjects during competitive games are often well described by reinforcement learning algorithms (Camerer, 2003; Lee, 2008). To test whether the choice behaviors of rhesus monkeys during the matching pennies games could be described by the same principle, we also applied the following reinforcement learning model to the same behavioral data described above. In the reinforcement learning theory (Sutton and Barto, 1998), β is the inverse temperature that controls the randomness of the animal's choices. When β=0, the animal chooses both targets with the same probabilities (p=0.5) regardless of the value functions, so its choices are completely random. As the value of β increases, the animal's choice becomes more deterministic, in that the animal always chooses the target with the larger value function. The value function for the target chosen by the animal in trial t was updated according to the reward prediction error, namely the difference between the reward in trial t and the value function for the chosen action. The following equation describes this update rule:

$$Q_{t+1}(x) = Q_t(x) + \alpha\{r_t - Q_t(x)\},$$

where r_t denotes the reward in trial t (0 and 1 for unrewarded and rewarded trials, respectively), and α the learning rate. The value function for the unchosen target was not updated. The two parameters of this reinforcement learning model (α and β) were estimated separately for each daily testing session using a maximum likelihood procedure (Pawitan, 2001; Lee et al., 2004; Seo and Lee, 2007, 2008).

If the animal's behaviors were well described by the reinforcement learning model, then the value of the learning rate should be between 0 and 1, and the inverse temperature should be larger than 0. Indeed, this was the case in the majority of testing sessions (269 of 319 sessions, 84.3%; Figure 12.3A). Across the entire data set, the average learning rate and inverse temperature were 0.27 and 0.84, respectively. A relatively small value of learning rate

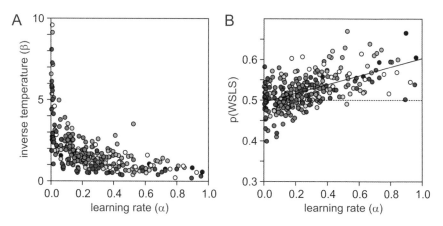

FIGURE 12.3 Parameters of reinforcement learning model. A. Inverse temperature (β) plotted against the learning rate (α) estimated from the same session. B. The probability that the animal would use the win-stay-lose-switch startegy is plotted against the learning rate in the reinforcement learning model. The circles filled in different gray scales indicate the results from different animals.

indicates that the animal's choice in a given trial was influenced by the outcomes of its previous choices in multiple trials. A relatively small value of the inverse temperature also indicates that the animal's choice was quite stochastic, as expected for the mixed strategy required in the matching pennies game. The learning rate and inverse temperature were strongly and negatively correlated ($r = -0.5532$, $p<10^{-20}$; Figure 12.3A). This is not surprising, since the animal's choice would become more predictable as the learning rate increases, which would then require a relatively small inverse temperature to prevent the animal's choices from becoming too predictable. In addition, a higher learning rate implies that the animal is more likely to choose its target according to the win-stay-lose-switch strategy. Indeed, there was a strong positive correlation between the learning rate and the probability of using the win-stay-lose-stay strategy ($r=0.5613$, $p<10^{-20}$; Figuer 12.3B).

Cortical Activity During the Matching Pennies Game

To investigate the neural mechanisms underlying the process of reinforcement learning and decision making during the matching pennies task, we recorded the activity of individual neurons in different cortical areas using a multi-electrode recording system. We have analyzed the activity of 322, 154, and 198 neurons recorded in the dorsolateral prefrontal cortex (DLPFC), dorsal anterior cingulate cortex (ACCd), and lateral intraparietal cortex (LIP) recorded during the matching pennies (Barraclough et al., 2004; Seo and Lee, 2007; Seo et al., 2007, 2009). Many of the neurons in these cortical areas modulated their activity according to the animal's choice, namely, it changed its activity differently depending on whether the animal chose the right-hand or left-hand target in a given trial. This was tested using a multiple linear regression model that included the animal's choices, the choices of the computer opponent, and the outcomes of the animal's choices in the current and three previous trials:

$$S_t = \mathbf{B}\left[1 \; u_t \; u_{t-1} u_{t-2} \; u_{t-3}\right]',$$

where S_t denotes the spike rate during a 0.5-s window defined relative to the target onset or the onset of the feedback ring, u_t a row vector consisting of the animal's choice in trial t (0 and 1 for the left-hand and right-hand target, respectively), the choice of the computer opponent (defined as for the animal's choice), and the outcome of the animal's choice (0 and 1 for unrewarded and rewarded trials, respectively), and $\mathbf{B}$ a vector of regression coefficients. Using this model, we found that the percentage of neurons that change their activity significantly during the fore-period according to the animal's upcoming choice was 12.1%, 18.4%, and 12.6% for the DLPFC, ACCd, and LIP, respectively. The corresponding percentages for the delay period were 19.9%, 17.5%, and 25.8% (Figure 12.4 top, Trial Lag=0). The majority of neurons recorded in the DLPFC and LIP changed their activity during the peripheral fixation period differently according to the animal's choice. Overall, 74.5% and 82.3% of the neurons in the DLPFC and LIP showed choice-related activity during the peripheral fixation period. The percentage of neurons in the ACCd that showed choice-related activity during the same period was 41.6% and therefore substantially lower than those in the DLPFC and LIP. The proportion of the neurons with choice-related activity decreased somewhat during the feedback period in all 3 areas tested in this study (Figure 12.4 top).

Neurons in the DLPFC and LIP often encoded signals related to the animal's choice in the previous trial. For example, during the fore period, 35.7% and 18.7% of the neurons in the DLPFC and LIP modulated their activity according to the animal's choice in the previous trial. The proportion of neurons with signals related to the previous choice increased somewhat in both areas, to 39.8% and 29.3%, during the delay period. For the ACCd, 11.0% and 18.2% of the neurons changed their activity during the fore period and delay period according to the animal's choice in the previous trial (Figure 12.4 top, Trial Lag=1). A relatively small proportion of neurons in the DLPFC and LIP also changed their activity according to the animal's choice two trials before the current trial. During the delay period, the percentages of neurons encoding the animal's choice made two trials ago were 11.2% and 8.6% for the DLPFC and LIP, respectively. Therefore, the signals related to the animal's choice arose gradually in all three cortical areas tested in this study during the fore period and delay period before the animal's choice was behaviorally manifested, and they decayed slowly in the next two or three trials. In reinforcement learning, the signals related to the animal's previous actions are examples of eligibility trace, which play an important role in linking the animal's choice and its corresponding outcome, especially when these two events are temporally separated (Walton et al., 2010). Therefore, the time course of signals related to the animal's choice in the DLPFC and LIP suggest that these cortical areas might be involved in updating the value functions for the actions chosen by the animal.

The analysis described above also revealed that the signals related to the outcome of the animal's choice were distributed broadly in multiple brain areas. During the feedback period, the percentages of neurons that changed their activity differently according to whether the animal was rewarded or not in the same trial were 68.9%, 81.8%, and 84.3% for the DLPFC, ACCd, and

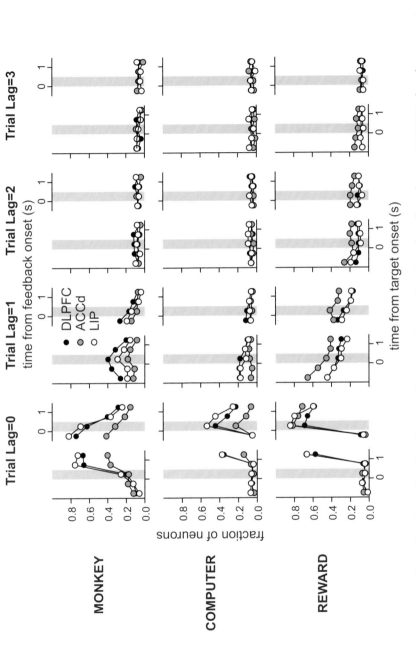

FIGURE 12.4 Comparison of neural activity related to choices and outcomes in the dorsolateral prefrontal cortex (DLPFC), dorsal anterior cingulate cortex (ACCd), and posterior parietal cortex (LIP). Each symbol indicates the fraction of neurons within a particular cortical area that significantly modulated their activity according to the animal's choice (top), the choice of the computer opponent (middle), and the reward in the current (Trial Lag=0) or previous trials (Trial Lag=1 to 3). The statistical significance for individual neurons was determined using a linear regression model applied to the spike counts in a series of non-overlapping 0.5-s windows aligned to target onset (left panels) or feedback onset (right panels). Gray background corresponds to the delay period (left panels) or feedback period (right panels).

LIP, respectively (Figure 12.4 bottom, Trial Lag=0). Similar to the signals related to the animal's choice, outcome-related activity decreased gradually in all three cortical areas, and many neurons in all of these areas modulated their activity during the fore period and delay period according to the outcome of the animal's choice in the previous trial. During the fore period, the percentages of the neurons that significantly modulated their activity according to the outcome of the animal's choice in the previous trial were 37.6%, 54.6%, and 37.4% for the DLPFC, ACCd, and LIP, respectively, whereas the corresponding percentages for the delay period were 32.9%, 45.5%, and 29.8% (Figure 12.4 bottom, Trial Lag=1). Many neurons also modulated their activity during the feedback period according to the outcome of the animal's choice in the previous trial, indicating that the feedback-related activity of the neurons tested in this study was often modulated by the animal's reward history (Seo and Lee, 2007; Seo et al., 2009). The activity of many neurons tested in this experiment also encoded the choice of the computer opponent. During the feedback period, 44.4%, 22.7%, and 53.5% of the neurons in the DLPFC, ACCd, and LIP changed their activity differently according to the choice of the computer opponent. The signals related to the choice of the computer opponent in the previous trial were found in some neurons in the DLPFC and LIP. During the fore period, 18.9% and 17.7% of the neurons in the DLPFC and LIP showed significant modulations in their activity related to the choice of the computer opponent in the previous trial. During the matching pennies game used in this study, the choice of the computer opponent determined the target the animal needs to choose to receive reward. Therefore, the signals related to the choice of the computer opponent might play an important role in updating the animal's decision-making strategy.

In the reinforcement learning model used to analyze the animal's behavior, the animal's choice is determined by the difference in the value functions for the two targets. Therefore, we tested whether the activity of neurons recorded in these cortical areas encoded the signals related to this decision variable, by applying the following regression model:

$$S_t = b_0 + b_1 c_t + b_2 \{Q_t(R) + Q_t(L)\} + b_3 \{Q_t(R) - Q_t(L)\},$$

where S_t denotes the spike rate during the delay period, c_t the animal's choice (0 and 1 for the left-hand and right-hand target, respectively), $Q_t(x)$ the value function for target x in trial t estimated by the reinforcement learning used to analyze the animal's choice data, and b_0 b_3 the regression coefficients. In this model, the activity related to the difference in the value functions was evaluated separately from the changes in activity related to the animal's choice and the sum of the value functions. In addition, the value functions estimated for successive trials are correlated, since they are adjusted gradually according to the reward prediction error. This violates the independence assumption in the regression analysis. Therefore, the statistical significance of each regression coefficient was evaluated using a permutation test. In this test, the spike counts of different trials were randomly shuffled and whether the magnitude of the resulting regression coefficient for each variable was larger than the magnitude of the regression coefficient estimated for the original data was tested. This procedure was repeated 1,000 times, and the proportion of shuffles in which the magnitude of the regression coefficient was larger than that of the original regression coefficient was used as the p-value.

The results of this analysis showed that the neurons in all three cortical areas often modulated their activity according to the sum of the value functions. Overall, 23.9%, 29.2%, and 21.7% of the neurons in the DLPFC, ACCd, and LIP showed significant modulations in their activity during the delay period according to the sum of the value functions, respectively (Figure 12. 5). In reinforcement learning, the sum of the value functions weighted by the probability of choosing each action corresponds to the state value function (Sutton and Barto, 1998), which provides the estimate for the future rewards expected from a particular state of the environment. The reinforcement learning model used to analyze the animal's choice behavior in the present study includes only one state, and therefore, the state value function in this model simply corresponds to the estimate of the overall reward probability. These results, therefore, suggest that the cortical areas tested in this study might all

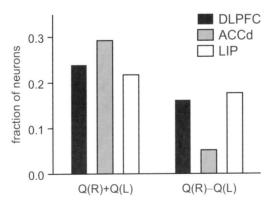

FIGURE 12.5 The proportion of neurons in the DLPFC, ACCd, and LIP that showed significant modulations in their activity related to the sum and difference of value functions (permutation test, p<0.05).

be involved in encoding the reward probability estimated from the animal's reward history (Seo and Lee, 2008; Seo et al., 2009). In addition, the neurons in the DLPFC and LIP often encoded the difference in the value functions, suggesting that they provide the signals necessary for the animal to choose its action in a given trial. The percentage of neurons that showed significant modulations in their activity related to the difference in the value functions was 16.2% and 17.7% for the DLPFC and LIP. Such neurons were relatively rare in the ACCd (5.2%) and did not differ significantly from the significance level used (p=0.05).

Variability in Cortical Activity During the Matching Pennies Game

Variability in the activity of cortical neurons places important constraints on information processing (Shadlen et al., 1996; Shadlen and Newsome, 1998; Churchland et al., 2010).The pattern of variability in neural activity associated with the animal's choice and its outcome during a free-choice task, such as the matching pennies game, however, has not been systematically investigated. In the present study, we compared the amount of variability in the activity of neurons in the DLPFC, ACCd, and LIP during multiple epochs throughout the matching pennies task. Similar to the analysis described above, this analysis was performed on the spike counts estimated for a series of 0.5-s windows defined relative to the target onset and feedback onset. We found that the mean spike counts tended to be larger in the LIP than in the DLPFC and ACCd (Figure 12.6A). During the fore period, for example, the mean spike counts (SEM) for the DLPFC, ACCd, and LIP were 2.84 (0.24), 2.83 (0.46), and 4.98 (0.36), respectively. Therefore, compared to the areas in the frontal cortex, the neurons in the LIP tended to display a higher level of activity. The mean spike counts were relatively stable and did not change much during the inter-trial interval and throughout the trial. In addition, the difference in the overall firing rate across different cortical areas was maintained.

In contrast to the mean spike counts, the variance of the spike counts in the DLPFC and LIP changed substantially during the course of a single trial, whereas the change in the spike count variance in the ACCd was relatively small. The spike count variances (SEM) in the DLPFC and LIP during the last 0.5 s of the inter-trial interval were 9.89 (1.02) and 18.44 (1.55), respectively, whereas they decreased to 7.20 (0.75) and 9.2 (0.88) during the delay period in the two cortical areas (Figure 12.6B). From the population mean and variance of the spike counts, we computed the variance-mean ratio, often known as the Fano factor, separately for each time window and cortical area. As expected, for

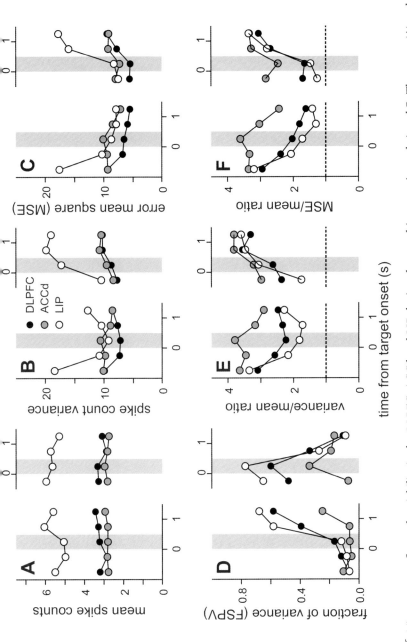

FIGURE 12.6 Time course of neural variability in the DLPFC, ACCd and LIP during the matching pennies task A and B. The mean (A) and variance (B) of spike counts were estimated for the same 0.5-s windows used in Figure 12. C. The error mean square (MSE) was computed using the regression model that included the animal's choices, the choices of the computer opponent, and the outcomes of the animal's choices in several trials as well as the sum and difference of the value functions. D. Fraction of supra-Poisson variance (FSPV) indicates how much of the variance beyond the value expected for Poisson spike trains were accounted for by the same regression model. E. Fano factors calculated from the population-averaged mean and variance of the spike counts. F. The ratio between the MSE and mean spike counts.

the DLPFC and LIP, the Fano factors decreased when the trial started. During the last 0.5 s of the intertrial interval, the Fano factors for DLPFC, ACCd, and LIP were 3.09, 3.64, and 3.35, respectively. The Fano factor for DLPFC and LIP decreased after the trial started, to 2.23 and 1.82 during the delay period, respectively, whereas for the ACCd, it did not change much (Fig 8.6E). Stochastic point processes that have a constant rate and no memory are referred to as Poisson, and it is often assumed that spike trains of cortical neurons are Poisson (e.g., Shadlen and Newsome, 1998). Whereas the Fano factor for a Poisson process is 1, the neurons in the cortical areas tested in this study showed more variability in their spike trains than expected for a Poisson process. This may not be surprising, since in the above analysis, the variance of spike counts was computed for the entire set of trials in which the spike rate was influenced by a number of factors, including the animal's choices and its outcomes in multiple trials.

To determine how much of the variance in the spike counts could be attributed to the factors known to influence the spike rates during the matching pennies task, we calculated the mean squared error (MSE) in the following regression model:

$$S_t = \mathbf{B}\,[1\ u_t\,u_{t-1}\,u_{t-2}\,u_{t-3}\,Q_\Sigma\,Q_\Delta]',$$

where $Q\Sigma = Q_t(R)+Q_t(L)$ and $Q\Delta = Q_t(R)-Q_t(L)$ denote the sum and difference of the value functions for the two targets, respectively. To obtain an unbiased estimate for the variance of error in the above regression model, the mean squared error (MSE) was computed as follows:

$$\mathrm{MSE}\ =\Sigma(S_t - \hat{S}_t)^2/\,(n-2)$$

where $\hat{S}_t$ denotes the estimate for the spike count obtained from the regression model described above, and n is the number of data points. Not surprisingly, MSE is generally smaller than the original spike count variance (Figure 12.6C). In addition, MSE for the spike counts in the DLPFC and LIP gradually decreased throughout the trial. We then computed the Fano factors, using MSE instead of the original spike count variance (Figure 12.6F). As expected, these modified Fano factors were substantially smaller than the original Fano factors, especially for the DLPFC and LIP. The difference was most dramatic during the fixation period for the chosen target. For this time window, the original Fano factors were 2.36 and 1.75 for the DLPFC and LIP, respectively, whereas they decreased to 1.71 and 1.26 when the Fano factor was computed using MSE (Figure 12.6F). Similar to the time course of MSE, the Fano factors for the DLPFC and LIP also decreased gradually throughout the trial.

For the neurons tested in this study, the spike counts were more variable than expected for Poisson processes. To test how much of this supra-Poisson variability was accounted for by the regressors included in the above regression model, we calculated the difference between the original spike count variance and MSE, and divided this by the difference between the original spike count variance and the mean spike count. This ratio, referred to as the fraction of supra-Poisson variance (FSPV), represents the proportion of the variance above the variance expected for the Poisson spike trains that was accounted for by the regression model:

$$\text{FSPV} = \left\{\text{var}(S_t) - \text{MSE}\right\} / \left\{\text{var}(S_t) - \text{mean}(S_t)\right\}$$

where mean (S_t) and var(S_t) refer to the mean and variance of the spike counts, respectively. FSPV would be close to 0 if the regression model does not accounts for any variability in the spike counts, namely if MSE is similar to var(S_t), whereas it would be close to 1 if the regression model reduces MSE to the value expected for the Poisson spike trains, namely mean (S_t). The results of this analysis showed that FSPV increased somewhat during the fore- period and delay period in the DLPFC and LIP, but not in the ACCd. FSPV further increased during the peripheral fixation period in the DLPFC and LIP, and reached the maximum value during the feedback period. During the feedback period, the FSPVs were 0.60 and 0.77 for the DLPFC and LIP, respectively, whereas they were 0.34 for the ACCd (Figure 12.6D). This suggests that the most of the supra-Poisson variability, especially during the feedback period, in the DLPFC and LIP, were due to the factors that can be observed or estimated from the observable events during the matching pennies task. The possible sources of the supra-Poisson variability for the spike counts in the ACCd, however, as well as the supra-Poisson variability in the DLPFC and LIP during the fore period, could not be determined in the present study.

Conclusions

Temporal sequences of action potentials, commonly referred to as spike trains, that are recorded from cortical neurons are highly stochastic. How such irregular spike trains underlie our seemingly orderly perceptual experience and can control our movements is a central question in neuroscience. Previous research on variability in neural activity has largely focused on how neural variability can be related to the process of sensorimotor transformation—namely, how the irregular spike trains generated in response to a variety of sensory stimuli can be transformed to the animal's behavioral responses (Britten et al., 1992;

Shadlen et al., 1996; Osborne et al., 2005; Churchland et al., 2006a, 2006b; Averbeck and Lee, 2006; Schoppik et al., 2008; Cohen and Newsome, 2009; Churchland et al., 2010). On the other hand, less is known about how such irregular spike trains of cortical neurons are related to the animal's choices when they are free to choose among multiple options only based on the animal's probabilistic knowledge of its environment. As a first step to address this question, we have utilized a behavioral task designed after competitive games that require the participating players to make stochastic choices. We found that similar to human subjects playing similar games, rhesus monkeys could learn to produce highly stochastic choices that approximate the optimal strategy during the matching pennies game (Barraclough et al., 2004; Lee et al., 2004; Seo and Lee, 2008). We also found that the spike count variance for the neurons recorded in multiple areas of the prefrontal cortex and parietal cortex substantially exceeded the level expected for the Poisson spike trains, especially during the inter-trial interval. This is likely due to the fact that the animal's behaviors and the resulting sensory inputs were not constrained during the inter-trial intervals. Moreover, spike trains of the neurons tested in this study displayed substantially more trial-to-trial variability than expected for Poisson processes even after the trial started., For the neurons in the DLPFC and LIP, however, much of this variability was due to the variability in the behavioral events that systematically influenced the activity of the neurons examined in this study. As a result, for the DLPFC and LIP, the variance of the residuals in the multiple regression model including a number of regressors related to the animal's choices, and their outcomes decreased and became more similar to the variance expected for Poisson processes once the trial was initiated by the animal and its behaviors became more consistent. Previous studies have found that the trial-to-trial variability in the activity of the neurons in the premotor cortex also decreased during the preparation of an upcoming movement (Churchland et al., 2006b). Indeed, the variability in neural activity tends to decrease after the onset of a sensory stimulus in many cortical areas (Churchland et al., 2010). In contrast, the estimates for the spike count variability for the neurons in the ACCd did not decrease much even when the same regression model was used to factor out the influence of the animal's previous and current choices and their outcomes. Instead, the residual variability in the spike counts for the neurons in the ACCd decreased largely towards the end of the trial when the outcome of the animal's choice was revealed. It has been shown that compared to the neurons in the DLPFC or LIP, ACC neurons might play a more important role in evaluating the outcomes of the animal's choices (Matsumoto et al., 2007; Seo and Lee, 2007; Hayden et al., 2009; Kennerley and Wallis, 2009). This suggests that the time course of the variability in the neural activity might be related to the information encoded by the population of neurons in a particular cortical area. Nevertheless, precisely how the animal's choices are influenced by the variability in the activity of cortical neurons, and how the variability in neural activity is controlled by the cortical network still remain largely unknown and should be further investigated in the future studies.

REFERENCES

Averbeck, B.B., Lee, D. (2006) Effects of noise correlation on information encoding and decoding. *J of Neurophysiology, 95*, 3633–3644.

Barraclough, D.J., Conroy, M.L., Lee, D. (2004) Prefrontal cortex and decision making in a mixed-strategy game. *Nat Neuroscience, 7*, 404–410.

Britten, K.H., Shadlen, M.N., Newsome, W.T., Movshon, J.A. (1992) The analysis of visual motion: a comparison of neuronal and psychophysical performance. *J of Neuroscience, 12*, 4745–4765.

Budescu, D.V. and Rapoport, A. (1994) Subjective randomization in one- and two-person games. *J Beh Decis Making, 7*, 261–278.

Camerer, C.F. (2003) *Behavioral game theory: experiments in strategic interaction.* Princeton, N.J.: Princeton University Press.

Churchland, M.M., Afshar, A., Shenoy, K.V. (2006a) A central source of movement variability. *Neuron, 52*, 1085–1096.

Churchland, M.M., Yu, B.M., Cunningham, J.P., Sugrue, L.P., Cohen, M.R., Corrado, G.S., Newsome, W.T., Clark, A.M., Hosseini, P., Scott, B.B., Bradley, D.C., Smith, M.A., Kohn, A., Movshon, J.A., Armstrong, K.M., Moore, T., Chang, S.W., Snyder, L.H., Lisberger, S.G., Priebe, N.J., Finn, I.M., Ferster, D., Ryu, S.I., Santhanam, G., Sahani, M., Shenoy, K.V. (2010) Stimulus onset quenches neural variability: a widespread cortical phenomenon. *Nat Neuroscience, 13*, 369–378.

Churchland, M.M., Yu, B.M., Ryu, S.I., Santhanam, G., Shenoy, K.V. (2006b) Neural variability in premotor cortex provides a signature of motor preparation. *J of Neuroscience, 26*, 3697–3712.

Cohen, M.R. and Newsome, W.T. (2009) Estimates of the contribution of single neurons to perception depend on timescale and noise correlation. *J of Neuroscience, 29*, 6635–6648.

Dean, A.F. (1981) The variability of discharge of simple cells in the cat striate cortex. *Exp Brain Res, 44*, 437–440.

Erev, I. and Roth, A.E. (1998) Predicting how people play games: reinforcement learning in experimental games with unique, mixed strategy equilbria. *Am Econ Rev, 88*, 848–881.

Estes, W.K. (1962) Learning theory. *Annu Rev Psych, 13*, 107–144.

Hanes, D.P. and Schall, J.D. (1996) Neural control of voluntary movement initiation. *Science, 274*, 427–430.

Hayden, B.Y., Pearson, J.M., Platt, M.L. (2009) Fictive reward signals in the anterior cingulate cortex. *Science, 324*, 948–950.

Henry, G.H., Bishop, P.O., Tupper, R.M., Dreher, B. (1973) Orientation specificity and response variability of cells in the striate cortex. *Vision Res, 13,* 1771–1779.

Kennerley, S.W. and Wallis, J.D. (2009) Evaluating choices by single neurons in the frontal lobe: Outcome value encoded across multiple decision variables. *Eur J Neuroscience, 29,* 2061–2073.

Kim, S., Hwang, J., Seo, H., Lee, D. (2009) Valuation of uncertain and delayed rewards in primate prefrontal cortex. *Neural Networks, 22,* 294–304.

Lee, D. (2008) Game theory and neural basis of social decision making. *Nat Neurosci., 11,* 404–409.

Lee, D., Conroy, M.L., McGreevy, B.P., Barraclough, D.J. (2004) Reinforcement learning and decision making in monkeys during a competitive game. *Cogn Brain Res, 22,* 45–58.

Lee, D., McGreevy, B.P., Barraclough, D.J. (2005) Learning and decision making in monkeys during a rock-paper-scissors game. *Cogn Brain Res, 25,* 416–430.

Lee, D., Port, N.L., Kruse, W., Georgopoulos, A.P. (1998) Variability and correlated noise in the discharge of neurons in motor and parietal areas of the primate cortex. *J of Neuroscience, 18,* 1161–1170.

Luce, R.D. (1986) Response times: their role in inferring elementary mental organization. Oxford: Oxford University Press.

Matsumoto, M., Matsumoto, K., Abe, H., Tanaka, K. (2007) Medial prefrontal cell activity signaling prediction errors of action values. *Nat Neuroscience, 10,* 647–656.

Mookherjee, D. and Sopher, B. (1994) Learning behavior in an experimental matching pennies game. *Games Econ Beh, 7,* 62–91.

Mookherjee, D. and Sopher, B. (1997) Learning and decision costs in experimental constant sum games. *Games Econ Beh, 19,* 97–132.

Nash, J.F. (1950) Equilibrium points in n-person games. *Proc Natl Acad Sci, 36,* 48–49.

Osborne, L.C., Lisberger, S.G., Bialek, W. (2005) A sensory source for motor variation. *Nature, 437,* 412–416.

Pawitan, Y. (2001) *In all likelihood: statistical modelling and inference using likelihood.* New York: Oxford University Press.

Rapoport, A. and Budescu, D.V. (1992) Generation of random series in two-person strictly competitive games. *J Exp Psychol General, 121,* 352–363.

Rieke, F., Warland, D., de Ruyter van Steveninck, R., Bialek, W. (1997) Spikes: exploring the neural code. Cambridge, Mass.: MIT Press.

Rose, D. (1979) An analysis of the variability of unit activity in the cat's visual cortex. *Exp Brain Res, 37,* 595–604.

Sally, D. (1995) Conversation and cooperation in social dilemmas: A meta-analysis of experiments from 1958 to 1992. *Ration Soc, 7,* 58–92.

Schoppik, D., Nagel, K.I., Lisberger, S.G. (2008) Cortical mechanisms of smooth eye movements revealed by dynamic covariations of neural and behavioral responses. *Neuron, 58,* 248–260.

Seo H, Lee D. (2007) Temporal filtering of reward signals in the dorsal anterior cingulate cortex during a mixed-strategy game. *J of Neuroscience, 27,* 8366–8377.

Seo, H. and, Lee, D. (2008) Cortical mechanisms for reinforcement learning in competitive games. *Philos Trans Roy Soc Lond B Biol Sci, 363,* 3845–3857.

Seo, H., Barraclough, D.J., Lee, D. (2007) Dynamic signals related to choices and outcomes in the dorsolateral prefrontal cortex. *Cereb Cortex, 17,* i110–i117.

Seo, H., Barraclough. D.J., Lee, D. (2009) Lateral intraparietal cortex and reinforcement learning during a mixed-strategy game. *J of Neuroscience, 29,* 7278–7289.

Shadlen, M.N., Britten, K.H., Newsome, W.T., Movshon, J.A. (1996) A computational analysis of the relationship between neuronal and behavioral responses to visual motion. *J of Neuroscience, 16,* 1486–1510.

Shadlen, M.N. and Newsome, W.T. (1998) The variable discharge of cortical neurons: implications for connectivity, computation, and information coding. *J of Neuroscience, 18,* 3870–3896.

Softky, W.R. and Koch, C. (1993) The highly irregular firing of cortical cells is inconsistent with temporal integration of random EPSPs. *J of Neuroscience, 13,* 334–350.

Sutton, R.S. and Barto, A.G. (1998) *Reinforcement learning: an introduction.* Cambridge, Mass: MIT Press.

Todorov, E. and Jordan, M.I. (2002) Optimal feedback control as a theory of motor coordination. *Nat Neuroscience, 5,* 1226–1235.

Tolhurst, D.J., Movshon, J.A., Dean, A.F. (1983) The statistical reliability of signals in single neurons in cat and monkey visual cortex. *Vision Res, 23,* 775–785.

Tomko, G.J. and Crapper, D.R. (1974) Neuronal variability: non-stationary responses to identical visual stimuli. *Brain Res, 79,* 405–418.

Walton, M.E., Behrens, T.E.J., Buckley, M.J., Rudebeck, P.H., Rushworth, M.F.S. (2010) Separable learning systems in the macaque brain and the role of orbitofrontal cortex in contingent learning. *Neuron, 65,* 927–939.

Part 4: Neuronal Variability and Brain Disorders

13

Circuit Mechanisms Underlying Behavioral Variability during Recovery of Consciousness following Severe Brain Injury

Nicholas D. Schiff

Disorders of Consciousness and Fluctuations of Behavioral Responsiveness following Severe Brain Injuries

Wide fluctuations of behavioral response are the *sine qua non* of recovery from coma following severe brain injuries. As argued below in this chapter, the varying levels of recovery following coma defined in different neurological syndromes ("disorders of consciousness") and the prominent behavioral fluctuations (i.e., variability in goal-directed ongoing behavior) seen after multifocal traumatic or nontraumatic brain injuries may arise from common mechanisms at the "circuit" level. Although severe brain injuries producing coma have many causes (see Posner et al., 2007, for a comprehensive review) an overlap of structural pathologies and functional disturbances isolated to specific cerebral structures has been noted (see below and Schiff and Plum, 2000, for review). At first glance, a consideration of the pathological, anatomical, and pathophysiological features of disorders of consciousness draws attention to the anterior forebrain, particularly the relationships of the brainstem and basal forebrain arousal systems, the central thalamus and frontostriatal pathways. This chapter reviews a circuit-level model that organizes several clinical observations of recovery of function following coma and severe brain injury (Schiff, 2009). The proposed model suggests mechanisms underlying prominent fluctuations in behavioral responsiveness seen in many patients.

Figure 13.1 organizes neurological disorders of consciousness on a two-dimensional grid that indexes the degree of impaired cognitive function against degree of motor function. At the bottom left of Figure 13.1, coma and vegetative state (VS) are both considered unconscious brain states as judged by the bedside behavioral exam. In both coma and vegetative state, patients do demonstrate responses to environmental stimuli or initiate goal-directed behaviors. In coma patients also show no state variation and usually remain closed eyes and show no response to the most vigorous stimulation. In VS, patients recover a cycling of irregular periods of eye opening and eye closure. This cyclical variation in behavioral state does not correlate with identifiable electroencephalographic (EEG) features of either sleep or normal wakefulness (Kobylarz and

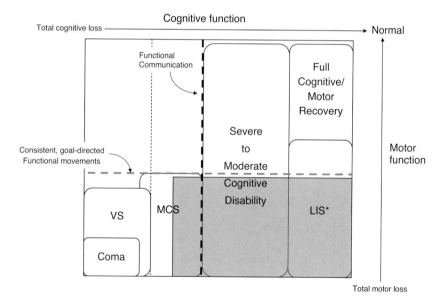

FIGURE 13.1 Correspondence of cognitive and motor impairment across outcomes following severe brain injurie VS, vegetative state; MCS, minimally conscious state; LIS, *-indicates locked-in state which is not a disorder of consciousness. Grey box shows large region of diagnostic uncertainty in establishing true cognitive level for patients who behaviorally cannot reliably signal through controlled goal-directed movements (dashed horizontal line).

Schiff, 2004). To the right on the diagram is the minimally conscious state (MCS) (Giacino et al., 2002). MCS patients demonstrate unequivocal but inconsistent evidence of awareness of self or the environment through a wide variety of behavioral response patterns that can be demonstrated at the bedside (Giacino and Whyte, 2005). For example, patients may track objects with their eyes, follow commands with small motor movements, or intermittent communication through verbal or gestural means of communication. The functional boundary indicating emergence from MCS is the demonstration of reliable verbal or gestural communication. Operationalizing this level of function is a topic of current research as even simple "yes" versus "no" communications can be difficult for brain-injured patients who retain confusion even though their level of overall function may considerably exceed the boundaries of MCS (see Nakase-Richardson et al., 2009). Fluctuation of behavioral responsiveness, however, is at the core of the definition of MCS and patients typically show marked variations in response with extremes of unresponsiveness and intermittent communication coexisting in many instances.

The large grey box in Figure 13.1 indicates the high-degree of uncertainty that attends efforts to identify the cognitive capacities of some patients who lack controllable motor output channels. The locked-in state (LIS; far right bottom of Figure 13.1) defines patients who retain total preservation of cognitive function but may appear no different than those in deep coma. While LIS typically arises in the context of neurological injuries selectively damage motor output pathways distal from their cortical origins or slowly reduce primary motor neuron function, complex brain injuries in some instances produce a highly problematic sets of patients who are unable to produce consistent goal-directed movements that allow for communication yet retain full consciousness. Such a patient might retain significant cognitive capacity near the normal range of cognitive function and yet be indistinguishable from MCS patients.

Recent studies have shown that the anatomic pathologies following severe injuries associated with vegetative state (Adams et al,. 2000), minimally conscious state (Jennett et al., 2001), as well as severe to moderate cognitive disability (Jennett et al., 2003) have several common features. Autopsy studies of patients remaining in vegetative state at the time of death have identified widespread neuronal death throughout the thalamus as the common finding following either anoxia or diffuse axonal injury producing widespread disruption of white matter connections (Adams et al, 2000). Of note, the severe bilateral thalamic damage after either trauma or anoxia in seen in permanent vegetative state is not invariably associated with diffuse neocortical neuronal cell death, particularly in traumatic brain injury where only approximately 10% show widespread neocortical cell death (Adams et al. 2000). These observations draw immediate attention to the thalamus as an essential structure supporting integrative functions of the forebrain. Specific subnuclei of the thalamus have further been identified as the site of most neuronal cell loss following global and multi-focal cerebral injuries produced by traumatic brain injuries (Maxwell et al., 2006). The central thalamic nuclei (intralaminar nuclei and related para-laminar nuclei) show the greatest degree of neuronal loss following severe traumatic brain injuries (Maxwell et al., 2006) with some evidence that similar pattern might be identified in hypoxic-ischemic injuries (cf. Kinney et al., 1994). In patients with only moderate disability following traumatic brain injury, neuronal loss is primarily identified within the central lateral nucleus, central medial, paracentralis nuclei of the anterior intralaminar group. Progressively severe disability grades with neuronal loss along a rostrocaudal axis with the anterior intralaminar and surrounding regions initially showing volume loss associated with moderate disability and ventral and lateral nuclei of the central thalamus (posterior intralaminar group) neuronal loss appearing with worsening disability associated with minimally conscious state and vege-tative state. The progressive and relatively specific involvement of the central thalamic nuclei is most likely a consequence of the unique geometry of these central thalamic neurons which have wide point to point connectivity across the cerebral hemisphere and are thus likely to integrate neuronal cell death across these large territories (van der Werf et al. 2002, Scannell et al., 1999).

Focal bilateral injuries to these regions of the central thalamus are associ-ated with global disorders of consciousness (coma, vegetative state and mini-mally conscious state) (Castaigne et al., 1981; Schiff and Plum, 2000). Typically, abrupt interruption of the central thalamus on both sides of the brain produces acute coma reflecting the key contribution of these cells to normal mechanisms of arousal regulation (Schiff, 2008). The central thalamus is strongly inner-vated by ascending projections from the brainstem/basal forebrain 'arousal systems' that control the activity of many cortical and thalamic neurons during the sleep-wake cycle. In addition, these same neurons receive descending projections from several frontal cortical regions (associated with "executive" functions) that support goal-directed behaviors. Collectively, these ascending and descending influences on the central thalamus serve to adjust the level of arousal associated with generalized alertness and variations in cognitive effort, stress, sleep deprivation, and other variables affecting the wakeful state (Kinomura et al., 1996, Paus et al. 1998, Nagai et al. 2004, Kinomura et al., 1996; Paus et al., 1997; van der Werf et al., 2002, reviewed in Schiff, 2008).

Neuromaging and electrophysiological studies correlate these anatomical specializations with evidence that the central thalamus selectively activates during tasks that either require a short-term shift of attention (Kinomura et al., 1996; Shah et al., 2009) sustained cognitive demands of high vigilance (Paus et al., 1997) or memory holds over extended time periods (Wyder et al., 2004, Shah et al., 2009). Both the anterior and posterior intralaminar nuclei and neurons in the mesencephalic reticular formation (these neurons have monosynaptically projections to both compartments of central thalamic neurons; Steriade and Glenn, 1982) activate during the short-term shifting of attention component of a forewarned reaction-time tasks (Kinomura et al., 1996). Central thalamic activation associated with varying levels of vigilance correlates with global cerebral blood flow (Kinomura et al., 1996) and specifically covaries within the anterior cingulate cortex (ACC) and pontomesecephalon (Paus et al., 1997). Activity in the ACC grades with increasing cognitive load and is recruited by wide range of cognitive tasks apparently reciprocally increasing activity along with, the central thalamus in response to increasing demands of cognitive effort (Paus et al., 1997, 1998). Large fluctuations in behavioral responsiveness are associated with direct injuries to the central thalamus with both unilateral (van der Werf et al., 1999; Mennemeier et al., 1997) or bilateral lesions (Gubermann and Stuss, 1983; Chatterjee et al., 1997). These fluctuations are very similar in appearance to the fluctuations seen in patients and animals following frontal lobe injuries (Robertson et al., 1998) reflecting close anatomical and functional relationships of the central thalamus and frontal lobe. Quantitative and qualitative similarity of behavioral variability produced by lesions of anterior intralaminar nuclei of the central thalamus and wide excision of frontal cortical regions has been demonstrated (Mair et al, 1998).

Possible Common "Circuit-Level" Mechanisms
Arising after Severe Brain Injuries

Following severe brain injuries, large-scale alteration of forebrain dynamics can arise as a result of widespread neuronal death and deafferentation of remaining neurons or secondary to dysfunction of large neuronal populations without overwhelming neuronal death. In either scenario, specific "circuit"-level functional disturbances may arise a result of the loss of these neuronal connections or alteration of cellular function that broadly affect cerebral network dynamics. As reviewed above, pathological studies provide evidence that the specific disconnection of the neurons within the central thalamus may play an important role in outcomes ranging from minimally conscious state to moderate disability (Maxwell et al., 2006). Figure 13.2 illustrates a key

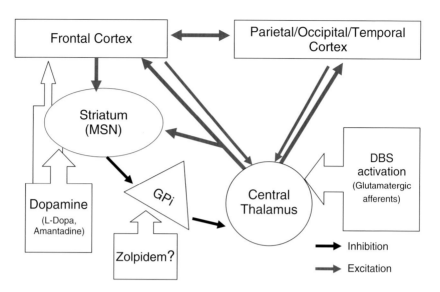

FIGURE 13.2 Possible "mesocircuit" linking behavioral fluctuations following severe brain injuries and improvements in response to interventions. A proposed 'mesocircuit' (cf. Bohland et al., 2009) underlying behavioral variability following severe brain injuries focuses on the modulatory role of the anterior forebrain in overall corticothalamic dynamics. As discussed in the text the anterior forebrain (frontal/prefrontal cortical-striatopallidal thalamocortical loop systems) is particularly vulnerable to large-scale dysfunction following multi-focal brain injuries that produce widespread deafferentation or neuronal cell loss. At least two mechanisms related to this "mesocircuit" appear to play a key role after severe injuries: (1) the high demands of striatum output neurons for background activity and dopaminergic innervations, and (2) the anatomical connections and physiological specializations of the thalamocortical projections from the central thalamus. These central thalamic neurons have a strong activating role strongly driving both cortical and striatal neurons and wide point-to-point connections that make them more sensitive reporters of global neuronal loss than other thalamic nuclei. Withdrawal of thalamocortical transmission from the central thalamus is known to associate with coma and other disorders of consciousness (see Schiff and Plum, 2000, for review). The thalamostriatal projection from the central thalamus contacts the medium spiny neurons (MSN) of the striatum (forming axodendritic (centromedian, Smith et al., 2009) or axospinous (central lateral, parafasicular Lacey et al. 2007) synapses. The MSNs in turn send inhibitory projections to the globus pallidus interna; without MSN output the globus pallidus interna tonically inhibits the central thalamus (Grillner et al., 2005). Thus, a suppression of MSN output resulting from a loss of dopaminergic modulation or marked reduction in background synaptic activity can potentially catalyze a shut down of the anterior forebrain. The mesocircuit model economically accounts for several clinical observations and aspects of normal physiology (see text for further discussion).

vulnerability of the anterior forebrain in the setting of such widespread deaf-ferentation and neuronal cell loss that may plausibly be associated with all severe brain injuries. This "mesocircuit" (Bohland et al., 2009) level model suggests that functional alterations across very large connected neuronal popu-lations of the anterior forebrain may arise primarily as a result of global decreases of excitatory neurotransmission (Schiff, 2009; Brefel-Courbon et al., 2007; Schiff and Posner, 2007). The majority of etiologies associated with coma and varying stages of recovery of consciousness diagrammed in Figure 1 effectively produce a broad decrease in background synaptic activity and excit-atory neurotransmission (e.g. diffuse axonal injury, anoxia, hypoxia-ischemia, cerebral vasospasm with strokes, etc; see Posner et al., 2007, for review).

As diagrammed in Figure 13.2 and reviewed above, the neurons in the central thalamus have wide point-to-point connections across all lobes of the cerebral hemisphere with a predominance of connections to frontal and pre-frontal cortices (van der Werf et al., 2002; Gronewegen and Berendse, 1994; Morel et al., 2005). In addition, these neurons have a unique connective topol-ogy having both direct (thalamostriatal) and indirect (corticostriatal) connec-tions with the striatum that return via projections from the globus pallidus. The thalamocortical projections from the central thalamus strongly innervate the frontal cortex (Morel et al., 2005) and anterior intralaminar thalamic neu-rons can have joint thalamostriatal projection (Deschenes et al., 1996). It has been demonstrated that thalamocortical projections to cortex produce a stron-ger driving excitation within the cortex than cortico-cortical projections (Rigas and Castro-Almancos et al., 2007) and down-regulation of the thalamic output can be expected to lead to very broad effects across cortical regions and the striatum. The projections from the central thalamus (both central lateral nucleus and parafasicularis nucleus) to the striatum innervate the medium spiny neurons (MSNs) and diffusely innervate the striatum (Lacey et al., 2007). The thalamostriatal projections use glutamate transmitters with a high proba-bility of synaptic release (Smith et al., 2009) and likely have a strong role in modulating background activity in the striatum.

The MSNs represent an important point of vulnerability in this anterior forebrain mesocircuit. These neurons have a "high threshold" UP state that keeps them below their firing threshold unless a high level of spontaneous background synaptic activity arising from excitatory corticostriatal and thalam-ostriatal inputs is present along with sufficient dopaminergic innervation (Grillner et al., 2005). The MSNs have a key role in maintaining activity in the anterior forebrain through their inhibitory projections to the globus pallidus interna which in turn inhibit the central thalamus (Grillner et al., 2005). In the setting of diffuse deafferentation or neuronal loss following brain injury it is proposed that broad withdrawal of both direct excitatory striatal projections from the central thalamus and corticostriatal inputs produce a marked reduction in synaptic background activity causing MSN output to shut down. Among frontal cortical regions that may strongly modulate the MSNs of the striatum, the anterior cingulate cortex receives strong inputs for the anterior intralaminar nuclei (central lateral nucleus, van der Werf et al., 2002) and also provides a very diffuse regulatory input across large territories of the rostral striatum (Calzavara et al., 2007).

Observations of regional changes in brain metabolism following severe brain injuries, specific responses to pharmacological and electrophysiological interventions in brain injured subjects, and normal variations in brain state are consistent with this mesocircuit model (see Schiff, 2009, for more comprehensive review). A consistent pattern of selective metabolic downregulation within the anterior forebrain has been shown to specifically grade with severity of behavioral impairment following diffuse axonal injury (Kato et al., 2007). Further consistent with the general model proposed, a common finding across different etiologies of severe brain injuries is a marked fluctuation to improved behavioral responsiveness following application of dopaminergic agents (Matsuda et al., 2003; Meythaler et al., 2002). These medications would facilitate both the output of the MSNs and direct modulately of mesial frontal cortical neurons possibly restoring anterior forebrain activity within the loop connections of the frontal cortex, striatum, pallidum and central thalamus.

Notably, another observation of paradoxical improvement of alertness and behavioral responsiveness with zolpidem (a nonbenzodiazepine hypnotic that potentiates GABA-A receptors also known as "Ambien") in some severely brain injured patients (Breufel-Courbon et al., 2007; Whyte and Myers, 2009; Shames and Ring, 2008; Cohen and Doung, 2008; Williams et al., 2009) can be interpreted within the model represented in Figure 13.2. Schiff and Posner (2007) have proposed that direct action of zolpidem on the globus pallidus interna may release a tonic inhibition of the central thalamus produced in the setting of a shut down of the inhibitory projection of the MSNs by a broad reduction in background excitatory neurotransmission (as seen for example following diffuse hypoxic-ischemic injury). Importantly, the MSNs are uniquely vulnerable to cellular dysfunction after hypoxia (Calabresi et al., 2000) and the majority of reported cases of marked improvement with zolpidem have occurred in the patients with hypoxic-ischemic injuries (Brefel Courbon et al., 2007; Shames and Ring, 2008; Cohen and Duong, 2008; Williams et al., 2009). The GABA-A alpha-1 subunit is expressed in large quantity in the globus pallidus interna and experimental studies support this mechanism of action (Chen et al., 2004).

In addition, the mesocircuit model of Figure 13.2 provides a framework for understanding observations that among the most statistically robust changes in regional cerebral blood flow during the transitions during the sleep-wake cycle, alteration of striatal blood flow is the most significant (Braun et al., 1997) and shows increases in during the transition from slow wave sleep to rapid eye movement sleep (REM) and decreases in the transition from wakefulness to non-REM sleep. This is likely simply a direct result of the broad change in excitability and background activity in the brain during the different non-REM stages of sleep compared to REM and wakefulness (Laureys et al., 2004) producing a shut of the MSNs that is easily reversed as the dynamics of sleep-wake cycle. Similar changes in metabolic activity specific to the anterior forebrain arise during early wakefulness and are associated with "sleep inertia" (Braun et al., 2002). Similarly, this mesocircuit model suggests an economical mechanism for the early selective metabolic downregulation in the mesial frontal and thalamic systems with different anesthetics (Alkire et al. 2008) that does not require a selective regional effect on the neurons of the thalamus or anterior forebrain and also accounts for a variety of specific changes across the induction and recovery from general anesthesia (see Brown et al., submitted).

The mesocircuit model proposed above, however, should be considered as primarily as a modulator of the dominant corticothalamic systems (Llinas et al., 2002; Llinas and Steriade, 2006; Jones 2001) which organize the overall dynamic architecture of sleep-wake cycles and cerebral integrative activity associated with perception, sensorimotor integration and presumably the contents of consciousness. The impairment of the anterior forebrain mesocircuit likely leads to instability in conscious behavior and awareness, perhaps like a flickering light or very dim illumination. Patients with direct injuries to the central thalamus and mesial frontal systems typically show slow, "akinetic", behavior (cf. Katz et al., 1987) but often remain quite conscious.

A Single Subject Study of Deep Brain Stimulation of the Central Thalamus in Minimally Conscious State

Another implication of the model shown in Figure 13.2 is that direct activation of the central thalamus may be common final path for facilitating behavioral responsiveness (and accounting for intermittent fluctuations in improved behavior arising across arousal state variations or in response to pharmacological interventions). Evidence that direct electrical stimulation of the central thalamus can produce behavioral facilitation is provided by the results of a single subject study of central thalamic deep brain stimulation (DBS) in the minimally conscious state (Schiff et al,. 2007). A 38-year-old man remained in

MCS for six years following a severe closed head injury following blunt trauma to the right frontal lobe. After three months in a vegetative state, the patient exhibited the first evidence of clear behaviors in response to sensory stimulation consistent with the minimally conscious state, MCS advancing to a best behavioral response of inconsistent command following and communication using eye movements without further recovery more than two years following injury. Four years at the time of the start of the DBS study the patient's formal behavioral assessment with the Coma Recovery Scale Revised (CRS-R) revealed no change in behavioral baseline. The patient entered into a study of central thalamic DBS (see Figure 13.3) which included a four-month quantitative behavioral assessment prior to placement of the DBS electrodes, followed by a two-month period with the electrodes remaining OFF to reassess the patient's post surgical behavioral baseline which did not change. Bilateral DBS electrodes were implanted in the anterior intralaminar thalamic nuclei (central lateral nucleus and adjacent paralaminar regions of the thalamus). Figure 13.3B shows the placement of the electrodes in situ. Two subsequent phases of the study focused on evaluation of DBS effects. First, a five-month titration phase of assessed tolerance to DBS and evaluated varying several stimulation parameters (contact geometry, frequency, intensity) and duration of stimulation period. Following the titration phase the patient entered into a six-month double-blind alternating crossover study. Throughout all phases of the study the patient received standard rehabilitation efforts amounting to three hours a day, four days per week.

Figure 13.3C tabulates the results of a 6-month double-blind alternating crossover study and comparison of pre-stimulation baselines of performance reflecting the overall impact of DBS compared to ~six months of ongoing rehabilitation efforts in the absence of exposure to DBS. The overall findings demonstrate marked improved behavioral responsiveness compared to pre-stimulation frequencies of the highest level behavioral response across six categories. The primary outcome assessments were prospectively chosen from the subscales of the CRS-R, a validated psychometric tool used in patients with disorders of consciousness that had shown variation during the pre-surgical baseline assessment. Notably, the CRS-R oral motor subscale was not chosen because no variation in this measure had been identified during the baseline assessment period. An object naming scale and two other tailored secondary measures were later developed during the titration phase after the patient's behavior demonstrated several changes that allowed the calibration of these secondary measurement scales. All six measures showed marked change from pre-stimulation baselines, with five of the six measurements showing higher level behaviors than seen prior stimulation whether the electrodes were ON or OFF.

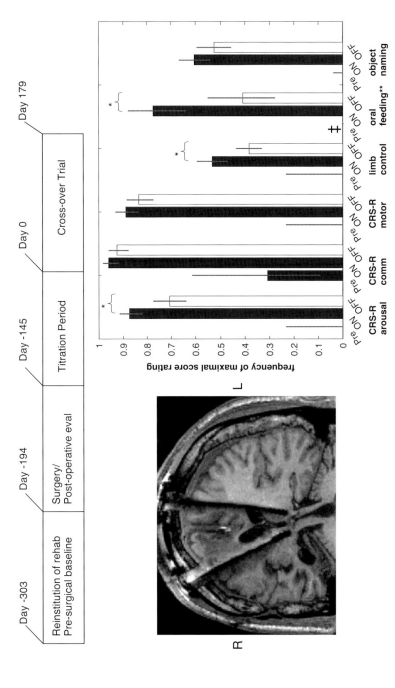

FIGURE 13.3 Central thalamic DBS in the minimally conscious state A. Study timeline. B. Electrode lead placements within central thalamus of patient's right (R) and left (L) hemispheres displayed in T1 weighted MRI coronal image. C. Comparison of pre-surgical baselines and DBS ON and DBS OFF periods during a six cross-over trial of central thalamic DBS in a patient with severe traumatic brain injury. (see text for further explanation). Figure elements adapted from Schiff et al. (2007) with permission.

For the secondary measures the lack of behavioral capacity for object naming, oral feeding and complex controlled goal directed movement set a frequency of zero for the pre-stimulation baseline (see Schiff et al., 2007, supplementary material). Three measures (one primary outcome measure, the CRS-R arousal subscale, and two secondary outcome measures, oral feeding and limb control) showed a statistically significant dependence on electrical brain stimulation during the six-month crossover trial as indicated by increasing the frequency of maximal score (Figure 13.3C). The top score for the CRS-arousal scale is achieved for no more than 3 non-response to an examiner across an assessment period and this score was significantly modulated ON versus OFF throughout the crossover trial. The functional limb control measure (demonstration of movements such as combing, drinking, etc.) and a scale measuring capacity for oral feeding (chewing, swallowing and completing meals compared to tube feeding) both demonstrated significant ON versus OFF effects. The continuation of improvements during the OFF periods of the cross-over trial compared to the pre-stimulation baselines indicates a carry-over effect of changes that occurred after exposure to DBS the titration period.

A recent detailed state–space analysis of the behavioral data indicates that during the OFF periods behavioral variability increased approximately two weeks into the OFF transition with marked declines in responsiveness during some DBS OFF transitions at this time (Smith et al., 2008). While these observations are limited to a single human subject and do not provide a guide to their generalizability (Victor and Schiff, 2008; Schiff et al., 2009) they are consistent with the proposed mesocircuit model suggested above. The carry-over of clinical improvements from the five-month titration period into the OFF DBS phases of the cross-over trial is supportive of at least two physiological time scales playing a role in of the observed CT/DBS effects: (1) a dynamical effect as suggested by the model in Figure 13.2, and (2) a the potential role for synaptic plasticity and normal learning and memory processes (Shirvalkar et al., 2006) or other mechanisms that could account for slow processes including structural alterations (see Chlovskii et al., 2004).

Among the most likely mechanisms playing a role in the patient's improved behavioral responsiveness is that DBS acted to partially reverse the markedly depressed cerebral global metabolism measured in this patient (Schiff et al., 2005) and also seen in other patients in minimally conscious state (Laureys et al., 2004). The depressed cerebral metabolism seen in MCS likely reflects both volume loss of neurons, deafferentation of remaining neurons, and neuronal functional impairments. All of these mechanisms may result in low firing rates of neurons in the neocortex, thalamus and striatum. The mesocircuit model shown in Figure 13.2 suggests that direct activation of the central thalamus in patients with such chronically downregulated background synaptic activity may produce excitatory output from central thalamic neurons that acts to partially normalize firing rates and possibly firing patterns within the cortico-striatopallidal-thalamocortical system.

Next steps

The suggested model in Figure 13.2 has several implications that can be either falsified or expanded upon in an effort to more systematically and rationally approach the management of severe brain injury. Specifically, if the anterior forebrain mesocircuit plays an important role in all severe injuries that associate with widespread neuronal death or disconnection, several pharmacological interventions can be predicted to have an impact and a systematic exploration should be possible. Similarly, it should be possible to study the metabolic and dynamical patterns associated with natural recovery and responses to effective interventions with measurements that can specifically look at the functional integrity of mesocircuit. Further research will elucidate the value of this organizational scheme.

Acknowledgments

The support of the Charles A. Dana Foundation and the NIH-NINDS NICHD are gratefully acknowledged.

REFERENCES

Adams, J.H., Graham, D.I., Jennett, B. (2000) The neuropathology of the vegetative state after acute insult. *Brain, 123*, 1327–1338.

Alkire M.T., Hudetz, A.G., Tononi, G. (2008) Consciousness and anesthesia. *Science, 322, 5903*, 876–880.

Balkin, T.J., Braun, A.R., Wesensten, N.J., Jeffries, K., Varga, M., Baldwin, P., Belenky, G, Herscovitch, P. (2002) The process of awakening: a PET study of regional brain activity patterns mediating the re-establishment of alertness and consciousness. *Brain, 125, (Pt 10)*, 2308–2319.

Bohland, J.W. et al. (2009) A proposal for a coordinated effort for the determination of brainwide neuroanatomical connectivity in model organisms at a mesoscopic scale. *PLoS Comput Biol., 5, 3*, e1000334.

Braun, A.R., Balkin, T.J., Wesenten, N.J., Carson, R.E., Varga, M., Baldwin. P., Selbie, S.,Belenky, G., Herscovitch, P. (1997) Regional cerebral blood flow throughout the sleep-wake cycle. An H2(15)O PET study. *Brain, 120, (Pt 7),* 1173–1197.

Brefel-Courbon, C. et al. (2007) Clinical and imaging evidence of zolpidem effect in hypoxic encephalopathy. *Ann Neurol., 62, 1,* 102–105.

Calabresi, P., Centonze, D., Bernardi, G. (2000) Cellular factors controlling neuronal vulnerability in the brain: a lesson from the striatum. *Neurology, 55, 9,* 1249–1255.

Calzavara, R., Mailly, P., Haber,S.N. (2007) Relationship between the corticostriatal terminals from areas 9 and 46, and those from area 8A, dorsal and rostral premotor cortex and area 24c: An anatomical substrate for cognition to action. *Eur J Neurosci., 26, 7,* 2005–2024.

Castaigne, P., et al. (1981) Paramedian thalamic and midbrain infarcts: clinical and neuropathological study. *Ann Neurol, 10, 2,* 127–148.

Chatterjee, A., Yapundich, R., Mennemeier, M., Mountz, J.M., Inampudi, C., Pan, J.W., Mitchell, G.W. (1997) Thalamic thought disorder: on being "a bit addled". *Cortex., 33, 3,* 419–440.

Chen, L, Savio Chan C, Yung WH. (2004) Electrophysiological and behavioral effects of zolpidem in rat globus pallidus. *Exp Neurol, 186,* 212–220.

Chklovskii, D.B., Mel, B.W., Svoboda, K. (2004) Cortical rewiring and information storage. *Nature, 431,* 782–788.

Cohen, S.I., Duong, T.T. (2008) Increased arousal in a patient with anoxic brain injury after administration of zolpidem. *Am J Phys Med Rehabil., 87, 3,* 229–231.

Deschenes, M., Bourassa, J., Parent, A. (1996) Striatal and cortical projections of single neurons from the central lateral thalamic nucleus in the rat. *Neuroscience., 72, 3,* 679–687.

Giacino, J.T., Ashwal, S., Childs, N., Cranford, R., Jennett, B., Katz, D.I., Kelly, J.P., Rosenberg, J.H., Whyte, J., Zafonte, R.D., Zasler, N.D. (2002) The minimally conscious state: definition and diagnostic criteria. *Neurology, 58,* 349–353.

Giacino, J.T., Whyte, J. The vegetative state and minimally conscious state: current knowledge and remaining questions. *J. Head Trauma Rehabilitation.*

Grillner S. et al. (2005) Mechanisms for selection of basic motor programs–roles for the striatum and pallidum. *Trends Neurosci, 28, 7,* 364–370.

Gronewegen, H., Berendse, H. (1994) The specificity of the "nonspecific" midline and intralaminar thalamic nuclei. *Trends in Neuroscience, 17,* 52–66.

Guberman, A., Stuss, D. (1983) The syndrome of bilateral paramedian thalamic infarction. *Neurology., 33, 5,* 540–546.

Jones, E.G. (2001) The thalamic matrix and thalamocortical synchrony. *Trends Neurosci, 24,* 595–601.

Kato T. et al. (2007) Statistical image analysis of cerebral glucose metabolism in patients with cognitive impairment following diffuse traumatic brain injury. *J Neurotrauma, 24, 6,* 919–926.

Katz, D.I., Alexander, M.P., Mandell, A.M. (1987) Dementia following strokes in the mesencephalon and diencephalon. *Arch. Neurol., 44,* 1127–1133.

Kinney, H.C., Korein, J., Panigrahy, A., Dikkes, P., Good, R. (1994) Neuropathological findings in the brain of Karen Ann Quinlan. The role of the thalamus in the persistent vegetative state. *N Engl J Med., 330, 21,* 1469–1475.

Kinomura, S., et al. (1996) Activation by attention of the human reticular formation and thalamic intralaminar nuclei. *Science, 271,* 512–515.

Lacey, C.J., Bolam, J.P., Magill, P.J. (2007) Novel and distinct operational principles of intralaminar thalamic neurons and their striatal projections. *J of Neurosciene, 27,* 16, 4374–4384.

Laureys, S., Owen, A.M., Schiff, N.D. (2004) Brain function in coma, vegetative state, and related disorders. *Lancet Neurol., 3, 9,* 537–546.

Llinas, R.R., Leznik, E., Urbano, F.J. (2002) Temporal binding via cortical coincidence detection of specific and nonspecific thalamocortical inputs: a voltage-dependent dye-imaging study in mouse brain slices. *Proceedings of the National Academy of Science, 99,* 449–454.

Llinás, R.R. and Steriade, M. (2006) Bursting of thalamic neurons and states of vigilance. *J of Neurophysiology, 95, 6,* 3297–3308.

Maxwell, W.L. et al. (2006) Thalamic nuclei after human blunt head injury. *J Neuropathol Exp Neurol, 65, 5,* 478–488.

Morel, A., et al. (2005) Divergence and convergence of thalamocortical projections to premotor and supplementary motor cortex: a multiple tracing study in the macaque monkey. *Eur J Neurosci, 21, 4,* 1007–1929.

Mair, R.G., Burk, J.A., Porter, M.C. (1998) Lesions of the frontal cortex, hippocampus, and intralaminar thalamic nuclei have distinct effects on remembering in rats. *Behav Neurosci., 112, 4,* 772–792.

Matsuda, W., Matsumura, A., Komatsu, Y., Yanaka, K., Nose, T. (2003) Awakenings from persistent vegetative state: report of three cases with parkinsonism and brain stem lesions on MRI. *J. Neurol. Neurosurg. Psychiatry, 74,* 1571–1573.

Meythaler, J.M., Brunner, R.C., Johnson, A., Novack, T.A. (2002) Amantadine to improve neurorecovery in traumatic brain injury-associated diffuse axonal injury: a pilot double-blind randomized trial. *J Head Trauma Rehabil, 17, 4,* 300–313.

Nakase-Richardson, R., Yablon, S.A., Sherer, M., Nick, T.G., Evans, C.C. (2009) Emergence from minimally conscious state: insights from evaluation of posttraumatic confusion. *Neurology, 73, 14,* 1120–1126.

Paus, T., et al. (1997) Time-related changes in neural systems underlying attention and arousal during the performance of an auditory vigilance task. *J. Cognitive Neurosci, 9,* 392–408.

Paus T, et al. (1998) Regional differences in the effects of task difficulty and motor output on blood flow response in the human anterior cingulate cortex: a review of 107 PET activation studies. *Neuroreport, 9, 9,* R37–47.

Posner, J., Saper C., Schiff, N., Plum, F. (2007) *Plum and Posner's Diagnosis of Stupor and Coma 4th Edition.* Oxford University Press.

Purpura, K.P. and Schiff, N.D. (1997) The thalamic intralaminar nuclei: role in visual awareness. *Neuroscientist, 3,* 8–14.

Rigas P. and Castro-Alamancos, M.A. (2007) Thalamocortical up states: Differential effects of intrinsic and extrinsic cortical inputs on persistent activity. *J of Neuroscience, 27, 16,* 4261–4272.

Robertson, I.H. et al. (1997) "Oops!": Performance correlates of everyday attentional failures in traumatic brain injured and normal subjects. *Neuropsychologia, 35,* 747–758.

Scannell, J.W. et al. (1999) The connectional organization of the cortico-thalamic system of the cat. *Cereb Cortex, 9, 3,* 277–299.

Schiff, N.D. (2008) Central thalamic contributions to arousal regulation and neurological disorders of consciousness. *Annals of New York Academy of Sciences,* 1129, 105–118.

Schiff, N.D. (2009) Recovery of consciousness after brain injury: a mesocircuit hypothesis. *Trends Neurosci. Nov 30.* [Epub ahead of print]

Schiff, N.D., Giacino, J.T., Fins, J.J. (2009) Deep brain stimulation, neuroethics, and the minimally conscious state: moving beyond proof of principle. *Arch Neurol., 66,* 6, 697–702.

Schiff, N.D., Giacino, J.T, Kalmar, K., Victor, J.D., Baker, K., Gerber, M., Fritz, B., Eisenberg, B., Biondi, T., O'Connor, J., Kobylarz, E.J., Farris, S., Machado, A., McCagg, C., Plum, F., Fins J.J., Rezai, A.R. (2007) Behavioral improvements with thalamic stimulation after severe traumatic brain injury. *Nature, 2007, 448,* 600–603.

Schiff, N.D., and Plum, F. (2000) The role of arousal and 'gating' systems in the neurology of impaired consciousness. *Journal of Clin. Neurophysiol, 17,* 438–452.

Schiff, N.D., and Posner, J.P. (2007) Another "Awakenings". *Annals of Neurology,* 62, 5–7.

Schiff, N.D. and Purpura, K.P. (2002) Towards a neurophysiological basis for cognitive neuromodulation through deep brain stimulation. *Thalamus and Related Systems,* 2, 55–69.

Schiff, N.D. et al. (2005) fMRI reveals large-scale network activation in minimally conscious patients. *Neurology, 64,* 514–523.

Shames, J.L., Ring, H. (2008) Transient reversal of anoxic brain injury-related minimally conscious state after zolpidem administration: a case report. *Arch Phys Med Rehabi, 89, 2,* 386–388.

Shah, S., Baker, J., Ryou, J.W., Purpura, K.P., Schiff, N.D. (2009) Modulation of arousal regulation with central thalamic deep brain stimulation. *Conf Proc IEEE Eng Med Biol Soc., 1,* 3314–3317.

Shirvalkar, P., et al. (2006) Cognitive enhancement with central thalamic electrical stimulation. *Proceedings of the National Academy of Sciences, 103, 45,* 17007–17012.

Smith, Y., Raju, D., Nanda, B., Pare, J.F., Galvan, A., Wichmann. T. (2009) The thalamostriatal systems: anatomical and functional organization in normal and parkinsonian states. *Brain Res Bull., 78, 2–3,* 60–68.

Steriade, M. and Glenn, L.L. (1982) Neocortical and caudate projections of intralaminar thalamic neurons and their synaptic excitation from midbrain reticular core. *J of Neurophysiology, 48,* 352–371.

Stuss, D.T. and Alexander, M.P. (2007) Is there a dysexecutive syndrome? *Philos Trans R Soc Lond B Biol Sci., 362, 1481,* 901–915.

Van der Werf, Y.D., Witter, M.P., Groenewegen, H.J. (2002) The intralaminar and midline nuclei of the thalamus. Anatomical and functional evidence for participation in processes of arousal and awareness. *Brain Res Brain Res Rev, 39, 2–3,* 107–140.

Van Der Werf, Y.D. et al. (1999) Neuropsychological correlates of a right unilateral lacunar thalamic infarction. *J. Neurol. Neurosurg. Psychiatry, 66,* 36–42.

Victor J.D. and Schiff, N.D. (2008) Meeting rigorous statistical standards in case reports. *Ann Neurol, 64, 5,* 592.

Williams, S, Conte, M.M., Kobylarz, E.J., Hersh, J., Victor, J.D., Schiff, N.D. (2009) Quantitative neurophysiologic characterization of a paradoxical response to zolpidem in a severely brain-injured human subject. *Society for Neuroscience Meeting* Abstract.

Whyte, J., Myers, R. (2009) Incidence of clinically significant responses to zolpidem among patients with disorders of consciousness: a preliminary placebo controlled trial. *Am J Phys Med Rehabil, 88, 5,* 410–8.

Wyder,M.T., Massoglia, D.P., Stanford, T.R. (2004) Contextual modulation of central thalamic delay-period activity: representation of visual and saccadic goals. *J of Neurophysiology, 91, 6,* 2628–2648.

14

Intermittent Vorticity, Power Spectral Scaling, and Dynamical Measures on Resting Brain Magnetic Field Fluctuations
A Pilot Study

Arnold J. Mandell, Karen A. Selz, Tom Holroyd,
Lindsay Rutter, and Richard Coppola

The Eyes Closed, Resting Record

The time dynamics of global brain electromagnetic field activity, recorded in humans as continuous, eyes-closed resting MEG (and EEG) records, are regarded by some as reflections of physiologically and psychologically relevant, emergent macroscopic behavior of nonlinearly coupled, cooperative brain systems (Basar et al., 1983; Bucolo et al., 2003; Chen et al., 2003; Friedrich et al., 1989; Haken, 1996; Mandell, 1983a). Others, more involved in neuronal current source localization studies of task or state-related magneto-encephalographic records (Cornwell et al., 2008; Fife et al., 2002; Garolera et al., 2007; Nolte et al., 2004) have treated the globally distributed, spontaneous neuronal current generated, brain magnetic field activity as "...high-ranked (leading eigen-valued) background activity... interfering magnetic fields generated from (not relevant) spontaneous brain activities...intrinsic brain noise..." (Sekihara et al., 1996; Sekihara et al., 2008;

Sekihara et al., 2006). Covariance matrix-derived beamformers from several minutes of the eyes-closed resting record have been used in "pre-whitening techniques," adding noise in order to get around linear dependency in the matrix if it is too low dimensional and to minimize interfering low dimensional intrinsic brain magnetic field noise (Sekihara et al., 2008; Zumer et al., 2007; Zumer et al., 2008).

Another view of spontaneous magnetic field fluctuations has been influenced by studies of spatial (neuroanatomical) brain localization using concomitant fMRI techniques. They have suggested the existence of spontaneous, regional, above-baseline activity in the normal eyes-closed, resting state. This activity is particularly pronounced in medial prefrontal, parietal and both posterior and anterior cingulate, and is suppressed during goal-directed behavior (Damoiseaus et al., 2006; Griecius et al., 2003; Gusnard and Raichle, 2001). Activity in this "network" has been labeled "default activation" by Raichle (Raichleet al., 2001).

The many second time scale of fMRI imaging demonstrated density variations that were characteristic for the normal eyes closed, resting condition (Biswal et al., 1995). Importantly, the spontaneous activity in the resting state also appears to involve neural network activity across several time scales (Honey et al., 2007).

In two-state, task–no task experimental designs, the resting activity, "default activation," has been speculated to reflect spontaneous, task-unrelated, images and thoughts (Greicius and Menon, 2004; Greicius et al., 2004; Raichle et al., 2001; Vincent et al., 2007). These transient mental events in the eyes closed, resting condition have also been called "daydreaming" (Singer, 1966), "task-unrelated-thoughts," TUTs (Giambra, 1989), "unrest at rest" (Buckner and Vincent, 2007), "wandering minds," and "stimulus independent thought" SITs (Gilbert et al., 2007).

Psychologists that have studied inner life subjectively, William James (1902) and Sigmund Freud (1914/1955 among many others, have focused on these autonomously arising transient streams of free associations and imagery. James analogized them to the turbulent eddies of the hydrodynamic flow of consciousness which he believed these transients to be among the universal properties of the conscious human brain. Examinations of a subject's spontaneous internal activity as exteriorized by the psychoanalytic instruction, "…say everything that comes to your mind…" has been central to the practice of psychoanalysis for over a Century {Fenichel, 1945 #8190).

It appears that the ostensibly resting "default brain activity" in the "default network" persists in monkeys through anesthesia-induced changes in states of consciousness (Vincent et al., 2007). This result is consistent with a several-decade history of research using priming, evoked potentials and task-recovery paradigms to demonstrate implicit, working memorial events that occur during even surgical anesthesia (Jordon et al., 2000). The implied relationship between 3–8 second, aperiodic epochs of MEG activation such as that seen below in Figure 14.5 as intermittent helical vortices (we call them *strudels*) and TUT or SIT-like subjective phenomena must remain entirely speculative.

General Premise and Hypothesis

It is the underlying premise of this pilot study of intrinsic brain magnetic field fluctuations that they manifest signatory *aggregate measure motion* conserving brain entropy and allowing the discrimination among global brain states. We examine this premise by isolating and qualitatively and quantitatively characterizing 12.5, 54, 180 or 240 seconds of eyes closed, resting spontaneous magnetic field activity in ten resting controls and ten medicated schizophrenic probands. One might anticipate from our our previous work in brain-related physiological systems (Mandell, 1979; Mandell, 1983b; Mandell, 1987; Mandell et al., 1982; Mandell and Selz, 1993), a more specific hypothesis would be suggested: *Compared with controls, magnetic field fluctuations in schizophrenic patients will demonstrate relatively higher values for some statistical indices of emergent dynamical structure and significantly lower values for an aggregate entropy measure measurable entropy manifold volume, memv, reflecting the dynamical entropy "used up" in their formation* (Mandell and Selz, 1997 Selz and Mandell, 1991; Selz et al., 1995; Smotherman et al., 1996).

A MEG-Derived Data Series: Symmetric
Sensor Difference Sequences, *ssds(i)*

Ten normal controls and ten age- and sex-matched schizophrenic proband subjects (see Subjects below) were studied in the National Institutes of Mental Health's Core MEG Laboratory in Bethesda, Md. A 275-channel, superconducting quantum interference device (SQUID radial gradiometer system from CTF Systems Inc.of Port Coquitlam, British Columbia, Canada (Anninos et al., 1986; Cohen, 1972; Rutter et al., 2009; Weinberg et al., 1984) was used in data collection (see Magnetoencephalographic Data Collection below).

Our approach to MEG-derived signals abrogates source orientation, localization, and inverse problem tools such as leadfield matrices (Dale and Sereno, 1993; Hamalainen et al., 1993), adaptive synthetic aperture magnetometer,

SAM, beamformer techniques, or projection onto Talairached MRI image reconstructed volumes (Dalal et al., 2008; Dalal et al., 2004). For these approaches to this data set, see Rutter et al (2009). In their study of spontaneous activity in the eyes-closed, resting state, they found a statistically significant decrement in the amplitudes of MEG recorded posterior regional gamma (30-70Hz+) activity in schizophrenic patients compared with normal controls (Rutter et al., 2009). In that study as well as these, a high pass, 0.6 Hz, as well as 60, 120, 180 and 240 Hz notch filters were routinely applied to the individual sensor records. These studies differed in that the application of filters was followed by a novel primary data transformation generating symmetric sensor difference sequences, ssds(i), (sequences of differences between two bilaterally symmetric sensor pairs.).

It is our presupposition that the "…spontaneous activity… all over the brain…" (Sekihara et al., 2008) reflects global and neurophysiologically meaningful patterns of complex neuronal activity-generated magnetic field fluctuations in interaction with MEG SQUID sensors (Barone A, and G., 1982; Braiman and Wiesenfeld, 1994). A magnetic flux applied to the SQUID magnetometer, gives rise to a circulating current, which in turn modulates the inductance of the autonomously oscillatory Josephson junctions (Landberg et al., 1966; Levi et al., 1977). The great sensitivity of the SQUID devices permits measuring changes in magnetic field associated with even a single flux quantum. If a constant biasing current is maintained in the SQUID device, it is the voltage which is modulated by changes in phase at junctions. Phase at Josephson junctions is sensitive to the quanta of magnetic flux.

We dismiss a common generalization of many MEG practitioners that most or all local polarities of the intrinsic magnetic field noise "cancel out." In the context of the somewhat analogous *magnetic dynamo problem*: "…given a flow in a conducting fluid, will a small seed magnetic field amplify exponentially with time…" and (Finn and Ott, 1988), we show below that ssds(i)s do—it was argued that the magnetic flux loops *nonuniformly* stretch and fold into themselves manifesting only *partial cancellation* and diffuse multiple scale oscillations, in a process which can be quantified by a fractional *cancellation exponent* (Ott et al., 1992) and measures made on temporal-spatial intermittency.

In addition, if some currents run parallel to magnetic fields, which is expected to be the case with multiple neocortical neuronal sources, the magnetic field lines may follow a variety of dynamical shapes in which the magnetic pressure gradient is balanced by the magnetic tension. For example, there may not be a Lorentz force, $J \times B = 0$, leading to a measurable field configuration without any net electrical current at all. We thus don't infer a particular neuronal current source (or event) for the data series. Characterizing the fluctuations allows the elucidation of patterns in the brain's global magnetic field flux dynamics without reference to anatomical location (Clarke, 1994). For example, we find a common dynamical pattern often involves intermittently appearing, multiple time scale helical vortices. We call them *strudels*, the German word for "whirlpools." In a none-turbulence related theoretical context, strudels might be seen as neocortical pyramidal-cell critical network *avalanches* (Beggs and Plenz, 2005; Levina et al., 2007).

In comparison with the several second time resolution of fMRI, the MEG's superior temporal resolution, ~ 1 ms, combined with its "underdetermined" weaknesses with respect to specific brain localization when used alone (Hamalainen et al., 1993; Im et al., 2005; Lee et al., 2007; Sarvas, 1987; Uutela et al., 1998), suited our goal of characterizing magnetic fields rather than inferring individual or network neuronal properties of what has been called intrinsic physiological brain noise (Nagarajan et al., 2006; Sekihara et al., 1997; Sekihara et al., 2005).

The use of *ssds(i)* exploits the approximate hemispheric symmetry of the human brain (Geschwind, 1970) and serves several purposes: (1) It imposes a natural gauge (distance from ~ zero mean) on the nonstationary MEG signal; (2) As such, it serves as a traveling, local normalization procedure; (3) The *ssdi(i)* reduces the penetrance of electromagnetic field correlates of blink, cough, and movement as well as the cardiac and respiratory artifacts that both symmetric sensors generally share; (4) Using ssds(i) instead of the raw MEG time series tends to cancel the symmetrically shared generic MEG (and EEG) Δ, Θ, α, β, and γ modes, as well as other sources of bihemispheric covariance; (5) Advantageous from the magnetic field point of view is the fact that using ssds(i) makes issues of neuronal current source location moot. The spatial sensitivity profile of a single pair recording a single *ssds(i)*,such as L- R C23 considered as a virtual sensor, includes over half of the three dimensional region including neocortical layers II and III in central, parietal, frontal and some temporal areas. The techniques similar to that used here of paired sensor difference series, *ssds(i)*, have been used to reduce or remove the mean and *double or more the higher moments* in analyses of nonstationary neural membrane conductance noise (Conti et al., 1980; DeFelice, 1977; Sigworth, 1981).

Our 600 Hz, (150 Hz acquisition cut off) three minute, eyes closed, resting data stream consists of 144,000 point, left minus right, *symmetric sensor difference sequences, ssds(i)*

$$\Sigma_i^n x(L) - \Sigma_i^n x(R) = \Sigma_i^n ssds(i) \qquad (1)$$

such that,

$$\Phi^t_{\Sigma ssds_i} \Omega_m \to \Omega_m \tag{2}$$

can be regarded as a dynamical system mapping an m-dimensional manifold, Ω_m onto itself (Bowen, 1978; Katok and Hasselblatt, 1995). As is the case with most nonlinear systems, our work consists of characterizing the solutions, not writing the equations, for the output of the (unknown) generating function, $\Phi^t\ ssds(i)$.

For a specific example of the MEG-derived data stream being studied, the output sequence of the right central C16 SQUID sensor is sequentially subtracted from that of the sequence recorded by the left central C16 sensor, the difference generating the C16, $\Phi^t\ ssds(i)$.

In Figure 14.1A, the red boxes indicate the physical locations of the symmetric central sensor pair generating the C16 $\Phi^t_{\Sigma ssds_i}$. In Figure 14.1A, the parietal sensor pair, P57, is indicated by green boxes; the temporal pair, T44, are marked by black boxes; the frontal, F14, by blue boxes. Figure 14.1B is a ~ 12.5 second segment of the three minute recording demonstrating the range of fluctuation amplitudes of 50 to 15 x $10^3\ fT$. Figure 14.1C is a graph of a segment of the C16 $\Phi^t_{\Sigma ssds_i}$ orbit in a three dimensional embedding of a $t, t+1, t+2$ phase-advance (~delay) plot. We see somewhat irregular, recursive patterns in phase delay space with a multiplicity of recurrence times. Figure 14.1D portrays the log-log frequency(power) spectrum of one minute of a C16 $ssds(i)$ with $f^{-\alpha}$, "self-similar" power law scaling of $\alpha = 1.54 \pm .28$. We computed the least square deviant linear slope of the middle third of the Fourier modular coefficients as α. This value is sometimes close to the universal power law scaling exponent of nonlinear systems in the state of self organized criticality, SOC, of -3/2. (see below). It can also, however, range well beyond the -5/3 Kolmogorov scaling of hydrodynamic turbulence.

Measures on Entropy Utilizing, Emergent Dynamical Structure: α, $W[\Psi_1\ (ssds(i))]$, U and k

A. The Slope of the Log-Log Power Spectra, Scaling Exponent α

Where $S(\omega)$ is the power spectrum of C16, $\Phi^t(ssds(i))$, with similarity parameters α (slope) and β (intercept), e the error term and brackets, < > indicating

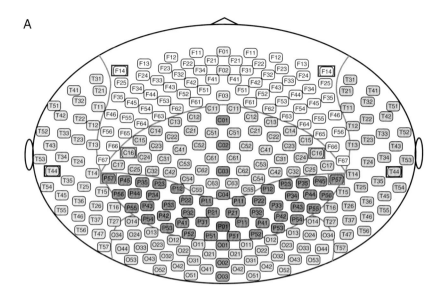

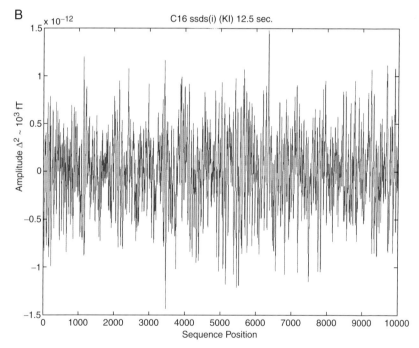

FIGURE 14.1 A: Color coded sensor pair locations; Central, C16, red; Parietal, P57, green; Temporal, T44, black; Frontal, F14, blue. B: 9920 point, Central, C16, symmetric sensor difference sequence, ssds(i) composing ~ 12.5 seconds of eyes closed, resting record. C: 300 point, Central, C16, phase delay (advance, n, n+1, n+2) portrait of ssds(i) embedded in R^3 and demonstrating irregular, recursive orbits with two t (top and bottom) local helical patterns wound into a multiplicity of recurrence times.

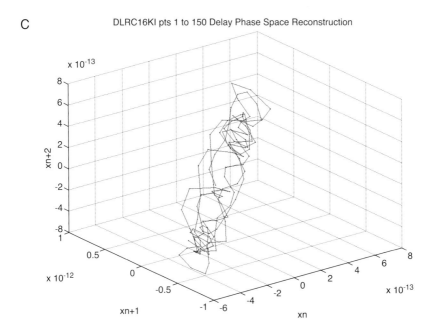

C DLRC16KI pts 1 to 150 Delay Phase Space Reconstruction

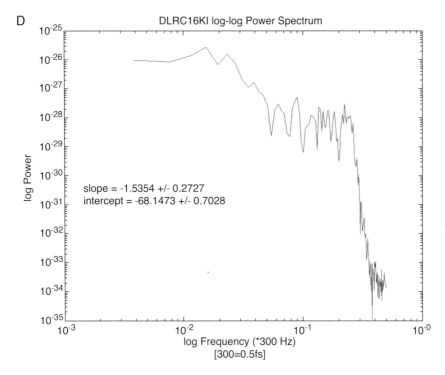

D DLRC16KI log-log Power Spectrum

slope = -1.5354 +/- 0.2727
intercept = -68.1473 +/- 0.7028

log Power

log Frequency (*300 Hz)
[300=0.5fs]

FIGURE 14.1 (Continued) D: Graph of a log-log frequency (power) spectral
transformation of 32,000 point (~54 seconds) ssds(i) of the Central, C16 resting record
demonstrating an $f^{-\alpha}$ "self similar" scaling with $\alpha = 1.54\pm28$. We compute the least
square deviant linear slope of the middle third of the Fourier modular coefficients as α.

averages over the range of frequencies, ω, we minimize the mean square deviation to estimate the slope, L

$$L = <[\log S(\omega) - \beta - \alpha \log \omega]^2>$$
$$e = L^{1/2} <|\log S(\omega)|>$$

(3)

Figure 14.1D shows an $f^{-\alpha}$ fractional power law, 1.54 ± 0.27 consistent with "self similar" dynamics manifesting a hierarchy of time scales, here from < 0.1 to > 120 Hz. The observable 150 Hz acquisition cutoff serves as the upper bound on the frequency range that can demonstrate the power spectral scaling. Figure 14.2 demonstrates the array of individually different log-log power spectra $f^{-\alpha}$ of ten control's C16 $ssds(i)$. The mean, median, standard deviation and variance of the $\alpha[ssds(i)]$ from the ten control subjects' C16 $\Phi^t_{\Sigma ssds_i}$ are, as averaged from the 10 control subjects' C16 $ssds(i)$, for $f^{-\alpha}$, the mean and s.d. α = 1.67± 0.43, median = 1.59 and variance = 0.18.

Table 14.1 summarizes the means and standard deviations of α values for the four regional sensor pairs, N = 10 in each group. Spectral fractional power law, "self-similar" behavior in human MEG signals has been reported by others as evidence consistent with intermittent turbulent flow(Novikov, 1990). More generally, the brain qualifies as a system with strong interactions and many degrees of freedom that characteristically demonstrate power law scaling (Novikov et al., 1997). Others have regarded power law spectra as evidence for intermittent, scale free "avalanches" of component activity and diagnostic of self organized criticality, SOC,(Kitzbichler et al., 2009; Tang andBak, 1988). Scale free (multiscale) critical behavior has been reported in studies of both computational and real cortical neural networks (Beggs and Plenz, 2005; Chialvo, 2004; Levina et al., 2007; Shin and Kim, 2006). From a more general point of view, we have studied turbulent intermittency as a common time dynamic in neurobiological systems from protein motion to global electromagnetic fields (Mandell and Selz, 1991; Mandell, 1983b; Mandell et al., 1991b).

In spite of the qualitative resemblance to avalanches, values for the scaling exponent α in Table 14.1 do not cluster around the universal exponent of SOC, -3/2 but rather seem closer to Kolmogorov's -5/3 scaling of wave number, $k^{-5/3,}$ the distribution of "energy" (in the inertial range) among eddies and vortices, as a function of vortex size in turbulent flows (Kolmogorov, 1941). This motivated the choice of the name, "strudels." The higher values of α in the proband's power spectra do *not* reach statistically significant. They are, nonetheless, in the direction one would predict for a higher α, "less white," more negatively sloped, log-log power spectrum with higher values for emergent dynamical

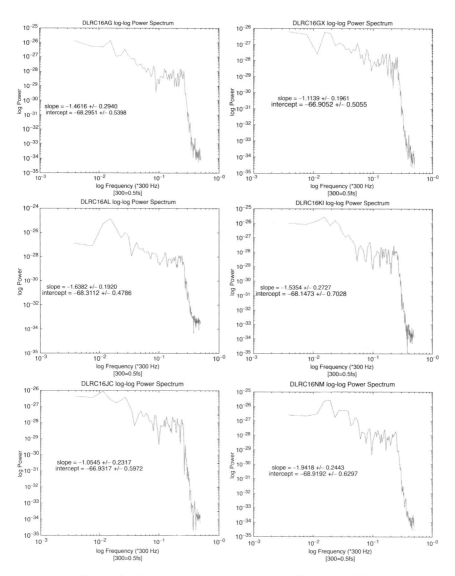

FIGURE 14.2 The log-log frequency (power) spectral transformation of the ten Central, C16, Control group's 32,000 point ssds(*i*) demonstrating a range of individual differences in *f* α scaling, $1.11 \leq \alpha \leq 2.35$. The mean and s.d. $\alpha = 1.67 \pm 0.43$, median = 1.59 and variance = 0.18. The average is closer to the universal -5/3 Kolmogorov scaling exponent of the log-log power spectra as the velocity structure function of the scaler fields of hydrodynamic turbulence.

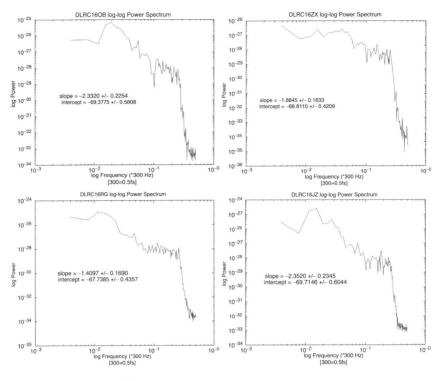

FIGURE 14.2 (Continued)

TABLE 14.1 Means and Standard Deviations of α (n = 10 in each group)

Sensor Pair	Controls	Probands
Central (C16)	1.67±0.43	1.89±0.67
Temporal (T44)	1.66±0.52	1.84±0.50
Parietal (T57)	1.97±0.25	2.28±0.54
Frontal (F14)	1.63±0.52	1.69±0.31

structure and lower values for a variety of measures of dynamical entropy, many of which are statistically significant (see below). It was initially speculated that this difference in α might reflect a higher density of intermittent helical events, more *strudels*, in the Probands. However, this issue remains unresolved since extending our n in more recent studies demonstrated a *relative decrease* in strudel count in many probands. This suggests that in the higher entropy measure manifesting controls, strudels, as turbulent eddies, might serve as a "mixing," source of brain entropy.

If *strudels* accompany TUTs or SITs (and we don't know that they do) we might speculate that, probands, with less of them, experience a relatively impoverished inner life. This finding would be consistent with the known *negative signs* of schizophrenia

Whereas there were no statistically significant differences between mean values of α in the $f^{-\alpha}$ of *ssds(i)* of C16, T44, P57 or F14, an analysis of variance did show statistically significant *individual differences* in the controls ($p = 0.0178$), but not in the probands. On the other hand, the schizophrenic probands had statistically significant *regional differences* in α (C vs T vs P vs F) ($p<0.0001$) that were not evident in controls. The uniformity in power law scaling in the probands may be explained by both their common disease and psychopharmacological treatment.

B. Leading BK Eigenfunction, Ψ_1, of ssds(i) and their Morlet Wavelet Transform, $W_M[(\Psi_1(ssds(i)))]$: Eigenzeit and its Intermittent Strudels

To explore the possibility of intermittent "avalanches" of $\alpha = -3/2$ SOC scaling, the vortices (*strudels*) with the $\alpha = -5/3$ turbulent eddies and other "heavy tailed" dynamics yielding fractional exponential power laws (Bendler et al., 2004), we made a more detailed examination of the behavior of *ssds(i)* in time (Strang, 1993). Searching the *ssds(i)* for dynamical patterns in time we have used Morlet wavelet transformations, W_M (Daubechies, 1992; Farge et al., 1993) of the leading Broomhead/King, B/K, eigenfunction, Ψ_1, $W_M[\Psi_1 (ssds(i))]$ which for reasons indicated below we call an *eigenzeit*. (Broomhead et al., 1987; Broomhead and King, 1986; Mandell et al., 2003; Mandell et al., 2000).

The *ssds(i)* sequence was used to generate an *M*-lagged data matrix from which the M x M Hermitean covariance matrix, *CM*, was computed with M chosen to approximate the autocorrelation decay of the *ssds(i)*. These *CM* were then decomposed into ordered eigenvalues and their associated eigenvectors formed. The leading eigenvector was sequentially composed with *ssds(i)* forming the leading Broomhead-King eigenfunction, Ψ_1. See previous applications for algorithmic details (Mandell et al., 1997; Mandell et al., 2000; Selz et al., 2004).

Figure 14.3 depicts four phase delay portraits of the Ψ_1 of increasing length: A. 250, B. 500, C. 750 and D. 1000 sequential points in R^3. The phase delay portraits are less irregular then in figure 14.1C, which displays the undecomposed *ssds(i)* from the same control subject. figures 14.3A, B, C, and D show patterns of recursive vortices, *strudels,* of various amplitudes and return times with a persistence of the "holes" around which the orbits of $\Psi_1(ssds(i))$ wind with increasing eigenfunction length.

A   DLRC16KI 1st Eigenfunction 1 to 250 Delay Phase Space Reconstruction

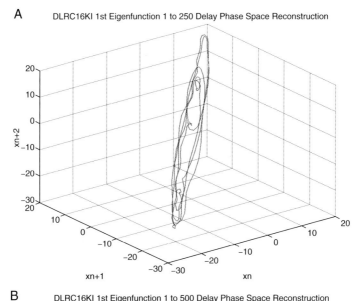

B   DLRC16KI 1st Eigenfunction 1 to 500 Delay Phase Space Reconstruction

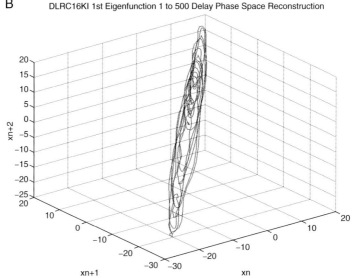

FIGURE 14.3 This figure depicts four phase delay (advance) portraits, *n, n+1, n+2*, of the leading B/K eigenfunction, Ψ_1, of increasing length: A. *i* = 250, B. *i* = 500, C. *i* = 750 and D. *i* = 1000 in an R^3 embedding of Control subject, KI' s Ψ_1 (ssds(*i*)). Helically recursive orbits of multiple length scales, *strudels*, wind around persistent "holes." The orbits of Ψ_1 (ssds(*i*)) are smoother than those in the comparable ssds(*i*) of Fig.14.1C.

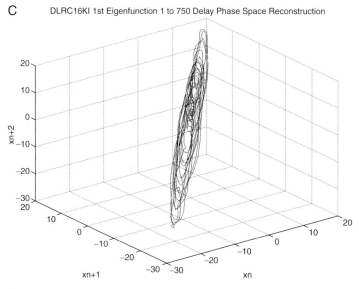

C   DLRC16KI 1st Eigenfunction 1 to 750 Delay Phase Space Reconstruction

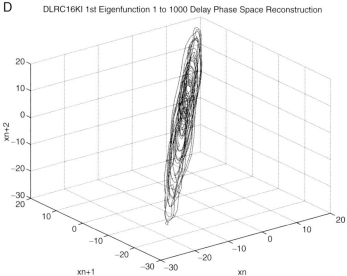

D   DLRC16KI 1st Eigenfunction 1 to 1000 Delay Phase Space Reconstruction

FIGURE 14.3 (Continued)

Continuous Morlet wavelet transformations of Ψ_1 ($ssds(i)$) were undertaken using standard algorithms (Daubechies, 1992; Strang, 1993; Wickerhauser, 1994). Generally, a Morlet wavelet transform, $W(a,b)$, of the Ψ_1 series of values, consists of decomposing the series into a translated, $f(n) \rightarrow f(n - b)$, and scaled, $f(n) \rightarrow f(n/a,)$ versions of itself as composed with the Morlet mother wavelet, w. (Grossman andMorlet, 1984). "Scale" as used here is analogous to the inverse radian frequency of a trigonometric function. The mother wavelet w is a waveform with an average value of zero ($\int w(n)dn = 0$). w is of finite duration and arbitrary regularity and symmetry. Across dilations, $f(n)/a$, and translations, $f(n - b. w)$ is convolved with Ψ_1 to generate, $W(\Psi_1)$ the *eigenzeit* ("its own time") sequence. w is a windowed, Gaussian, sine transformation maximized with respect to the trade-off in resolution between dilation (ordinate, "mother wavelet wavelength") and translation (abscissa, Ψ_1, $i...n$ sequence position). We call the $W(\Psi_1)$ an *eigenzeit* because it's composed of the Ψ_1 sequence along the abscissa in place of time and the ordinate indicating the scaling metric on the Ψ_1 sequence, not as time sequence. An *eigenzeit* ("its own time") brings its own time scaling structure to the observation.

Figure 14.4 contains four graphs of Morlet wavelet transforms, W_M, of the $\Psi_1(ssds(i))$, $W[\Psi1(ssds(i))]$. We call them *eigenzeits*. Roughly 12.5 seconds of the sequence is shown on the abscissa. The Ψ_1 mother wavelength scaling is shown along the ordinate and Morlet mother wavelet, w, convolution is color coded for modular amplitude as indicated. The modular amplitudes are normalized for each scale. The *eigenzeit*, $W[\Psi_1(ssds(i))]$, over its sequence and modular amplitude, inscribes the same intermittently recursive helicity of the *strudels* seen in the embedded phase delay studies of Ψ_1 of increasing lengths (Figure 14.3A-D.). The *strudels* manifest a pattern of expanding, multiscale and intermittent vorticity in the fluctuations of $\Psi_1(ssds(i))$. The resulting power law spectra (Figures 14.1D and 14.2) are known to be associated with the intermittency and anomalous diffusivity of Josephson junction dynamics (Gaspard and Wang, 1988; Geisel et al., 1985; Shlesinger and Klafter, 1985).

One might also notice in Figure 14.4 that the intermittent and sometimes almost regular, smallest scale magnetic field activity (smallest scales being at the bottom of the graph) appears to seed the expansion of the *strudels* "upward" into longer, mother wavelet wave lengths, in the upper part and beyond of the wavelet graphs. As noted above, these electromagnetic dynamics are similar to those observed in studies of the magnetic dynamo problem in the low resistivity domain (Finn and Ott, 1988; Ott et al., 1992). This problem as stated is "...given a flow in a conducting fluid, will a small magnetic field seed amplify exponentially with time..." (Finn and Ott, 1988). It seems that the measures on the *ssds(i)* below are consistent with expansive dynamics.

Figure 14.5, a graph of Morelet wavelet transformations of Central, C16, eigenfunction, $\Psi(ssds(i))$ during a transient, petite mal, absence epileptic episode. The *eigenzeit* demonstrates more definitive evidence for a (here rhythmic) small scale seeding and driving the expansion of magnetic field fluctuations into *strudels* of larger scale, longer mother wavelet wavelength.

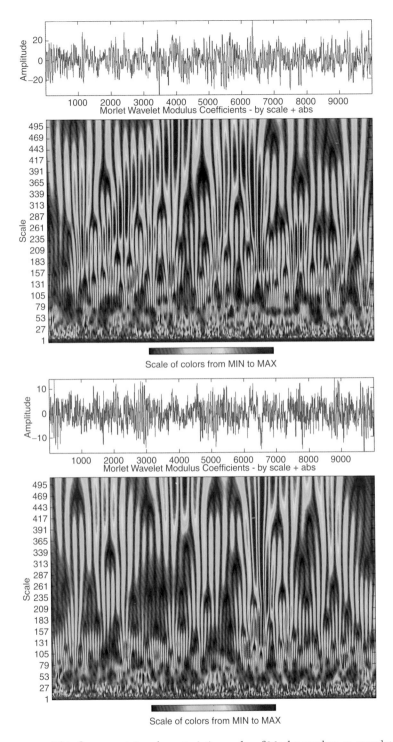

FIGURE 14.4 This figure contains characteristic graphs of Morlet mother, w, wavelet transformations, W, of the leading B/K eigenfunctions, Ψ_1, of four ~12.5 second ssds(i), W[Ψ_1(ssds(i))]. They are called *eigenzeits* ("own time") because the sequence is not in

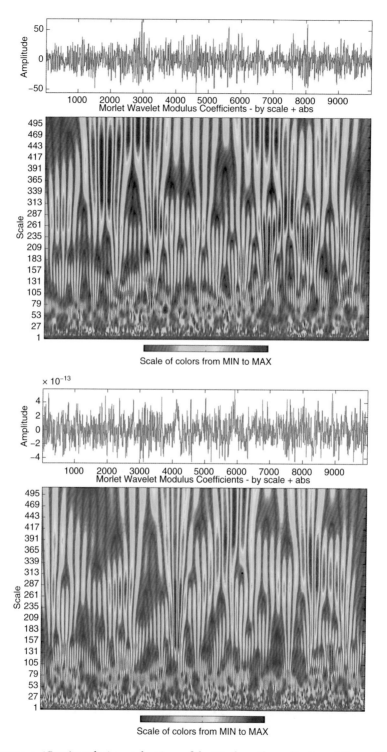

FIGURE 14.4 (Continued) time, t, but in n of the Ψ_1 along the ordinate and the scaling of Ψ_1's n along the abscissa. In comparable time, the wavelet scales range roughly from 0.001 to almost one second. Modular amplitudes, *by scale,* are color coded as indicated.

FIGURE 14.4 (Continued) The event time keeping of the reddish, tan *strudels* of the *eigenzeits* emerge in a pattern of intermittent, small scale to large scale, expanding vorticity apparently driven by the fast small scale activity which only intermittently becomes a full scaling *strudel*. Note that the duration of some *strudels,* 2–5 seconds, are in the range of TUTs, "task unrelated thoughts" (Giambra, 1989) and "stimulus independent thoughts," SITs (Gilbert et al., 2007).

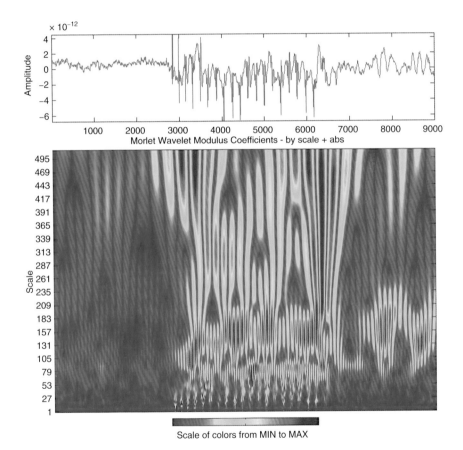

Scale of colors from MIN to MAX

FIGURE 14.5 This figure is derived from the transformation, $W[\Psi_1(ssds(i))]$, of a Central, C16 sensor pair of an opportunistically obtained MEG record while the subject manifested a transient *petite mal* (*petite absence*, *"staring spell"*) epileptic episode. The associated *eigenzeit* demonstrates more clearly than in Fig. 14.4, regular, very small scale fast driving, the intermediate scale 1-3 Hz "waves" and the intermittent emergence of longer mother wavelet wavelength, hierarchically scaling, helical *strudels* from some but not all fast and intermediate scale events.

313

C. Intermittent Helical Scaling Structures, Strudels*; Their Relative
Unwinding Numbers, U(c) and U(p) in Controls and Probands*

The unwinding number, $U(c,p)$, of helical *strudels* is defined as the number of
sequential lags in the phase delay space required to reach within one standard
deviation of the asymptotic value of the capacity dimension, D_C as embedded
in R^3 (see Figure 14.6). To define D_C, if $n(\varepsilon)$ is the minimum number of covers
of diameter $\le \varepsilon$, then $n(\varepsilon)$ is proportional to ε^{-D} as $\varepsilon \to 0$:

$$D_C \simeq \lim \frac{\ln\ n(\varepsilon)}{\ln\ (\varepsilon)} \tag{4}$$

The sequential lags unwind the putative helical *strudels,* increasing the
relative occupancy of phase delay space as indicated by an increase in D_C to an
asymptotic value. As an example from sensor pair F14, the top row of Figure
14.6 demonstrates the unwinding of *strudels* in phase delay space of a control
subject. The unwinding to the D_C asymptotic value $\pm$ 1 SD is completed in two
lags, $U(c) \sim 2.0$. The phase delay space of this F14 proband subject displayed in
the second row of Figure 14.6 shows more resistance to unwinding of *strudels,*
requiring $U\ (p) \ge 8.0$. Though often not the case, this proband's *ssds(i)* is more
dense in helicity *"strudelness"* than the ssds(i) of the control.

Table 14.2 is a summary of the mean and standard deviations of the
unwinding numbers, $U(c,p)$ as determined for the indicated pairs in which, for
each result, n = 10. The differences between control and proband subjects
failed to achieve statistical significance (as in ***Table 14.1***).

D. Kurtosis, k, An Extremal of the Probability Distribution, p(ssds(i))

Although in equilibrium statistical mechanical systems, there is no necessary
relationship between characteristics of the Fourier transformed frequency
(power) spectrum, (such as the similarity exponent α) and those of the probability
density distribution, *p(ssds(i))*, this is not the case in many variable systems

TABLE 14.2 Average unwinding number, U(c, p); Phase delay Lags to asymptotic
D_C (n = 10 for each group)

Sensor Pair	U(c) Controls	U(p) Probands
Central (C16)	3.6±1.83	6.1±2.84
Temporal (T44)	2.2±0.63	5.0±1.56
Parietal (P57)	3.8±1.66	6.6±2.8
Frontal (F14)	2.4±0.83	4.8±1.70

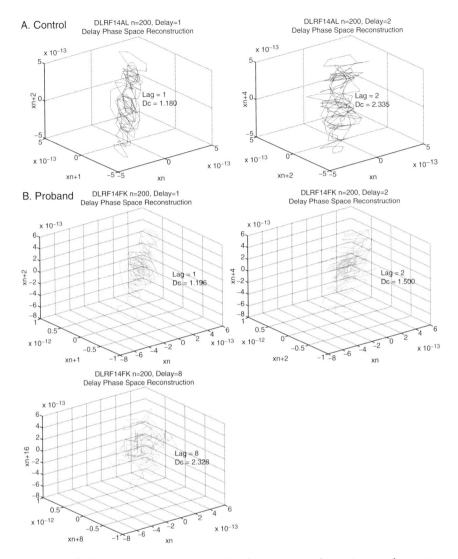

FIGURE 14.6 This figure portrays the results of computational experiments that test our conjecture, drawn from the phase portraits of Figures 14.1C and.14.3 and the *eigenzeits* of Figure.14.4, that intermittent scaling *strudels* are differentially helical. Sequential lags are used to "unwind" the putative helical *strudels,* increasing the relative occupancy of phase delay space in R^3 as indicated by an increase in D_C to within one standard deviation of its asymptotic value. The top row of Figure 14.6 demonstrates the unwinding of 200 point *strudels* in phase delay space of an F14 ssds(i) control subject. The unwinding to the D_C asymptotic value $\pm$ 1 SD is completed in two lags, the *unwinding number,* U(c) ~ 2.0. The phase delay space of an F14 ssds(i) Proband subject displayed in the bottom row of Fig 6 appears to be wound more tightly as evidenced by more resistance to the lag-unwinding of 200 point *strudels* such that U (p) $\geq$ 8.0. Table II summarizes the values for U(c) and U(p) by sensor pair region. See text.

TABLE 14.3 Mean and median values of k (n = 10 for each group)

Sensor Pair	Controls	Probands
Central (C16)	0.315±0.27	0.8216±1.28
Mean; Median	0.232	0.390
Temporal (T44)	0.338±0.26	0.266±0.20
Mean; Median	0.201	0.223
Parietal (P57)	0.369±0.42	0.750±1.19
Mean; Median	0.225	0.386
Frontal (F14)	0.316±0.19	0.770±0.674
Mean; Median	0.270	0.477

with strong interactions, such as in hydrodynamic turbulence (Monin and Yaglom, 1975). As in statistical studies of turbulence(Pope, 2000) and a variety of brain systems (see www.cieloinstitute.org; *Neuroscience*), α scaling of the log-log power spectrum, varies with an index of the peakedness and, particularly, the weight in the tail of "heavy tailed" distribution (Adler et al., 1998), as estimated here by the kurtosis, k:

$$k = \Sigma_i^n \left[\frac{ssds(i) - av(ssds)}{s.d.(ssds)} \right]^4 - 3 \tag{5}$$

Table 14.3 summarizes the values for the mean, standard deviation and median of k in a comparison of ten schizophrenic probands and their age and sex matched controls. In this pilot study, probands evidence higher values for k than the controls. The large individual variation in k, as was the case for α and U (Figure 14. 2, Table 14.1 and Table 14.2) may be responsible for the failure of these differences to achieve statistical significance. As was the case for α and U, the results of the large n study, currently underway, will be required before we can make claims for the statistical significance (or lack thereof) of any of these control-proband differences and relationships among α, U and k.

Measures of Entropy Generation and Support: h_T, Λ_1 and D_C

The theoretical frame of reference for this part of the work derives from the confluence of Poincare's geometric theory of differential equations and Boltzmann's statistical mechanics. It has evolved into the modern ergodic theory of dynamical systems (Arnold, 1983; Arnold andAvez, 1968; Eckmann andRuelle, 1985; Kolmogorov, 1957). In this context, real valued time series can be reconstructed on smooth manifolds for geometric, topological and statistical characterization (Bowen, 1978; Sinai, 1970; Smale, 1967)as in Figures 14.1C and 14.3. Entropies arise as statistically invariant (from any initial condition), "ergodic" measures (Cornfield et al., 1982) on single orbit dynamics on these manifolds (Weiss, 1995a). The symmetric MEG sensor difference sequences, $ssds(i)$ are treated as the output of a differentiable dynamical system, a smooth map Φ^t on an n-dimensional manifold as in Eq. 2.

There is an important family of theorems applicable to $\Phi^t(ssds(i))$ as a non-uniformly, exponentially divergent, "hyperbolic", (*i.e.* no norm = 1) dynamical system (Eckmann and Ruelle, 1985). With respect to measure, it has been proven that for the behavior of nonlinear dynamical systems, entropy is the *only* invariant (Ornstein, 1989; Ornstein, 1974). Unfortunately, the descriptions and proofs of this theorem include no instructions about how to estimate such unique entropy in the data of real world observations. In their place are an array of related entropies that emphasize different aspects of dynamical behavior (Dinaburg, 1971). We approach this problem by developing a more intuitive, three dimensional, extensive, entropy volume measure, *measureable entropy manifold volume, memv,* as a Cartesian product of its components: the topological entropy, h_T, the leading Lyapounov exponent, Λ_1 and the capacity dimension, D_C, $\prod[h_T \Lambda_1 D_C] = memv$.

A. Topological Entropy

The term entropy, in addition to its formal, though sometimes "enigmatic," role as a companion of lost energy and generated heat in the Second Law of thermodynamics (Capek and Sheehan, 2005), is also commonly used as a description of disorder, missing information, redundant multiplicity and/or freedom of action (Burgers, 1954; Darrow, 1944; Jaynes, 1957; Styer, 2000). Without further specification, the ambiguity of the common "disorder" interpretation of systems decay toward maximum entropy, Boltzmann's descent into the "...disordered most probable state..." (Boltzmann, 1964 (1896)), can lead to errors of incompleteness. For example, crystal formation or protein folding in solution looks like an increase in order while it fails to account for the global and large entropic increase in the degrees of freedom of the solvent (water is structured like "ice" at the surface of the protein's hydrophobic moieties) in what is considered to be temperature dependent, "entropy driven" processes.(Leffler, 1955; Lumry and Rajender, 1970). The entropy of "missing information," though well defined (Jaynes, 1957; Shannon, 1948), fails to connect neurobiological phenomena with thermodynamic time, space and possibly the felt psychic energy of brain dynamical systems (Freud, 1927).

In place of the intuitions of "disorder" or "missing information" for entropy in our analyses of $\Phi^t(ssds(i))$, we invoke both the images of orbit creation (Adler et al., 1965) and spreading (Leff, 1996; Yomdin, 1987). The latter intuition includes both separation among neighboring points, what Clausius called disgregation (Clausius, 1862), and growth in both entropy manifold volume (Tsallis et al., 2005; Yomdin, 1987) and its dimension. Recall that the manifold, Ω_m, is the locally Euclidean, m-dimensional surface upon which the action of $\Phi^t(ssds(i))$ takes place.

With respect to rate of orbital creation, if $\Phi^t_{ssds_i}$ $\Omega_m \rightarrow \Omega_m$ is a transformation that conserves the probability measure μ on manifold Ω_m, then the general measure theoretic entropy, h_μ, is here replaced with the lim sup of the entropies, the *topological entropy*, h_T (Adler and Marcus, 1979; Mandell and Selz, 1997) which measures the logarithmic (exponential) rate of emergence of new orbits, "information," $exp(m,h_T)$, such as the appearance of new recursive points in Ω_m (Adler and Marcus, 1979; Adler et al., 1965; Kolmogorov, 1958). Topological entropy, h_T, is a non-negative real number which describes the exponential growth rate of the number of distinct orbits as $t \rightarrow \infty$. Conditioned by a smooth, differentiable manifold that is a compact metric space and $r(n,\varepsilon)$ the maximum cardinality (size) of a n,ε separated set, the topological entropy, h_T, can be written:

$$h_T = \lim_{\varepsilon \rightarrow 0, n \rightarrow \infty} \ \limsup \frac{1}{n} \log(r,(n,\varepsilon)) \tag{6}$$

Computationally, h_T can be estimated as the growth rate of the trace, the Frobenius-Perron eigenvector, of the exponentiated $n \times n$ matrix transfer operator, derived from the partitioning of the symbolic dynamic sequence space. In our studies of $ssds(i)$, the partition is an arbitrary two dimensional six-equipartition, such that the assignment of symbol sequences to trajectories is consistent across control and proband conditions (Cornfield et al., 1982; Hirata et al., 2004; Paulus et al., 1990; Sinai, 1970). The partition is fixed so that variation in the partition doesn't use up the variation that we would want to observe as real number differences in h_T.

B. The Leading Lyapounov Exponent, Λ_1

In addition to an entropy-relevant measure of creation, h_T, a complementary entropy measure can be made on the rate of orbital spreading, a geometric measure on the rate of separation of neighboring points and coming together of far away points and their mixing (getting out of order). In the discussion above, we have suggested that the intermittently appearing *strudel* may play a role in this mixing. In the dynamics of $\Phi^t(ssds(i))$, the rate of expansion can be quantified using a non-zero, leading positive Lyapounov characteristic exponent, Λ_1. This constant quantifies the exponential rates of divergence and convergence along the dominant orbital eigendirection. of the linear decomposition of Φ^t, the unstable manifold, Ω_u of $\Phi^t(ssds(i)$ as a (perhaps nonuniformly) hyperbolic system (Oseledec, 1968). It is also the case that the sum of the positive Lypounov exponents, $\Sigma \Lambda_i > 0$, can serve as another estimate of the entropy (Cornfield et al., 1982; Eckmann and Ruelle, 1985).

In the interest of getting a geometric intuition for Λ_1: Under the expansive actions of $\Phi^t(ssds(i))$, an infinitesimally small, n dimensional hypersphere of initial conditions in n dimensional phase space (imagine a very small magnetic seed of an emergent magnetic dynamo (Finn and Ott, 1988)) deforms into an hyper-ellipse. A measure on the rate of expansion of the *principle axis*, L_1, of the hyper-ellipse in time, $L_1(t)$, yields an estimate of Λ_1.

$$\Lambda_1 = \lim_{t \to \infty} \log\left[\frac{L_1(t)}{L_1(0)}\right] \tag{7}$$

If v represents a vector tangent to the expansive, unstable manifold, Ω_u, at some initial value for $ssds(i)$, then iterating $\Phi^t(ssds(i))$ and averaging its derivative D will yield another estimate of Λ_1:

$$\Lambda_1 = \lim_{t \to \infty} \frac{1}{t} \log \| D\Phi^t(t)(ssds)v \| \tag{8}$$

C. The Capacity Dimension, D_C

On a compact manifold, Ω_m, with (conserved) probability measure, μ, let $B(ssds(i), r)$ denote a ball of radius r about the $ssds(i)$. Then (as in Eq. 4 and attendant discusssion), with ε indicating the cover on m of diameter $\leq \varepsilon$, the dimension of m, dim (m) is equal to D_C, the *capacity dimension*

$$D_C = \lim_{\varepsilon \to 0} \frac{\log \ m(B(ssds), \varepsilon)}{\log \ (\varepsilon)} \tag{9}$$

TABLE 14.4 Means of 10 Controls and 10 Probands: h_T, D_c and Λ_1 and the p values for their one tailed tests of significance

Sensor Pair	h_T	D_c	Λ_1
C16:Controls	0.42	2.31	0.59
Probands	0.36	2.05	0.46
p(1-tail)	0.038	0.069	0.074
T44:Controls	0.37	2.46	0.54
Probands	0.24	2.39	0.49
p(1-tail)	0.06	0.146	0.071
P57:Controls	0.92	2.13	0.64
Probands	0.71	1.82	0.53
p(1-tail)	0.026	0.007	0.085
F14:Controls	0.89	2.31	0.53
Probands	0.80	2.05	0.46
p(1-tail)	0.013	0.014	0.022

More generally, D_C represents the log-log ratio of the rate of the convergence of the measurement to the measure, as the measure $\rightarrow 0$ in an appropriate embedding space.

Table 14.4 summarizes the results of the comparison of Control and Proband groups with respect to two measures reflecting rates of entropy generation, h_T and Λ_1, and the capacity dimension of their support, D_C. These values reflect dynamical creation and expansion in the $\Phi(ssds(i))$ of four paired sensor magnetic fields (Eqs. 4, 6, 7, 8, 9). We compute Λ_1 with an R^3 embedding using the algorithm of Wolf et al (1985), D_C was estimated with an R^4 embedding using the algorithm of Farmer et al (1983). We have described our computations of h_T in previous work. The transition matrices were computed on a six equipartition of the $ssds(i)$ in R^2 (Mandell and Selz, 1997c; Paulus et al., 1990).

The F14 Frontal sensor pair (Figure 14.1A blue) most consistently demonstrated a $p < 0.05$ difference between Controls and Probands in all three measures. These statistically significant differences in the measures of the proband's F14 frontal paired sensor field are consistent with the prominence of the frontal lobe in recent neuropathological research in schizophrenia (Fuster, 1980; Liddle andMorris, 1991; Paea et al., 2004; Roth et al., 2004; Yacubian et al., 2002).

In contrast, the T44 Temporal sensor pair (Figure 14.1A, black) showed no significant difference in any of the three measures. Parietal pair, P57

(Figure 14.1A, green) was $p < 0.05$ in two of the measures, h_T and D_C. The Central pair, C16 (Figure 14.1A, red), showed statistically significant differences in one, h_T. Note that the topological entropy discriminated Controls from Probands in three of the four symmetric pairs of MEG sensor fields. Though these results were certainly promising, a large number of subject's records from both groups (currently on-going) will be required before definitive claims can be made for a decrement in measures of the dynamical entropy in probands, as hypothesized and suggested by the observed differences in h_T, D_c and Λ_1 and *memv* (see below) in this pilot study.

The Measureable Entropy Manifold Volume, *memv*

For smooth system $\Phi^t (ssds(i)) \, \Omega_m \to \Omega_m$ which conserves probability measure, Pesin (Pesin, 1977) proved for Hausdorf-like capacity dimension, D_C, in expansive dynamical systems that

$$h_T[\Phi^t(ssds(i))] = \Lambda_1[\Phi^t(ssds(i))] \bullet D_C[\Phi^t(ssds(i))] \tag{10}$$

It is the multiplicative, aggregate entropic processes which we have conjectured involve the actions of orbital creation, h_T, and spreading composed of separation, Λ_1, of orbits and/or expansion of the dimension of their support, D_C. In Figure 14.7 the heuristic graphs of Control and Proband *memv*s portray logarithmic volumes derived from Cartesian products of the exponential entropy expansion indices, $\Pi[h_T \Lambda_1 D_C]$ = the *measureable entropy manifold volume, memv*, of $\Phi^t(ssds_i)$ (Mandell and Selz, 1997; Manning, 1981; Young, 1982; 1998). As the divergent orbits in the *memv* expansion are reinjected into the dynamical system, $\Phi^t(ssds(i))$, the *memv* increases with time. The entropy volume differences in Figure 14.7, viewed from the perspective of the thermodynamic formalism, is the result of differences in *topological pressure* resulting from an increasing rate of creation of new orbits (Bowen andRuelle, 1975; Eckmann and Ruelle, 1985; Ruelle, 1978). Intuitively the volume of *memv* reflects the amount available of what psychoanalysts have called *psychic energy,* and we think of as *psychic entropy*.

Figure 14.7 portrays the volumes of a three dimensional implicit function representation of *memv* (Gowers et al., 2008), the Cartesian product of the components of the Pesin-Young equality in Eq 10 which generates a three dimensional volume.

$$memv = \Pi \, [h_T \bullet \Lambda_1 \bullet D_C] \tag{11}$$

**REDUCED *MEMV* IN REPRESENTATIVE EYES CLOSED,
RESTING PROBANDS VERSUS CONTROLS (Frontal F14 Pairs)**

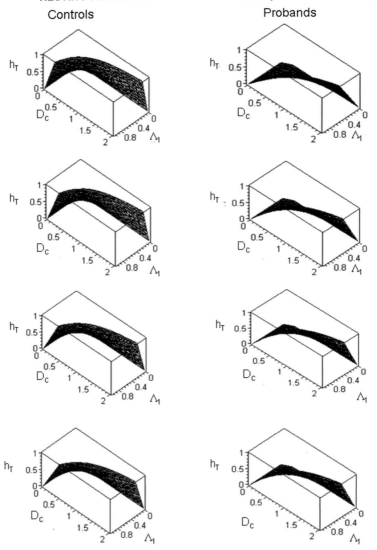

FIGURE 14.7 This figure contain graphs of R³ implicit function representations of
$\Pi[\Lambda_1 D_C h_T] = memv$ computed on the F14 ssds(i) of four Controls and four Probands.
They demonstrate graphically the reduced *memv* in Probands compared with Controls.
Table V summarizes the results for all subjects and the four regions studied which
show ~ 40–50% reductions in entropy volumes in the Probands.

TABLE 14.5 Cartesian products, $\prod[\Lambda_1 D_C h_T] = memv$ in log units by regional sensor pair and the percent differences between Controls and Probands

Sensor pair regions	Control group (10)	Proband group (10)	Percent Differences
C16 "central"	0.572	0.339	↓ 40.7%
P57 "parietal"	1.254	0.685	↓ 45.4%
F14 "frontal"	1.387	0.754	↓ 50.5%
T44 "temporal"	0.484	0.283	↓ 41.4%

Figure 14.7 graphically portrays the lower values of *memv* in a comparison of the F14 frontal sensor pairs' *ssds(i)* in four Control and four Probands subjects. Decreases in orbital creation and spreading is reflected in lower measureable entropy manifold volume, *memv*, yielding a space of reduced possibilities for $\Phi^t(ssds(i))$ in the creation of emergent dynamical structure. In the ergodic theory of dynamical systems, loss of an entropy volume measure (Yomdin, 1987) (roughly analogous to *memv*) occurs concomitant with losses in hyperbolicity (Young, 1982; 1998).

Table 14.5 summarizes the application of Eq. 10 to the four regional sensor pairs in Control and Proband subjects demonstrating the generality across regions of the differences in entropy volumes, *memv*, as portrayed graphically for four F14 records in Figure 14.7. *Memv* is in logarithmic units. the results of the Cartesian products of three exponents.

As noted, the *memv*, an extensive entropy thermodynamic parameter, is reminiscent of one of the main concepts in the architecture of the *thermodynamic formalism* (Ruelle, 1978). Topological pressure (Bowen, 1978) is a quantity which belongs to the thermodynamic formalism, which is itself a generalization of the concepts of statistical physics to the area of ergodic theory of dynamical systems(Walters, 1982). Topological pressure can be seen as a generalization of topological entropy, h_T. The *memv* as an aggregate extensive entropy parameter is even a more general representation of the same intuitive idea: *The volume of the "dynamical entropy box" appears to be shrunken in the Probands relative to the Controls.*

Discussion

We and many others have, for several decades, been concerned with the functional implications of changes in various estimates of the entropy of neurobiological dynamical systems as computed on human brain-relevant time series

(Basar, 1990; Dulawa et al., 1999; Mandell, 1983a; Mandell et al., 1982; Mandell and Selz, 1997 Paulus et al., 1990; Pezard et al., 1996; Russo, 2007; Smotherman et al., 1996; Watanabe et al., 2003). It remained at issue whether the decay of integrative brain function with injury, aging or disorders such as schizophrenia is associated with the more classical, statistical thermodynamic notions of loss of functionality through an entropy *increase* (*memv*)(Benzinger, 1956; Boltzmann, 1964 (1896); Drachman, 2006; Glansdorff and Prigogine, 1971; Hill, 1964) or from spontaneously emergent aberrant dynamical structure eating up the available entropy. This would indicate an information generation and transport abnormality signaled by a *decrease in memv* (Costa et al., 2005; Lipsitz and Goldberger, 1993; Mandell, 1987; Mandell and Shlesinger, 1990; Paulus et al., 1996; Tonga et al., 2003).

Recent studies suggest that the applications of ergodic-statistical measures to quantification of continuous MEG activity are promising (Blank et al., 1993; Fell et al., 2000; Gomez et al., 2008; Hornero et al., 2008; Stam, 2006; Tecchio et al., 2006; van Walsum et al., 2003). For example, in a study of continuous MEG measures during a resting state versus those associated with the completion of three simple arithmetic or verbal mental tasks, it was found that only entropy measures on time dependent sequences of amplitudes were discriminating between tasks. An entropy measure made on MEG amplitude series was significantly higher during short, simple arithmetic and verbal tasks than during the eyes closed, resting condition (Fell J et al., 2000).

Consistent with existing theory and findings of our previous studies of entropic measures in neurobiologically relevant dynamical systems (Mandell et al., 1991a; Mandell, 1987; Mandell et al., 1984; Mandell andSelz, 1993; Mandell andSelz, 1995), we have predicted that the MEG $ssds_i$ from the medicated schizophrenic proband group (secondary to the medication, the underlying pathology or both) would demonstrate a decrease in *memv* compared with matched normal controls (Figure 14.7, Table 14.5). A secondary prediction, based on recent neuropathological findings in schizophrenia, was that the difference in *memv* will be more marked in the proband's frontal than in their central or parietal sensor regions (Fuster, 1980; Liddle andand Morris, 1991; Paea et al., 2004; Roth et al., 2004; Yacubian J et al., 2002). In this pilot study we find that the reduction in *memv* in the Proband group occurs in all four sensor pairs, in the central, parietal, frontal and temporal symmetric sensor difference sequences.

Although we did not find consistent, statistically significant Control-Proband differences in the separate indicators of emergent dynamical structure, power law scaling measure α, helical unwinding number, U, distributional extremal measure k. We should note that the direction of the differences were consistent with our hypothesis. In addition, that characteristic differences in orbital patterns within the dynamics of similar, even equivalent scaling measures, such as α, are known (Cornfield et al., 1982; Katok and Hasselblatt, 1995; Mandell and Selz, 1997 Young, 1998). Our most recent results have been more consistent with a decrease in *strudel* density in the Probands, an issue that remains to be resolved.

The indicators of dynamical entropy generation, h_T, Λ_1 and D_C were more promising with respect to differentiating Probands and Controls in this pilot study. The results of all three measures on the *ssds(i)* from the Frontal, F14 (Figure 14.1, blue), sensor pair were statistically significantly different as were most of the measures in Central, C16 (Figure 14.1, red), and Parietal, P57 (Figure 14.1, green) pairs. Only the Temporal pair, T44 (Figure 14.1, black) failed to reveal statistically significant differences in any of the three measures related to entropy generation. The aggregate entropy volume, the Cartesian product, $memv = \prod[\Lambda_1 D_C h_T]$ showed comparable Control/Proband differences in all four of regional symmetric sensor pairs, a finding in favor of our dynamical entropy decrement hypothesis.

Summary

It remains our conjecture that quantitative measures of emergent dynamical structure as well as the entropy-related indices derived from the ergodic theory of single orbit dynamics (Adler and Weiss, 1967; Weiss, 1995b; Young, 1982) and the thermodynamic formalism (Eckmann and Ruelle, 1985; Ruelle, 1978) applied to the *ssds(i)* of brain magnetic flux fluctuations will discriminate global states of dysfunction from normal states of the human brain. Current work involves extending this pilot study by increasing the number of Probands and Controls by more than ten fold. This, will allow a more definitive examination of the usefulness of the *ssds(i)* derivative of the magnetoencephalography data and the measures on: (1) Their emergent dynamical structure: log-log power spectral scaling exponent α, the *strudels* of *eigenzeits* $W[\Psi_1 (ssds(i))]$, unwinding number, U and kurtosis, k; (2) Indices of dynamical entropy generation: topological entropy h_T, the leading eigenfunction, Λ_1 the capacity dimension, D_C and their Cartesian product, the measureable entropy manifold volume, $memv = \prod[\Lambda_1 D_C h_T]$.

We are developing an quantitative theory of these phenomena using elements of perturbed Josephson junction dynamics (Levi et al., 1977; Owen and Scalapino, 1967), the nonlinear dynamics of the magnetic dynamo problem (Ott et al., 1992) theories of intermittency (Berge, 1984)and the strange (only marginally chaotic) attractors of quasiperiodically driven nonlinear oscillators

(Bondeson et al., 1985; Ding et al., 1989). Topologically, the available orbital "choices" between local and global recurrences seen in the phase portraits suggest a topological manifold of a two holed torus. In numerical simulations, we have observed co-dimension two, parameter sensitive dynamics that demonstrate power spectral scaling, intermittent *strudels* in their *eigenzeits,* increases in the values of the indices of emergent dynamical structure and inverse changes in measures of dynamical entropy (In preparation).

Subjects

Data collection occurred as part of the Clinical Brain Disorders Branch/National Institute of Mental Health Genetic Study of Schizophrenia (National Institutes of Health Study ID NCT00001486). Initial screening required that applicants had to be aged between 18 and 60 years, have a premorbid IQ score greater than 70, and be able to give informed consent. Applicants were disqualified if they had alcohol or drug abuse in the past six months, dependence in the past year, or more than a five-year history of abuse or dependence. Healthy subjects were recruited from the community and through the National Institutes of Health (NIH) Normal Volunteer Office and were screened with an additional criterion that they did not have a first-degree relative with schizophrenia. Schizophrenic outpatients and their siblings were recruited from local and national sources.

All procedures were approved by the National Institute of Mental Health (NIMH) Institutional Review Board. For more details on participant recruitment, evaluation, and potential ascertainment biases, see Egan et al. (2000). In the current study, all subjects were right-handed as determined by the Edinburgh Handedness Questionnaire (Oldfield, 1971). From the data collected under the Sibling Study, we randomly chose ten schizophrenic patients from a pool of thirty-eight from whom we had relatively artifact free MEG resting recordings. We then chose ten healthy control datasets that best matched the age and gender profile of the clinical datasets from the large NIH pool available to us.

Magnetoencephalographic Data Collection

The MEG recordings were carried out in the National Institutes of Mental Health's Core MEG Laboratory in their magnetically shielded room with a whole-head, 275-channel, superconducting quantum interference device (SQUID), radial gradiometer system from VSM MedTech Ltd., makers of CTF MEG Systems Inc. Port Coquitlam, BC, Canada. MEG signals were continuously

recorded using a SQUID sensor array consisting of 275 radial first-order gradi-
ometers uniformly distributed over the inner surface of a whole-head helmet.
Real-time head positions inside the magnetometer were determined by digitiz-
ing the position of reference coils that were attached to the nasion and bilateral
preauricular points of each subject. Thermal and electrical sensor noise and
external power line and room noise were subject to noise cancelation algorithms. (Fife et al., 2002). The three fiducial points were also photographed for
each participant as a means to coregister their MEG signals and their anatomical MRI (3T General Electric MRI scanner) data onto a common coordinate
system. Sensor locations relevant to brain locations used in this study have
been reported elsewhere (Rutter et al., 2009).

Acknowledgments

Appreciation is expressed for helpful discussions with Frank Moss, Michael
Shlesinger, Adi Bulsara, Hal Puthoff, Paul Gailey and Markus "Tino" Procida.
This work was supported, in part, by the Fetzer-Franklin Trust, DARPA
(Microtechnology Office) and Space and Naval Warfare Center Grant # N66001-
09-1-2051.

REFERENCES

Adler, R. J., Feldman, R. E. and Taqque, M. S. (1998). A practical guide to heavy tails;
statistical techniques and applications. Boston: Birkhauser.

Adler, R. L., Konheim, A. G. and McDndrew, M. H. (1965). Topological entropy. *Trans
AMS, 114,* 309–319.

Adler, R., L. and Marcus, B. (1979). Topological entropy and equivalence of dynamical
systems. *Mem. Amer. Math. Soc,* 219, 114–126.

Adler, R. L. and Weiss, B. (1967). Entropy, a complete metric invariant for
automorphisms of the torus. *Proc. Natl. Acad. Sci.,* 57, 1573–1576.

Anninos, P. A., Kokkinidis, M., Hoke, M., Pantev, C., Lehnertz, K. and Lutkenhoner,
B. (1986). MEG measurements with SQUID as a diagnostic tool for epileptic
patients. *Brain Res Bull, 16, 4,* 549–551.

Arnold, V. I. (1983). Geometrical methods in the theory of ordinary differential
equations. NY: Springer-Verlag.

Arnold, V. I. and Avez, A. (1968). *Ergodic problems of classical mechanics.* Reading, MA:
Addison-Wesley.

Barone, A. and G., P. (1982). *Physics and applications of the Josephson effect.* New York:
John Wiley and Sons.

Basar, E. (Ed) (1990). *Chaos in brain function.* Berlin: Spinger.

Basar, E., Flohr, H., Haken, H. and Mandell, A. (Eds) (1983). *Synergetics of Brain*. Berlin: Springer.

Beggs, J. and Plenz, D. (2005). Neuronal avalanches are diverse and precise activity patterns that are stable for many hours in cortical slices. *J. Neuosci, 24*.

Bendler, J., Fontenella, J. and Shlesinger, M. (2004). Sources of exponents. *Physica D, 193*, 67–72.

Benzinger, T. H. (1956). Equations to obtain, for equilibrium reactions, free- energy, heat and entropy changes from two calorimetric measurements. *Proc. Natl. Acad. Sci., 42*, 109–113.

Berge, P., Pomeau, Y. and Vidal, C. (1984). *Order and chaos*, N.Y: John Wiley and Sons.

Biswal, B., Yetkin, F., Haughton, V. and Hyde, J. (1995). Functional connectivity of the motor cortex of resting human brain using echo-planar MRI. *Magn Reson Imaging, 34*, 537–554.

Blank Hr, Frank M and G. M. (1993). Dimension and entropy measures of MEG time series of the alpha rhythm. *Zeitschrift für Physik. B., 91*, 251–22556.

Boltzmann, L. (1964 (1896)). *Lectures in gas theory*. Berkeley (Leipzig): University of California Press (Barth).

Bondeson, A., Ott, E. and Antonsen, T. M. (1985). Quasiperiodically forced damped pendula and Schrodinger equations with quasiperiodic pontetials; implications of their equivalence. *Phys. Rev. Lett, 55*, 2103–2106.

Bowen, R. (1978). On Axiom A diffeomorphisms. CBMS Regional conference series in mathematics. Vol 35. Providence, RI: A.M.S. Publications.

Bowen, R. and Ruelle, D. (1975). The ergodic theory of Axiom A flows. *Invent Math., 29*, 181–202.

Braiman, Y. and Wiesenfeld, K. (1994). Global stabilization of a Josephson-junction array. *Phys Rev B Condens Matter, 49, 21*, 15223–15226.

Broomhead, D. S., Jones, R. and King, G. P. (1987). Addenda and correction. *J Phys. A, 20*, L563–L569.

Broomhead, D. S. and King, G. P. (1986). Extracting qualitative dynamics from experimental data. *Physica D, 20*, 217–236.

Buckner, R. L. and Vincent, J. B. (2007). Unrest at rest; default activation and spontaneous network correlation. *Neuroimage, 37*, 1091–1096.

Bucolo, G., Bucolo, M., Frasca, M., La Rosa, M., Shannnahoff-Khalsa, D. and Sorbello, M. (2003). Spatial modes in magnetoencephography, spatio-temporal evolution. *Proc. IEEE EMBS*, Cancun, Mexico Meeting, 2705–2711.

Burgers, J. (1954). Entropy and disorder. *Br. J. Philos. Sci., 5*, 70–71.

Capek, V. and Sheehan, D. P. (2005). Challenges to the second law of thermodynamics theory and experiment. Dordrecht: Springer.

Chen, Y., Ding, M. and Kelso, J. A. (2003). Task-related power and coherence changes in neuromagnetic activity during visuomotor coordination. *Exp Brain Res, 148, 1*, 105–116.

Chialvo, D. (2004). Critical brain networks. *Physica A, 340*, 756–765.

Clarke, J. (1994). SQUIDS. *Scientific American, 271*, 46.

Clausius, R. (1862). On the application of the theorem of the equivalence of transformations to the internal work of a mass of matter. *Philos. Mag., 24,* 81–97.

Cohen, D. (1972). Magnetoencephalography: detection of the brain's electrical activity with a superconducting magnetometer. *Science, 175, 22,* 664–666.

Conti, F., Neumcke, B., Nonner, W. and Stampfli, R. (1980). Conductance fluctuations from the inactivation process of sodium channels in myelinated nerve fibres. *J Physiol, 308,* 217–239.

Cornfield, I., Fomin, V. and Sinai, Y. (1982). *Ergodic theory.* Berlin: Springer-Verlag.

Cornwell, B. R., Carver, F. W., Coppola, R., Johnson, L., Alvarez, R. and Grillon, C. (2008). Evoked amygdala responses to negative faces revealed by adaptive MEG beamformers. *Brain Res, 1244,* 103–112.

Costa, M., Goldberger, A. L. and Peng, C. K. (2005). Multiscale entropy analysis of biological signals. *Phys Rev E Stat Nonlin Soft Matter Phys, 71, 2 Pt 1,* 021906.

Dalal, S. S., Guggisberg, A. G., Edwards, E., Sekihara, K., Findlay, A. M., Canolty, R. T., Berger, M. S., Knight, R. T., Barbaro, N. M., Kirsch, H. E. and Nagarajan, S. S. (2008). Five-dimensional neuroimaging: localization of the time-frequency dynamics of cortical activity. *Neuroimage, 40, 4,* 1686–1700.

Dalal, S. S., Zumer, J. M., Agrawal, V., Hild, K. E., Sekihara, K. and Nagarajan, S. S. (2004). NUTMEG: a neuromagnetic source reconstruction toolbox. *Neurol Clin Neurophysiol, 2004,* 52.

Dale, A. and Sereno, M. (1993). Improved localization of cortical activity by combining EEG and MEG with MRI surface reconstruction: a linear approach. *J. Cogn. Neurosci, 5,* 162–176.

Damoiseaus, J., Rombouts, S., Brakhof, F., Scheltens, P. and Stam, C. J. (2006). Consistent resting-state networks across healthy subjects. *Proceedings of the Nationall Academy of Science, 103,* 13848–13853.

Darrow, K. K. (1944). The concept of entropy. *Am. J. Phys, 12,* 183–196.

Daubechies, I. (1992). Ten Lectures on Wavelets. Philadelphia: SIAM.

DeFelice, L. J. (1977). Fluctuation analysis in neurobiology. *Int. Rev. Neurobiol, 20,* 169–208.

Dinaburg, E. I. (1971). On the relations among various entropy characteristics of dynamical systems. *Math. USSR-Isv, 5,* 337–378.

Ding, D. C., Grebogi, C. and Ott, E. (1989). Evolution of attractors in quasiperiodically forced systems:from quasiperiod to strange nonchaotic to chaotic. *Phys. Rev. A, 39,* 2593–2598.

Drachman, D. A. (2006). Aging of the brain, entropy and Alzheimer's disease. *Neurology, 67,* 1340–1352.

Dulawa, S. C., Grandy, D. K., Low, M. J., Paulus, M. P. and Geyer, M. A. (1999). Dopamine D4 receptor-knock-out mice exhibit reduced exploration of novel stimuli. *J of Neuroscience, 19, 21,* 9550–9556.

Eckmann, J. P. and Ruelle, D. (1985). Ergodic theory of chaos and strange attractors. *Rev. Mod. Phys., 57,* 617–656.

Egan, M. F., Goldberg, T. E., Gscheidel, T., Weirich, M., Bigelow, L. B. and Weinberger, D. (2000). Relative risk of attention deficits in sibblings of patients with schizophrenica. *Am. J. Psychiat., 157,* 1309–1316.

Farge, M., Hunt, J. C. R. and Vassilicos, J. C. (1993). Wavelets, fractals and Fourier Transforms: Detection and analysis of structure. *In Wavelets, Fractals and Fourier Transforms.* Farge, M., Hunt, J. C. R. and Vassilicos, J. C. (Eds). Oxford: Clarendon Press.

Farmer, J. D., Ott, E. and Yorke, J. (1983). The dimension of chaotic attractors. *Physical, D7,* 153–162.

Fell J, Röschke J, Grözinger M, Hinrichs H and Heinze., H. (2000). Alternations in continuous MEG measures during mental activity. *Neuropsychobio., 42,* 99–106.

Fenichel, O. (1945). Psychoanalytic Theory of Neurosis. NY: Norton.

Fife, A., Vrbe, J. and Coppola, R. 2002. (2002). A 275 channel whole-cortex MEG system. *Proceedings 13th International Conference on Biomagnetism,* 912–915.

Finn, J. M. and Ott, E. (1988). Chaotic flows and magnetic dynanamos. *Phys. Rev. Lett., 60,* 760–763.

Freud, S. (1914/1955). *On Narcissism.* London: Hogarth Press.

Freud, S. (1927). *The Ego and the Id.* London: Hogarth Press.

Friedrich, R., Fuchs, A. and Haken, H. (1989). Synergetic analysis of spatio-temoral EEG patterns. In *Nonlinear Wave Processes in Excitable Media.* (ed. A. Holden). NY: Plenum.

Fuster, J.M. (1980). *The prefrontal cortex.* New York: Raven Press.

Garolera, M., Coppola, R., Munoz, K. E., Elvevag, B., Carver, F. W., Weinberger, D. R. and Goldberg, T. E. (2007). Amygdala activation in affective priming: a magnetoencephalogram study. *Neuroreport, 18, 14,* 1449–1453.

Gaspard, P. and Wang, W.-J. (1988). Sporadicity; Between periodic and chaotic dynamical behaviors. *Proceedings of the Nationall Academy of Science, 85,* 4591–4595.

Geisel, T., Nierwetberg, J. and Zacherl, A. (1985). Acclerated diffusion in Josephson Junctions and related chaotic systems. *Phys. Rev. Lett., 54,* 616–620.

Geschwind, N. (1970). The clinical syndromes of the cortical connections. *Mod Trends Neurol, 5, 0,* 29–40.

Giambra, L. (1989). Task-unrelated-thought frequency as a function of aging:a laboratory study. *Psychology and Aging, 4,* 136–143.

Gilbert, S., Dumontheil, I., Simons, J., Frith, C. D. and Burgess, P. W. (2007). Comment on "wandering minds," default network and "stimulus independent thought". *Science, 317(July 7),* 43b.

Glansdorff, P. and Prigogine, I. (1971). *Thermodynamic Theory of Structure, Stability and Fluctuations.* London: Wiley-Interscience.

Gomez, C., Mediavilla, A., Hornero, R., Abasolo, D. and Fernandez, A. (2008). Use of the Higuchi's fractal dimension for the analysis of MEG recordings from Alzheimer's disease patients. *Med Eng Phys.* Aug 1. 1350–4533.

Gowers, T., Barrow-Green, J. and Imre, L. (Eds.) (2008). *The Princeton Companion to Mathematics.* Princeton, N.J.: Princeton University Press.

Greicius, M. D. and Menon, V. (2004). Default-mode activity during a passive sensory task: uncoupled from deactivation but impacting activation. *J Cogn Neurosci, 16, 9,* 1484–1492.

Greicius, M. D., Srivastava, G., Reiss, A. L. and Menon, V. (2004). Default-mode network activity distinguishes Alzheimer's disease from healthy aging: evidence from functional MRI. *Proceedings of the Nationall Academy of Science,* 101, 13, 4637–4642.

Griecius, M., Krasnow, B., Reese, A. and Menon, V. (2003). Functional connectivity in the resting brain: a network analysis of the default mode hypothesis. *Proceedings of the Nationall Academy of Science,* 100, 253–258.

Grossman, A. and Morlet, J. (1984). Decomposition of Hardy functions into square integrable wavlets of constant shape. *SIAM J. Math. Anal., 15,* 723–736.

Gusnard, D. A. and Raichle, M. E. (2001). Searching for a baseline:functional imaging and the resting human brain. *Nat. Rev. Neurosci., 2,* 685–694.

Haken, H. (1996). *Principles of Brain Function.* Berlin: Springer.

Hamalainen, M., Hari, R., Ilmoniemi, R. J., Knutilla, J. and Lounasamaa, O. V. (1993). Magnetoencephalography-theory, instrumentatioon and application to noninvasive studies of the working human brain. *Rev. Mod. Phys., 65(#2).*

Hill, T. L. (1964). *Thermodynamics of Small Systems.* New York: Benjamin.

Hirata, Y., Judd, K. and Kilminster, D. (2004). Estimating a generating partition from an observed time series; symbolic shadowing. *Phys. Rev. E, 70,* 016215.

Honey, C., Kotter, R., Breakspear, M. and Sporns, O. (2007). Network structure of cerebral cortex shapes functional connectivity on multiple time scales. *ProcEedings Of The Nationall AcadEmy Of SciEnce, 104,* 10240–10245.

Hornero, R., Escudero, J., Fernandez, A., Poza, J. and Gomez, C. (2008). Spectral and nonlinear analyses of MEG background activity in patients with Alzheimer's disease. *IEEE Trans Biomed Eng, 55, 6,* 1658–1665.

Im, C. H., Lee, C., Jung, H. K., Lee, Y. H. and Kuriki, S. (2005). Magnetoencephalography cortical source imaging using spherical mapping. *IEEE Trans Magn, 41,* 1984–1987.

James, W. (1902). *Varieties of religious experience: A study in human nature.* New York: Dover.

Jaynes, E. (1957). Information theory and statistical mechanics. *Phys. Rev., 106,* 120–630.

Jordon, C., Vaughan, D. J. and Norton, D. E. (Eds). (2000). *Memory and Awareness in Anesthesia IV (I-IV).* London: Imperial College Press.

Katok, A. and Hasselblatt, B. (1995). *Introduction to the Modern Theory of Dynamical Systems.* Cambridge: Cambridge University Press.

Kitzbichler, M. G., Smith, M. L., Christensen, S. R. and Bullmore, E. (2009). Broadband criticality of human brain network synchronization. *PLoS Comput Biol, 5,* 3, 1–13.

Kolmogorov, A. N. (1941). The local structure of turbulence in viscous incompressable fluid at very large Reynold's numbers. *Dokl Akad Nauk SSSR, 30,* 301–305.

Kolmogorov, A. N. (1957). General theory of dynamical systems and classical mechanics. *Proc. Internat. Cong. Math.,* 3155–3333.

Kolmogorov, A. N. (1958). A new invariant for transitive dynamical systems. *Dokl. Acad. Nauk. SSSR, 119,* 861–864.

Landberg, D., Scalapino, D. and Taylor, B. N. (1966). The Josephson effects. *Sci Am,* 21, 30–39.

Lee, C., Chang-Hwan, I., Choi, K. and Jung, H.-K. (2007). Estimation of solution accuracy from leadfield matrix in magnetoencephalogrphy. *IEEE Trans Mag., 43,* 1701–1704.

Leff, H. S. (1996). Thermodynamic entropy: the spreading and sharing of energy. *Am. J. Phys, 64,* 1261–1271.

Leffler, J. (1955). The enthalpy-entropy relationship and its implications for organic chemistry. *J Org. Chem, 20,* 1202–1231.

Levi, M., Hoppensteadt, F. and Miranker, W. L. (1977). Dynamics of the Josephson junction. *Quarterly Applied Math, July,* 167–198.

Levina, A., J, H. and Geisel, T. (2007). Dynamical synapses causing self-organized criticality in neural networks. *Nature Physics, 3,* 857–860.

Liddle, P. F. and Morris, D. L. (1991). Schizophrenic syndromes and frontal lobe performance. *Brit. J. Psychiat., 158,* 340–345.

Lipsitz, L. A. and Goldberger, A. L. (1993). Loss of "complexity" and aging: Potential applications of fractals and chaos theory to senescence. *JAMA, 267,* 1806–1809.

Lumry, R. and Rajender, S. (1970). Enthalpy-entropy compensation phenomena in water solutions of proteins and small molecules: a ubiquitous property of water. *Biopolymers, 9, 10,* 1125–1227.

Mandell, A. and Selz, K. A. (1991). Nonthermodyanmic formalism for biological information systems; hierarchical lacunarity in partition size of intermittency. In Self-Organization, Emerging Properties and Learning. Babloyantz, A. (Ed)., New York: Plenum Press. 255–266.

Mandell, A., Selz, K. A. and Shlesinger, M. F. (1991a). Some comments on the weaving of contemporaneous minds. In *Chaos in the Brain,* Duke, D.W. and Pritchard, W.S. (Eds)., Hong Kong: World Scientific Press. 174–190.

Mandell, A. J. (1979). The Sunday syndrome: a unique pattern of amphetamine abuse indigenous to American professional football. *Clin Toxicol, 15, 2,* 225–232.

Mandell, A. J. (1983). From intermittency to transitivity in neuropsychobiological flows. *Am. J. Physiol. (Reg. Integ.Compar. Physiol.), 245, 14,* R484–R494.

Mandell, A. J. (1987). Dynamical complexity and pathological order in the cardiac monitoring problem. *Physica D, 27,* 235–242.

Mandell, A. J., Knapp, S., Ehlers, C. and Russo, P. V. (1984). The stability of constrained randomness: lithium prophylaxis at several neurobiological levels. In *Neurobiology of mood disorders.* Post. R.M. and Ballenger, J.C. (Eds)., Baltimore, Md.: Williams And Wilkins. 744–776.

Mandell, A. J., Russo, P. V. and Knaoo, S. (1982). Strange stability in hierarchically coupled neuropsychobiological systems. In *Synergetics*. Haken, H. (Ed). New York: Springer-Verlag.

Mandell, A. J. and Selz, K. A. (1993). Brain stem neuronal noise and neocortical "resonance". *J. Stat. Physics, 70*, 355–373.

Mandell, A. J. and Selz, K. A. (1995). Nonlinear dynamical patterns as personality theory for neurobiology and psychiatry. *Psychiatry, 58, 4*, 371–390.

Mandell, A. J. and Selz, K. A. (1997). Entropy conservation as h(T) = lyapounov x (capacity) dimension. *Chaos, 7*, 67–81.

Mandell, A. J., Selz, K. A., Owens, M. J. and Shlesinger, M. F. (2003). Broomhead-King hydrophobic modes in receptor-targeted peptide design: how to find modes in short data sequences. In *Unsolved Problems of Noise and Fluctuations*. Bezrukov, S.M. (Ed)., Melville, N.Y.: American Institute of Physics Press. 553–559.

Mandell, A. J., Selz, K. A. and Shlesinger, M. F. (1991). Some comments on the weaving of contemporaneous minds. In *Proceedings of the Conference on Measuring Chaos in the Brain*. Duke, D.W. and Pritchard, W.S. 136–155. Singapore: World Scientific.

Mandell, A. J., Selz, K. A. and Shlesinger, M. F. (1997). Mode matches and their locations in the hydrophobic free energy sequences of peptide ligands and their receptor eigenfunctions. *Proceedings of the Nationall Academy of Science*, 94, 25, 13576–13581.

Mandell, A. J., Selz, K. A. and Shlesinger, M. F. (2000). Predicting peptide-receptor, peptide-protein and chaperone-protein binding using patterns in amino acid hydrophobic free energy sequences. *J Physical Chem. B., 104*, 3953–3959.

Mandell, A. J. and Shlesinger, M. F. (1990). Lost choices; paralellism and topological entropy decrements in neurobiological aging. Washington, D C.: AAAS.

Manning, A. (1981). A relation between Lyapounov exponents, Hausdorff dimension and entropy. *Ergod. Theor. Dyn. Syst., 2*, 451–459.

Monin, A. S. and Yaglom, A. M. (1975). *Statistical Fluid Mechanics; Mechanics of Turbulence; Volume I; Volume II*. Cambridge, Mass.: MIT Press.

Nagarajan, S. S., Attias, H. T., Hild, K. E., 2nd and Sekihara, K. (2006). A graphical model for estimating stimulus-evoked brain responses from magnetoencephalography data with large background brain activity. *Neuroimage, 30, 2*, 400–416.

Nolte, G., Holroyd, T., Carver, F., Coppola, R. and Hallett, M. (2004). Localizing brain interactions from rhythmic EEG/MEG data. *Conf Proc IEEE Eng Med Biol Soc, 2*, 998–1001.

Novikov, A. (1990). The effects of intermittency on statistical characteristics of turbulence and scale similarity of breakdown coeficients. *Phys. Fluids, 2*, 614–620.

Novikov, E., Novikov, A., Shannahoff-Khalsa, D., Schwartz, B. and Wright, J. (1997). Scale-similar activity in the brain. *Phys. Rev. E, 56*, R2387–R2389.

Oldfield, R. C. (1971). The assessment and analysis of handedness: The Edinburgh handedness inventory. *Neuropsychologia, 9,* 97–113.

Ornstein, D. (1989). Ergodic theory, randomness and chaos. *Science, 243,* 182–187.

Ornstein, D. S. (1974). *Ergodic Theory, Randomness and Dynamical Systems.* New Haven: Yale University Press.

Oseledec, V. I. (1968). The multiplicative ergodic theorem: Liapunov characteristic numbers of dynamical systems. *Trans. Moscow Math. Soc., 19,* 197–231.

Ott, E., Du, Y., Sreenivasan, K. R., Juneja, A. and Suri, A. K. (1992). Sing-singular measures: fast magnetic dynamos and high Reynolds-number fluid turbulence. *Phys. Rev. Lett., 69,* 2654–2657.

Owen, C. S. and Scalapino, D. (1967). Vortex structure and critical currents in Josephson junctions. *Phys. Rev., 164,* 538–544.

Paea, C. U., Choe, B. Y., Kima, T. S., Yooc, S. S., Choid, B.-G., Kima, J.-J., Leea, S.-J. I.-H., Paika, I. H. and Lima H.-K. (2004). Neuronal dysfunction of the fontal lobe in schizophrenia. *Neuropsychobiology, 50,* 211–215.

Paulus, M. P., Geyer, M. A. and Braff, D. L. (1996). Use of methods from chaos theory to quantify a fundamental dysfunction in the behavioral organization of schizophrenic patients. *Am J Psychiatry, 153, 5,* 714–717.

Paulus, M. P., Geyer, M. A., Gold, L. H. and Mandell, A. J. (1990). Application of entropy measures derived from the ergodic theory of dynamical systems to rat locomotor behavior. *Proceedings of the National Academy of Science, 87, 2,* 723–727.

Pesin, Y. (1977). Characteristic Lyapounov exponents and smooth ergodic theory. *Russ Math. Surveys, 32,* 55–114.

Pezard, L., Martinerie, J., Muller, J., Varela, F. and Renault, B. (1996). Entropy quantification of human brain spatio-temporal dynamics. *Physica D, 96,* 344–354.

Pope, S. B. (2000). *Turbulent Flows.* Cambridge: Cambridge University Press.

Raichle, M. E., Macleod, A. M., Snyder, A. Z., Powers, W. J., Gusnard D.,Shulman G. L. (2001). A default mode of brain function. *Proceedings of the National. Academy of Science, 98,* 676–672.

Roth, R. M., Flashman, L. A., Saykin, A. J., Mcallister, T. W. and Vidaver, R. (2004). Apathy in schizophrenia: reduced frontal lobe volume and neuropsychological deficits. *Am. J. Psychiat., 161,* 157–159.

Ruelle, D. (1978). *Thermodynamic Formalism.* Reading, Mass.: Addison Wesley.

Russo, O. (2007). Entropy changes in brain function. *Int. J. Psychophys., 64,* 75–80.

Rutter, L., Carver, F. W., Holroyd, T., Nadar, S. R., Mitchell-Francis, J., Apud, J., Weinberger, D. and Coppolla, R. (2009). Magnetoencephalographic gamma powerreduction in patients with schizophrenia duringresting condition. *Hum. Brain Map.,* In Press.

Sarvas, J. (1987). Basic mathematical and electromagnetic concepts of the biomagnetic inverse problem. *Phys. Med. Biol., 32,* 11–22.

Sekihara, K., Abraham-Fuchs, K., Stefan, H. and Hellstrandt, E. (1996). Suppression of background brain activity influence in localizing epileptic spike sources from biomagnetic measurements. *Brain Topogr, 8, 3,* 323–328.

Sekihara, K., Hild, K. E., Dalal, S. S. and Nagarajan, S. S. (2008). Performance of prewhitening beamforming in MEG dual experimental conditions. *IEEE Trans Biomed Eng, 55, 3,* 1112–1121.

Sekihara, K., Hild, K. E. and Nagarajan, S. (2006). A novel adaptive beamformer for MEG source reconstruction when large background brain activities exist. *IEEE Trans Biomed Eng, 53, 9,* 1755–1764.

Sekihara, K., Poeppel, D., Marantz, A., Koizumi, H. and MiyashitA, Y. (1997). Noise covariance incorporated MEG-MUSIC algorithm: a method for multiple-dipole estimation tolerant of the influence of background brain activity. *IEEE Trans Biomed Eng, 44, 9,* 839–847.

Sekihara, K., Sahani, M. and Nagarajan, S. S. (2005). A simple nonparametric statistical thresholding for MEG spatial-filter source reconstruction images. *Neuroimage, 27, 2,* 368–376.

Selz, K. A. and Mandell, A. J. (1991). Bernoulli partition equivalence of intermittent neuronal discharge patterns. *Int. J. Bifurcation and Chaos1:–Bifurcation and Chaos, 1,* 717–722.

Selz, K. A., Mandell, A. J., Anderson, C. C., Smotherman, W. and Teicher, M. (1995). Distribution of local Mandelbrot-Hurst exponents: motor activity in cocaine treated fetal rats and manic depressive patients. *Fractals, 3,* 893–904.

Selz, K. A., Mandell, A. J., Shlesinger, M. F., Arcuragi, V. and Owens, M. J. (2004). Designing human m1 muscarinic receptor-targeted hydrophobic eigenmode matched peptides as functional modulators. *Biophys J, 86, 3,* 1308–1331.

Shannon, C. E. (1948). A mathematical theory of communication. *Bell System Tech J., 1948,* 379–423; 623–656.

Shin, C. W. and Kim, S. (2006). Self-organized criticality and scale free properties in emergent functional neural networks. *Phys. Rev. E, 74,* 045101.

Shlesinger, M. and Klafter, J. A. (1985). Comment on "Accelerated diffusion inJosephson Junctions…". *Phys. Rev. Lett., 54,* 2551.

Sigworth, F. J. (1981). Interpreting power spectra from nonstationary membrane current fluctuations. *Biophys J, 35, 2,* 289–300.

Sinai, Y. (1970). Dynamical systems with countably-multiple Lebesgue spectrum. *Trans AMS, 68,* 34–88.

Singer, J. (1966). *Daydreaming: An Introduction to the experimental study of inner experience.* New York: Random House.

Smale, S. (1967). Differentiable dynamical systems. Bull. *AMS, 73,* 747–817.

Smotherman, W. P., Selz, K. A. and Mandell, A. J. (1996). Dynamical entropy is conserved during cocaine-induced changes in fetal rat motor patterns. *Psychoneuroendocrinology, 21, 2,* 173–187.

Stam, C. J. (2006). *Nonlinear Brain Dynamics.* New York: Nova.

Strang, G. (1993). Wavelet transformation versus Fourier transformation. Bull. *AMS*, *28*, 288–305.

Styer, D. (2000). Insight into entropy. *Am. J. Phys*, *(68)*, 1090–1096.

Tang, C. and Bak, P. (1988). Critical exponents and scaling relations for self-organized critical phenomena. *Phys. Rev. Lett.*, *60*, 2347–2350.

Tecchio, F., Zappasodi, F., Tombini, M., Oliviero, A., Pasqualetti, P., Vernieri, F., Ercolani, M., Pizzella, V. and Rossini, P. M. (2006). Brain plasticity in recovery from stroke: an MEG assessment. *Neuroimage*, *32, 3*, 1326–1334.

Tonga, S., Bezerianosa, A., Malhotraa, A., Yisheng, Z. N. and Thakor, N. (2003). Parameterized entropy analysis of EEG following hypoxic–ischemic brain injury. *Phys. Lett. A*, *314*, 354–361.

Tsallis, C., Gell-Mann, M. and Sato, Y. (2005). Asymptotically scale-invariant occupancy of phase space makes the entropy, S_q, extensive. *Proceedings of theNationalAcademy of Science*, *102*, 15377–15382.

Uutela, K., Hamalainen, M. and Salmelin, R. (1998). Global optimization in the localization of neuromagnetic sources. *IEEE Trans. Biomed. Eng*, *45*, 716–723.

Van Walsum, A. C., Pijnenburg, Y., Berendse, H., Van Dijk, B. D., Knol, D., Scheltens, P. and Stam, C. J. (2003). A neural complexity measure applied to MEG data in Alzheimer's disease. *Clin. Neurophysiol*, *114*, 1034–1040.

Vincent, J., Patel, G., Fox, M., Synder, A., Baker, J. and Raichle, M. E. (2007). Intrinsic functional architecture in the anesthetized monkey brain. *Nature*, *447*, 83–86.

Walters, P. (1982). *An introduction to ergodic theory*. Berlin: Springer.

Watanabe, T. A., Cellucci, C. J., Kohegyi, E., Bashore, T. R., Josiassen, R. C., Greenbaun, N. N. and Rapp, P. E. (2003). The algorithmic complexity of multichannel EEGs is sensitive to changes in behavior. *Psychophysiology*, *40,1*, 77–97.

Weinberg, H., Brickett, P. A., Vrba, J., Fife, A. A. and Burbank, M. B. (1984). The use of a squid third order spatial gradiometer to measure magnetic fields of the brain. *Ann N Y Acad Sci*, *425*, 743–752.

Weiss, B. (1995a). *Single Orbit Dynamics*. Providence, R I: Am. Math. Soc. (Reg. Conf. # 95).

Weiss, B. (1995b). *Single Orbit Dynamics*. Providence, R I: Am. Math. Soc.

Wickerhauser, M. V. (1994). *Adapted Wavelet Analysis from Theory to Software*. Wellesley, Mass.: A.K. Peters.

Wolf, A., Swift, J., Swinney, H. L. And Vastano, J. A. (1985). Determining Lyapounov exponents from a time series. *Physica D*, *16D*, 285–317.

Yacubian, J., De Castro, C.C., Ometto, M., Barbosa, E., D., Camargo, C.P., Tavares, H., Cerri, G.G. and Gattaz, W.F. (2002). 31P-spectroscopy of frontal lobe in schizophrenia: Alterations in phospholipid and high-energy phosphate metabolism. *Schizophr Res*, *58*, 117–122.

Yomdin, Y. (1987). Volume growth and entropy. *Israel J. Math.*, *87*, 285–301.

Young, L.-S. (1982). Dimension, entropy and Lyapounov exponents. *Ergod. Theor. Dyn. Syst.*, *2*, 123–138.

Young, L.-S. (1998). Statistical properties of dynamical systems with some hyperbolicity. *Ann. Math., 147*, 585–650.

Zumer, J. M., Attias, H. T., Sekihara, K. and Nagarajan, S. S. (2007). A probabilistic algorithm integrating source localization and noise suppression for MEG and EEG data. *Neuroimage, 37,* 102–115.

Zumer, J. M., Attias, H. T., Sekihara, K. and Nagarajan, S. S. (2008). Probabilistic algorithms for MEG/EEG source reconstruction using temporal basis functions learned from data. *Neuroimage, 41, 3,* 924–940.

15

Population Variability and Bayesian Inference

Terran Lane

Introduction

Variability is a critical issue in understanding neuroscience data. It appears at all scales, from single-electrode recordings to entire brain imaging scans to entire populations, at time scales ranging from millisecond to years. It is both a friend and an enemy: without some variation, there is no signal to detect, no information to analyze. Too much variation, however, can swamp us with uncertainty and make it hard or impossible to recover the signal we care about.

The purpose of this chapter is to examine variability as a *statistical* and *computational* problem within the field of neuroscience. In so doing, we want to illustrate that we can make some sources of variability—those due to latent or confounding variables—work for us.

Scientists and engineers invest enormous amounts of effort in controlling and minimizing variability: designing experiments to control confounding variables, building instruments to maximize signal-to-noise ratios, and so on. While these efforts have been quite successful, and their practice is key to many advancements in neuroscience, they address only half the story.

At its roots, variability stems from one of three different sources:

1. **Noise:** Data variability stemming from some truly random or effectively unmodelable process, such as

thermal noise, randomness in neural firing rates, or complicated cognitive processes that are only dimly observed in imaging data streams.

2. **Nonstationarity**: Variability due to a change in the system under study over time, such as the effects of learning or adaptation, fatigue, maturation over a longitudinal study, and so on.

3. **Latent variables**: Variability due to a variable that cannot (conveniently) be directly observed, such as the set of diseases that a subject may have, a subject's genetic signature, or idiosyncratic neural connectivity.

Setting aside nonstationarity, there is a tension between noise and latent variables: the first should be suppressed to the extent possible, while the second can be very informative. Latent variables (a.k.a., hidden variables or confounds) express crucial distinctions among populations. We need to incorporate them explicitly into statistical models for two reasons: first, because ignoring them can lead us to draw poor or even erroneous conclusions (e.g., due to Simpson's paradox (Casella and Berger, 1990; Pearl, 2000)); and second, because they help us isolate populations and draw conclusions about the behavior of those populations.

For example, consider the case of inferring the structure of brain activity networks from data drawn from subjects suffering from a mental illness versus healthy controls (Section 2.1). A cartoon example of such a scenario is given in Figure 15.1, which illustrates a hypothetical memory circuit in which (for the healthy population), the amygdala (AM), and hypothalamus (HYP) together mediate the entorhinal cortex (ERC), whose activity in turn mediates the hippocampus (HIP). In the ill population, on the other hand (Figure 15.1b), the normal circuits from HYP → ERC and ERC → HIP are disrupted, and instead AM directly drives both HYP and HIP.

Clearly, we want our models to depend on the "healthy vs. ill" variable (Figure 15.1 a and b) – neglecting this variable by pooling the two populations would yield a single network model that does not tell us anything specific about either population (Figure 15.1c). Indeed, it represents only an "average network" that misleadingly combines behavior from the two populations, while missing facets of each. In Figure 15.1c, for example, the inferred network includes the AM → HYP influence from the ill population and the ERC → HIP from the healthy, while it misses the HYP → ERC and AM → HIP influences. Thus, the average network conflates two populations and ends up representing neither well.

On the surface, this example appears trivial – the first rule of empirical science is to control significant variables. Statistically, this usually means splitting

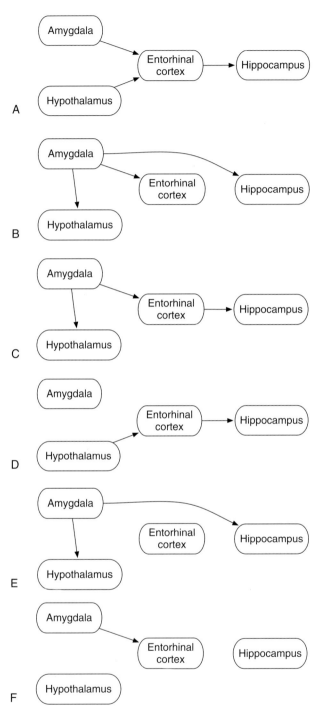

FIGURE 15.1 Cartoon examples of the influence of a latent variable (ill vs. healthy) on inferred brain activity network models Boxes represent activity in different regions of the brain, while arrows represent modulatory connections inferred from functional

FIGURE 15.1 (Continued) imaging data. (a) Network inferred from healthy population data alone. (b) Network inferred from ill population data alone. (c) Network inferred from both populations, collected into a single pool. (d) Healthy-specific network component. (e) Illness-specific network component. (f) Shared network component.

the data into separate pools, corresponding to the states of our independent variable (healthy vs.ill). When the illness state of each subject is known, the data can easily be separated into pools and analysis performed on each pool independently. This example, however, is more complex than first meets the eye.

For one thing, splitting data is expensive and inefficient. When only one variable must be controlled, splitting the total subject set halves the amount of data available for each of two models. If we have to control other variables as well (e.g., drug use, gender, etc.), successively splitting the data leaves us with exponentially small subject sets. After not too many splits, we haven't enough data to parametrize any single model.

Another challenge is that in many cases, we do not know, a priori, to which population a given subject belongs. This is common when dealing with mental illnesses that exhibit closely related symptoms – such as bipolar illness and major depression – or when dealing with commonly comorbid conditions, such as schizophrenia and drug abuse. In such cases, we first have to guess or statistically infer a subject's category before we can even meaningfully partition the data.

A more subtle issue arises as well: simply splitting data does not capture the true complexity of structures like brain activity networks. Splitting subject data into separate pools and developing network models independently for the pools asserts, statistically, that the brain activity networks for the two populations are completely independent – that the presence or absence of a network connection in one population does not give us any information about whether that connection is present or absent in another population.

In practice, however, many (indeed, most) brain activities are common among populations. Thus, even when the disease variable is known, a more detailed analysis will reveal that each edge falls into one of three possible networks: that associated with the healthy population only (Figure 15.1d), that associated with the ill population only (15.1e), and that associated with both (15.1f).

Again, it might seem that the solution is straightforward: infer separate models for the distinct populations and then subtract the models to find the population-specific differences; anything cancelled by the subtraction is shared.

This is a fine procedure and is roughly what is done by a traditional, frequentist hypothesis test. It turns out, however, that this approach is only an approximation to a more rigorous, and more efficient, Bayesian reasoning process.

The real lesson of the toy example of Figure 15.1 is that the system is replete with latent variables. Essentially, every edge is associated with a hidden, trinary variable that indicates whether that edge is associated with the healthy condition, the ill condition, or both. An efficient statistical inference procedure will take advantage of this latent variable structure to work from the combined data pool, dynamically estimating the membership of each network component and drawing on the correct, membership-dependent, subset of data to learn and parametrize that component. While complex, such a simultaneous inference process is well defined in a Bayesian framework. It offers the potential to make the best possible use of data for each network component of the brain, while revealing structures that might be missed by a simple subtractive model.

The goal of this paper is to lay out the Bayesian inferential reasoning framework to carry out such reasoning about condition-dependent brain activity networks. Along the way, we introduce necessary mathematical background on Bayesian inference for latent variable systems and hierarchical models (Section 2). We give, as an examples of such reasoning, our own previous work in network identification (Section 2.1) and an example of hierarchical Bayesian reasoning from the literature (Section 3.1). Finally, we lay out our framework for inferring condition-dependence of network components (Section 4) and give some preliminary results on the necessary reasoning and optimization processes (Section 4.3).

Background: Latent Variables and Hierarchical Models

The prototypical latent variable model is classical point clustering (Mitchell 1997; Hastie et al., 2001; Duda et al., 2001; Bishop, 2006). In this problem, sketched in Figure 15.2, we are given a set of observational data, denoted X, and are asked to assign each point to a cluster, c. The cluster identity of each point is the hidden variable, and the inference problem is to estimate $p(c|X; \theta)$ via Bayes's rule applied to the generative, or forward, model, $p(X|c; \theta)$, where θ is the set of parameters associated with the model. Typically, both θ and c are unknown, so we face a simultaneous inference/estimation problem to identify both the latent variable and parameters. Most commonly, this problem is solved with the Expectation-Maximization (EM) algorithm (Dempster et al., 1977; Moon, 1996; Bishop, 2006).

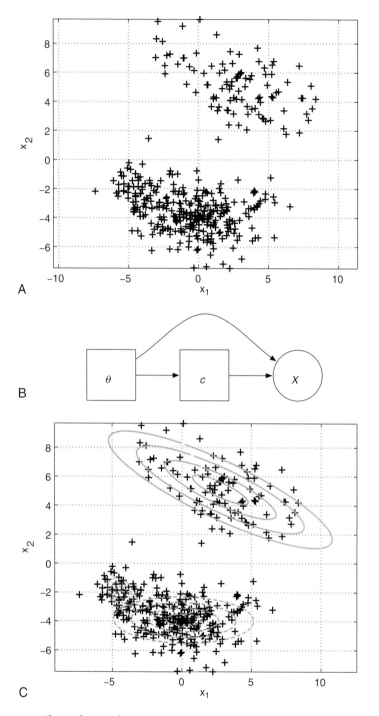

FIGURE 15.2 Classical point clustering in 2 dimensional Euclidean space (a) Example data set (synthetic data): 3-cluster Gaussian mixture model in 2-dimensional real space. (b) Generative model for the clustering data. Circular nodes represent observable variables, while square ones represent hidden variables. Arrows represent

FIGURE 15.2 (Continued) statistical dependencies. (c) Result of clustering inference. Ellipses illustrate the isopotential lines for the different clusters identified by inference on the model of (b); the posterior probability of membership in a given cluster for each point is given by that point's potential with respect to the given cluster.

At a conceptual level, the inference and parameter estimation problem remains the same for more sophisticated latent variable models: the core operations remain:

1. Define the forward probability model that links latent and observable variables,
2. Use Bayes's rule to invert the forward model into an inference model for the latent variable, given observed, and
3. Use EM to simultaneously infer the hidden variable and estimate the system parameters.

The same schematic can be applied to virtually all latent variable inference problems. The straightforwardness of this process, however, belies the complexity of carrying out this agenda in practice for more sophisticated models – the art is in resolving the computational and statistical barriers to implementing this schematic for a given problem.

For example, popular time-series models such as hidden Markov models (Rabiner, 1989; Rabiner and Juang, 1993; Lane and Brodley, 2003) or Kalman filters (Russell and Norvig, 2002) involve multiple, coupled hidden variables (one for each time point, coupled by a Markov chain or a linear-Gaussian dynamical process, respectively). For these models, naive implementation of Bayes's rule would seem to require an exponentially large summation or integral to marginalize over all possible histories. It requires some clever algebra and computational thinking to show that these seemingly intractable forms can be rearranged into polynomial-time operations. Extensions of those insights lead to efficient algorithms for a broad class of multivariate time-series models with high-order hidden- and observable-variable dependencies, known as Dynamic Bayesian Networks (DBNs) (Smyth et al., 1997; Murphy, 2002).

Case Study: Inference of Latent Connectivity Structure

Latent variables need not be restricted to only a single condition (as in the clustering example of Figure 15.2) or a sequence of temporally-chained variables (as in an HMM or DBN). A particularly powerful use of the Bayesian latent variable viewpoint is to infer the *connectivity* or *structure* of a brain activity network.

In this approach, we specify an activity network via a statistical graphical model that defines a probability distribution over observable data (Pearl, 1988; Charniak, 1991; Murphy, 2002; Neapolitan, 2003). These models comprise two parts: a graph structure that defines statistical (in)dependence relations among variables, and a quantitative component that defines the conditional probability relationships among variables in the context of the graph. Figure 15.1 illustrates the structural components of such models, specifying, for example, that region of interest (ROI) HIP is statistically dependent on the ERC ROI, while it is (conditionally) independent of regions AM and HYP (Figure 15.1a). The quantitative component (not shown in Figure 15.1) would determine the exact functional form of the interaction among those three variables, for example, conditional-Gaussian or multinomial.

To identify a network structure from data, we treat the graph structure component itself as a latent variable. That is, we hypothesize that there is some graph that interconnects the regions of the brain, but we cannot image this interconnection directly. We observe the graph only via its effect on observable data, such as blood oxygenation level-dependent (BOLD) response. This effect is represented by the quantitative part of the model and can be treated as a forward model in the sense required by Step 1 from Section 2. Thus, we can follow Steps 2 and 3 to infer the hidden variable, i.e., the graph structure, from the observed data. The details of doing so can be a bit tricky and mathematically dense, but a number of reasonable approaches are well known in the literature (Friedman, 1998; Heckerman, 1999; Friedman and Koller, 2003; Burge and Lane, 2006; Roy et al., 2009). We will return to some of the computational issues of learning such networks in Section 4.

Our research team applied such methods to elicit networks associated with dementia (Burge et al., 2009) and schizophrenia (Kim et al., 2008). Figure 15.3, for example, shows fragments of networks inferred from an archival dementia data set (Buckner et al., 2000). One key finding of this study was the differential activity of the amygdala between demented elderly subjects and healthy elderly control subjects: in the healthy population, the amygdala (AMY) statistically influences only itself, while in the dementia population, the amygdala influences many more regions. This finding agrees with a number of previous behavioral and imaging findings in dementia. A predominant behavioral symptom of dementia is agitation, which includes a high state of anxiety and motor restlessness. The amygdala is central to the perception and expression of anxiety in humans and other primates (Sander et al., 2003), with a diminution of its influence with normal aging (Bauman et al., 2004). The present findings

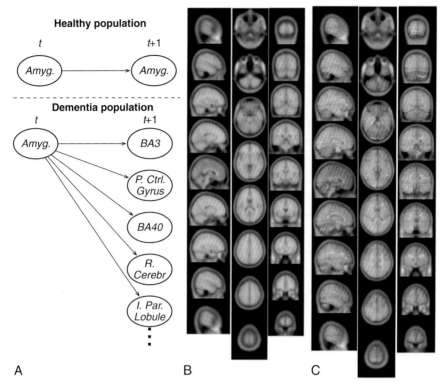

FIGURE 15.3 (a) Fragments of DBN structural models for healthy elderly (top) and demented elderly (bottom) subjects. Circles indicate variables encoding ROI activity and arrows represent statistical dependencies. These temporal models encode the evolution of the activity from time step t to t+1 (columns of variables). (b) Map of ROIs statistically dependent on the amygdala in the healthy population. (c) Map of ROIs statistically dependent on the amygdala in the dementia population.

suggest that the agitation associated with dementia may result from a greater influence of the amygdala.

The drawback to this approach, as posed, is that to find population-specific networks (e.g., schizophrenia-specific networks) requires separating the healthy control and ill test populations' data, building separate network models for each, and then subtracting the networks to find the structural differences between them. This is somewhat unwieldy, given the size of the networks involved (hundreds of nodes), but more critically, as argued in Section 1, it is inefficient of data and is likely to miss important features of networks. We can realize some improvements by adjusting the optimization criterion for inferring networks (Burge and Lane, 2005), but the most rigorous solution is to re-examine the set of latent variables involved in the system, as we shall do in Section 4. First, however, we must introduce the notion of hierarchical Bayesian models.

Hierarchical Models

The model given in Figure 15.2b models only a single, unobservable facet of the data (cluster membership of each data point). Similarly, models like HMMs and Kalman filters posit a single latent variable that influences the observable time series. In many neuroscience data analysis tasks, however, there are many more latent factors that could bear on the data. For example, genetic factors, gender, handedness, age, drug use/abuse, family history: all can factor into the etiology of a mental illness and, therefore, into observable data. Such complex sets of interacting factors create a profusion of potential sub-populations and it is difficult or impossible to model them with single latent variables.

A common approach to handling such complexity is the *hierarchical Bayesian model,* in which a hidden variable influences another hidden variable which, in turn, influences the observable data. For example, a specific genetic allele might influence the development of axonal tracts, which, in turn, influences brain connectivity and observable neuroimaging data. The choice of allele determines populations and the development of specific tracts within that determines sub-populations (perhaps representing the development of mental illness versus not).

In Bayesian terms, we think of such hierarchical relationships as forming a chain of random variables. A similar, though more intricate, inference process to that used in the example of Figure 15.2 is used to infer the layers of latent variables. For example, Blei, Jordan and colleagues have recently demonstrated a hierarchical Bayesian model for clustering with an unknown/non-fixed number of clusters, and they have shown how to use this process to perform document clustering (Blei et al., 2003; Blei et al., 2003). In the neuroscience realm, Stephen et al. have used this form of hierarchical Bayesian reasoning to make inferences about sub-population-based variance in functional neuroimaging studies.

Case Study: Sub-population Inference in Dynamic Causal Models

In the neuroimaging community, a familiar temporal latent-variable model is the Dynamic Causal Model (DCM) (Friston et al., 2003; Friston et al., 2006). DCMs use a set of hidden state variables that represent (average) neural activity in tissue regions. These are coupled to observable data sources, such as BOLD response or magnetodynamics, via forward models such as the balloon model (Friston et al., 2003) or a lead-field matrix-based random process (Sarvas, 1987). The system dynamics are encoded at the hidden variable layer by a linear differential equation model (a first-order Taylor series approximation to a general nonlinear process) given by a connectivity matrix. Task stimulus affects the system via a bilinear modulation of connectivity among the hidden variables (the stimulus-dependent derivative terms in the Taylor expansion). This model is structurally similar to an input-output HMM (IOHMM), albeit a sophisticated one that is carefully designed for the neuroimaging domain.

DCMs can, in principle, be fit to either subject or population data. Attempting to fit a single DCM model to an entire population, however, suffers from trying to incorporate large degrees of data heterogeneity (due to population variability) in a single model. Stephan et al. (2009) therefore propose a hierarchical Bayesian inference model in which a separate DCM is fit to each subject's data and a hierarchical model couples the per-subjects models into a population model.

In this framework, whose generative model is sketched in Figure 15.4, the population is assumed to be divided into one of k "model classes", $c_1,...,c_k$ (analogous to the k clusters of the classical Gaussian mixture model of Figure 15.2). The prior probabilities of the model classes are given by a multinomial distribution parametrised with a vector r: $p(c_i|r) = r_i$. r itself is presumed to be

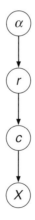

FIGURE 15.4 Example hierarchical Bayesian model for group-level model inference of DCMs (following Stephan, et al. 2009) α_ denotes the hyperparameter of a Dirichlet distribution from which a random vector, r, is drawn.

r is taken to be the parameter of a multinomial distribution that describes the prior distribution of k classes, c. Each class is associated with a single DCM model, DCM(c), that generates observable data X.

drawn from a Dirichlet prior distribution with parameter α. Each model class is associated with a single DCM model structure, which, in turn, generates observable data, X (e.g., fMRI imaging data). The complete "generative pipeline", then, reads: Pick a random vector r according to α. For each subject, pick a category for that subject according to r. For each category, pick a model, c. For each subject, generate imaging data according to the corresponding category model. When run in reverse, via Bayesian inference, this assigns subjects to categories and develops category-specific models.

Stephan et al. use this model to demonstrate that they can differentiate sub-populations in a mixed sample. For example, in a ventral-stream processing task, they examine two DCM structures: one in which intra-hemispheric connections are modulated by a letter-decision task alone, while inter-hemispheric connections are modulated by task and visual field stimulus (c_1), and one in which the modulatory influences are reversed (c_2). They showed that a traditional, frequentist analysis would be inclined toward model c_2, but that this is largely due to a single outlier subject who heavily favors that model. Using the hierarchical Bayesian model of Figure 15.4, they were able to partition the subjects correctly and determine that the majority of the population favors model c_1.

Condition-Specific Network Variability: A Proposal

In this section, we lay out a proposed framework for simultaneous inference of brain activity networks and disease conditions. We focus in particular on *comorbidity*: the simultaneous presence of multiple conditions in a single subject. By conditions, we mean both mental illnesses (such as psychotic spectrum and depression spectrum illnesses, which often co-occur and may present similar delusion or hallucination symptoms (American Psychiatric Association, 2000)) and non-illness confounding factors (such as drug use, genetic variates, gender, family history, etc.). Some such conditions are directly observable, but often (as in the case of differential or joint diagnosis) we need to infer some or all conditions from the observable data. In the context of network analysis (Section 2.1), we are particularly interested in the influence of such condition variables on network structure, as in Figure 15.1.

Specifically, the core analytic problems that we are trying to address here are:

1. **Diagnosis:** Which condition(s) does a given subject have, given observed symptoms and functional neuroimaging data?
2. **Network inference:** Which functional activity networks are present? Which are condition-correlated or condition-differential?

Our approach to all of these problems is fundamentally Bayesian. The generative framework underpinning our proposal is diagrammed in Figure 15.5. We will describe the notation and the model precisely presently, but the high-level overview is:

- A subject has a set of illnesses or conditions, denoted χ in Figure 15.5 (left center), comprising a subset of the possible conditions, $c_1 \ldots c_k$,
- The set of illnesses/conditions influences the brain activity effective connectivity network (N, center),
- The brain network specifies which parameters (θ, right center) are possible. The set of conditions influences the parameters themselves, and
- Together with applied stimulus signal (u), if any, the parameters drive the observed imaging data, X.

Let the set of ROIs be $\mathbf{R} = \{R_i\}_{i=1}^p$. An *effective connectivity network* (or simply brain network) models the local activity relationship among a set of these ROIs. Such a network is defined by two components. First is the set of ROIs

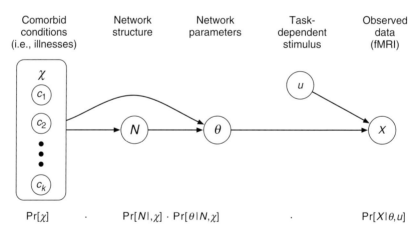

FIGURE 15.5 Generative model underlying our approach to analyzing comorbid conditions As in Figure 15.1, nodes indicate random variables and arrows denote statistical dependency. Unlike Figure 15.1, however, some of the nodes here are not scalar. The $(\chi)_-$ node comprises k "condition bits" (indicated by circles), while the N node comprises a network model (not pictured). The probability terms of the generative model are given beneath the corresponding nodes. Altogether, the model represents the statistical relationship between a set of comorbid conditions (χ_-), an effective connectivity network (N (υ)), a set of network parameters (θ_-), and an observed BOLD signal (X), given an input sensory stimulus (u).

that participate in the network, $N = \{R_i\}_{i \in I} \subseteq \mathbf{R}$, where I is some index set.[1] Examples of such local effective connectivity networks are given in Figure 15.1. For example, in Figure 15.1a, $N_{\mathrm{HIP}} = \{\mathrm{HIP, ERC}\}$, while in 15.1b, $N_{\mathrm{HIP}} = \{\mathrm{HIP, AM}\}$. (Of course, these sets can be larger than two ROIs – they can potentially involve an arbitrary number of ROIs.) The set of all possible such ROI sets will be the power set of $\mathbf{R}$, $\mathcal{N} = 2^{\mathbf{R}}$.

The second component defining a brain network is a *potential function* that describes the functional relationship among the ROIs in the network. For example, if we use Bayesian network framework (Pearl, 1988; Jordan, 1999; Neapolitan, 2003) for modeling networks, then the potentials are given by conditional probability distributions, while in the Markov random field (MRF) framework (Geman and Geman, 1984; Jensen, 2001), the potentials are denormalized joint probability. Regardless of the specific formulation, the local potentials are specified by some set of parameters, which we will denote θ.

A *condition* is a variable that can be either present or absent and that affects the brain's activity and symptoms[2]. Let the set of possible conditions be $\mathbf{C} = \{c_i\}_{i=1}^{k}$ and the power set of $\mathbf{C}$ be denoted $\mathcal{C}$. $\mathbf{C}$ represents all possibly comorbid or co-occurring conditions that we might need to handle. For example, $\mathbf{C}$ might include potentially co-occurring illnesses such as schizophrenia, depression, and substance abuse. The notion of "condition" here is quite general, however, and could include not only illnesses but also, say, different classes of medications that the subject might be currently taking or other potential confounding factors.

$\mathcal{C}$, in turn, represents all possible ways that a single subject could have some combination of these conditions. For example, one subject could have schizophrenia and nicotine addiction while being treated with atypical neuroleptic medication, while a second has both schizophrenia and chronic depression and is unmedicated, and yet a third subject has none of these conditions (i.e., a healthy control). Note that $\mathcal{C}$ is quite large: $|\mathcal{C}| = 2^{|\mathbf{C}|}$. That is, we can

---

[1] Formally, this and the following discussion only describe a single *Markov blanket* (MB) – essentially, the set of influences on a single ROI. For notational simplicity, we will only discuss a single MB in this chapter. There are important issues involved in searching for a complete brain network, involving multiple MBs (Friedman, 1998; Heckerman, 1999; Friedman and Koller, 2003; Burge, 2007), but for this discussion it is sufficient to think about a single MB.

[2] This is, of course, an oversimplification of real diseases, which often have many subtypes and complicated confounds. Fortunately, the Bayesian framework we use is flexible about the types of variables in the model, so in practice we will use multi-valued categorical variables or perhaps even continuous variables to represent the spectrum of some diseases. For this discussion, though, we use the simplest choice – binary variables – for clarity.

think of an element $\chi \in C$ as a k-element bit vector, where each bit tells us the presence or absence of a given condition.

Let $\chi_i \in C$ be a random variable giving the set of conditions that the ith subject has. In general, some of these may be known (e.g., current medications, nicotine use), but many are unknown (e.g., specific illnesses, facets of family history, genetics). For the sake of generality we will assume for the moment that they are all unknown (hidden).

Let X_i be the imaging data for the ith subject. For notational simplicity, we will think of this as fMRI data under a single imaging run. But the techniques we propose are not limited to this setting – in principle, any measurable quantity can be included in X.

Finally, the stimulus presented during the imaging session is denoted u. Both u and X are time series, so the full model will actually be a dynamic Bayesian model, as in Section 2.1. We have omitted the temporal component from Figure 5 and from our notation for simplicity of description, but it remains a key facet of this model.

The model of Figure 15.5 gives a hierarchical generative model for observed neuroimaging data that roots in the set of illnesses or conditions that a subject has. Specifically, it asserts a complete joint distribution over illnesses, network, parameters, and observed data:

$$p(\chi, N, \theta, X) = p(\chi)p(N \mid \chi)p(\theta \mid N, \chi)p(X \mid u, \theta) \tag{1}$$

In principle, with (1) in hand, we can infer anything we wish about the system. For example, we can get the probability of the set of illnesses from the observed data by conditioning on X and marginalizing over N and θ. From there, we can construct a Bayes-optimal classifier for χ via a likelihood ratio test (Fukunaga, 1990; Duda et al., 2001).

In practice, however, this is an aggressively complex model. Making it work in the real world involves both fundamental research and practical engineering and calibration. Here we outline possible approaches to tractable and accurate inference in this model.

Dual Diagnosis of Comorbid Conditions

Our goal here is to infer χ_i from observed data. That is, we wish to estimate $p(\chi_i|X_i)$. A Bayesian estimate integrates over all possible network models and over all possible parameter settings for each network:

$$p(\chi_i \mid X_i) = \frac{1}{Z} p(X_i \mid \chi_i)p(\chi_i)$$

$$= \frac{1}{Z} p(\chi_i) \sum_{n \in \mathcal{N}} \int_\theta p(X_i \mid \theta) p(\theta \mid n, \chi_i) p(n \mid \chi_i) d\theta, \tag{2}$$

where $Z = p(X_i)$ is a normalizing scale factor. (We omit the external stimulus, u, henceforth because it presents no difficulty but clutters notation.)

There are two drawbacks to this basic Bayesian formulation:

1. The integral and sum in (2) are intractable in most real cases (and, therefore, it is also intractable to compute the normalizing factor Z), and
2. The variable χ_i is a k-element bit vector from an exponentially large (in k) space. Thus, representing the full posterior for (or even conditioning on) χ_i is not simple.

There are relatively standard approaches to the first difficulty, including:

- Neglect interactions among comorbid conditions and assume statistical independence (Roy et al., 2009). That is, assume that $p(\chi_i \mid X_i) = \prod_{c_j \in \chi_i} p(c_j \mid X_i)$, which dramatically simplifies the conditionals in (2).
- Approximate the exact integrals by numerical expectations over a sample drawn, for example, via Markov chain Monte Carlo (MCMC) sampling (Gilks, 1995; Schmidt et al, 1999; Bertrand et al., 2001; Friedman and Koller, 2003).
- Directly approximate the posterior of χ_i with a Monte Carlo approach such as particle filters (Doucet et al., 2001; Somersalo et al., 2003; Roy et al., 2006; Murray and Storkey, 2008; Daunizeau et al., 2007).
- Use a variational method to approximate $p(\chi_i|X_i)$ directly, avoiding the need to carry out the integrals (Jordan et al., 1999; Penny et al., 2003; Woolrich et al., 2004; Woolrich and Behrens, 2006).
- Give up on a full Bayesian posterior altogether and seek only a point estimate. For example, maximum a posteriori (MAP) estimates remove the need for Z.
- Further along the previous line, we can take a frequentist point estimate by, for example, taking a maximum likelihood estimate of n and θ and picking the maximizing χ_i given those fixed parameters (Casella and Berger, 1990).

Such techniques are generally well understood and provide us a variety of angles toward solving the first obstacle. The really significant problem presented by (2), however, is the second: dealing with the cardinality of the set of possible condition combinations, $|C|$. Addressing that requires a novel approach to inference.

Fast Approximate Inference for Large State Spaces

Handling the cardinality of $|C|$ is basically a problem of statistical inference in very large state spaces (i.e., exponentially large). Again, there are a few popular approaches to doing so:

- Assume statistical independence among the components of the state (i.e., the bits of χ_i).
- Again, use a sampling approach, such as MCMC, to draw a sample from the posterior of χ, trusting the chain to explore the "important" parts of the exponential space.
- Assume some very compact parametric form for the conditional distributions, $p(n|\chi)$ or $p(\theta|n,\chi)$.

None of these are ideal, however – inference in exponential state spaces remains an open and active area of research in machine learning and statistics.

Independence assumptions allow us to factor the state space and estimate distributions in independent subspaces separately. For example, we can assume that each condition's presence and influence is independent of each other's. This is essentially the assumption made by multivariate linear regression, pairwise correlation-based, and similar models. Such methods have been quite successful, but their assumptions are strong – they neglect population disease correlations and synergistic/epistatic interactions among illnesses, for example.

MCMC methods take an unknown period of time to converge and will still sample only a very small fragment of the state space. And MCMC is unlikely to sample much of the "interesting" structure of the posterior, except for particularly simple distributions (ones in which most of the probability mass of the posterior is concentrated near the mode, for example).

Finally, parametric forms (e.g., Gibbs or maximum entropy distributions), are very effective but dramatically constrain the possible models that can be located. (And, therefore, bias the effort to identify comorbid illnesses.)

We propose a fundamentally new approach to estimating conditional and posterior probability distributions in exponentially large spaces. Recent advances in graph theory (Chung, 1997) and topological methods (Kondor and

Lafferty, 2002; Mahadevan, 2005; Coifman and Maggioni, 2006) provide us a way to perform a direct, empirical estimate of the high-dimensional distribution. Our approach exploits the fact that while it is extremely difficult to represent the *entire*, exponentially large posterior, it is considerably more tractable to measure the posterior for *individual* values of χ. Given a small sample of such empirical posteriors, we use regression techniques to approximate the posterior on all other states of the distribution.

For example, consider the problem of estimating the posterior probability distribution, $p(\chi_i|X)$, over three conditions: schizophrenia, chronic depression, and Asperger's syndrome. That is, $\mathbf{C} = \{S, D, A\}$ and $|C| = 2^3 = 8$ (for all possible combinations of these three conditions). The three conditions are pictured in Figure 15.6a.

We can think of each possible combination of conditions as being a bit vector. In turn, we think of each of these vectors as a node itself in a "meta-graph"': a graph over all condition assignments (Figure 15.6b). The edges of this meta-graph are single bit flips: two nodes (bit strings) are connected in the meta-graph iff they differ by a single bit flip. Thus, the distance between any pair of nodes in the meta-graph is given by the Hamming distance, and the entire meta-graph itself is the Hamming hypercube (Cormen et al., 1990).

Given a fixed data set, X, Equation (2) is function, f, that assigns a non-negative real scalar value to each node of this meta-graph, $f : C \rightarrow \chi$. Thus, our posterior estimation problem reduces to a scalar regression problem on the meta-graph.

Graph theory and graph-based machine learning (Kondor and Lafferty, 2002; Smola and Kondor, 2003; Zhou and Schölkopf, 2004; Corona et al., 2008) provide powerful approaches to estimating scalar functions on graphs from a limited data sample. They work by constructing a regression model of the sample from a linear combination of nonlinear basis functions defined over the whole graph. The graph Laplacian, $\mathcal{L}$, (Mohar, 1991; Chung, 1997) gives us an ideal set of such basis functions.

Briefly, the graph Laplacian is a discrete generalization of the usual Laplacian operator, $\Delta = \partial^2/\partial x^2 + \partial^2/\partial y^2 + \partial^2/\partial z^2$, that is widely used, for example, in the heat and wave equations (Ramo et al., 1994; Kondor and Lafferty, 2002). The graph Laplacian is an extension of the familiar form from Euclidean real space to arbitrary discrete manifolds (such as the meta-graph of Figure 15.2b). It is a second derivative operator, so $f'' = \mathcal{L} f$. Thus its eigenvectors, $\{\phi_i\}_{i=1}^{|C|}$, form a basis for the L_2 space on the graph (the set of smooth, square-integrable functions). The low-order eigenvectors, $\{\phi_i\}_{i=1}^{k}$ ($k = |C|$, corresponding to the k smallest-magnitude eigenvalues) are the most "smooth"

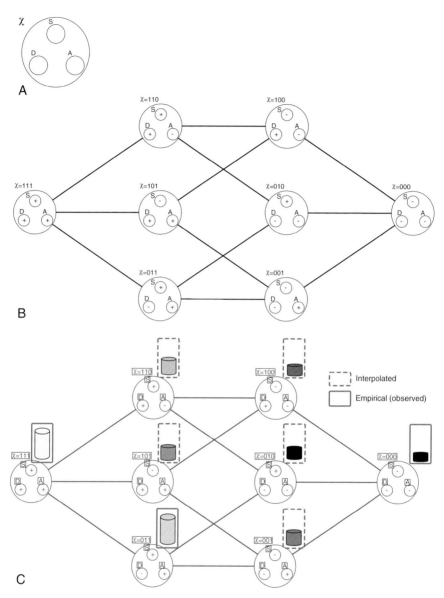

FIGURE I5.6 Sketch of the graph theoretic approach to comorbid condition inference for a simple example of three potential conditions. (a) The set of conditions: S: schizophrenia, D: depression, A: Asperger's syndrome. Altogether, the bits representing the three conditions make up a single instance of the random variable χ_-. (b) The meta-graph over the complete state space of all combinations of presence (+) or absence (–) of each condition. (c) Interpolated posterior probability of condition sets using the Laplacian regression framework. Cylinder heights and grayscale indicate posterior probability for the corresponding condition set. Cylinders outlined in solid indicate directly computed empirical

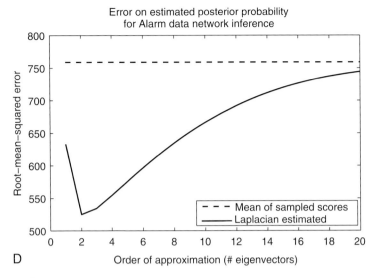

D

FIGURE 15.6 (Continued) posterior probability (_ = 111; 011; or 000); dashed outlines indicate estimated posterior probability using Laplacian interpolation (all other nodes). Total RMSE for this example is _ 6%. (d) Performance of Laplacian estimation on a more challenging posterior estimation problem: posterior probability estimation on the Alarm network. The horizontal axis shows the order of the regression model (number of Laplacian eigenvectors used in the regressor; right is a more complex model); the vertical axis gives RMS estimation error (down is good). The solid line shows that with a small number of eigenvectors and only 1000 samples of the posterior, we can attain a small error on a held-out sample of the network space. Compare to the dashed line, which shows the error of the estimate obtained with a simple average of the same 1000 sampled posterior values.

basis vectors, corresponding to low-frequency components in which most of the signal lives. Conversely, the high-order eigenvectors (corresponding to the largest-magnitude eigenvalues) are the high-frequency, "jagged" basis functions, in which most of the noise lives. Therefore, we can form an effective estimator for f of the form:

$$f \approx \hat{f} = \sum_{i=1}^{k} w_i \phi_i,$$ (3)

where w_i are the weights for the linear model.

The approximator in (3) is a classical general linear model (GLM), however; it is designed to operate on the meta-graph rather than on the real,

Euclidean space. Like the GLM, the optimal w_i are available in closed form via regularized least-squares estimation (Hastie et al., 2001):

$$W = \arg_{\Pi^k} \min \|f - \Phi W \Pi\|^2 + cW^T \Lambda^b W \qquad (4)$$

$$\Rightarrow W = (\Phi^T \Phi + c\Lambda^b)\Phi^T f, \qquad (5)$$

where W is the vector of the k target w_i values, Φ is the rectangular matrix whose columns are the k lowest-order eigenvectors of $\mathcal{L}$ and whose rows correspond to the observed points, Λ is the diagonal matrix of the corresponding eigenvalues, and f is the vector of observations (the evaluations of Equation (2)) at a subset of the nodes of $\mathcal{C}$, given imaging data X). c and b are regularization parameters that control the total smoothness of the final approximator and the relative influence of low- and high-order eigenvectors, respectively.

The important thing about the approximator given in (3) is that its solution in (5) does not require enumeration of the entire meta-graph. So long as individual entries of the eigenvectors can be computed in closed form, (5) requires only $O(k|f|)$ entries to compute and can be solved in $O(k^3)$ time (in the worst case). Fortunately, for regular topologies, such as the Hamming cube, closed forms are available for these eigenvectors (Kondor and Lafferty, 2002; Yackley et al., 2009). Thus, it is possible to estimate complicated functions, like the posterior density, over exponentially large spaces using a bounded amount of computation and data.

The quality of the approximation will depend on the order of the model chosen (k), the number of prototype models used for training (vertices of the meta-graph), and the choice of regularization parameters. The latter can be found using standard techniques such as cross-validation (Hastie et al., 2001; Bishop, 2006). In other, recent work we have shown that the training data sets can be quite small (hundreds to thousands of sampled meta-graph nodes), so long as the sampling is done in keeping with prior beliefs about model space (Anderson and Lane, 2009).

To examine dependence on order of the approximator, we applied this approach to a preliminary problem: estimation of posterior densities for network structure space on the standard Alarm network (Beinlich et al., 1989). This is a thirty-seven-node network inference problem, corresponding to a meta-graph with $2^{\binom{37}{2}} \approx 10^{200}$ nodes. The results are shown in Figure 15.6d, where we see that by sampling only 1000 networks (far fewer than the total number of possibilities), we can achieve a strong estimate of the posterior probability landscape using only two eigenvectors of $\mathcal{L}$.

It remains to assemble the parts: to combine the graph Laplacian-based function estimator of Equations (3)–(5) with the posterior likelihood for the condition-dependent network framework of Equation (2). The result is Algorithm 1. This algorithm begins by sampling the configuration space of possible condition sets ($\mathcal{C}$) in Lines 3–6. It evaluates each of these samples according to Equation (2) using one of the methods mentioned in Section 4.1. It then constructs the eigenvector and value matrices Φ and Λ (Lines 8–13). It is important to note that the full graph Laplacian, $\mathcal{L}$, is never explicitly constructed, nor are the full eigenvalues and eigenvectors. For the special case of the Hamming hypercube that arises here, we can exploit closed form solutions for the eigenvectors and values. Finally, we solve the GLM model using the standard least-squares solution of Equation (5) (Line 14).

While we have been successful with this method on small test cases and benchmark data sets to date (Yackley et al., 2009; Anderson and Lane, 2009), the full implementation for the complexity of neuroscience network data is considerably more complex. We are currently developing the code to implement this method for the system of Equation (2).

Condition-Specific Networks and Population Variability

The careful reader will have noted that we have departed a bit from our planned goal. Rather than estimating condition-specific networks, we have so far only addressed the condition sets themselves. That is, Equation (2) provides us *diagnosis* of conditions, but not assessment of the *network substrates* of those conditions.

Getting to networks, while not precisely simple, at least presents no conceptual challenges beyond those of Section 4.1. While Equation (2) tells us how to infer unknown conditions from known data, in this case we are interested in unknown networks given known data:

$$p(N \mid X) = \frac{1}{Z} \sum_{\chi \in \mathcal{C}} p(\chi) p(N \mid \chi) \int_{\theta} p(\theta \mid N, \chi) p(X \mid \theta) d\theta. \tag{6}$$

This requires marginalization over the exponential space $\mathcal{C}$ rather than function estimation on it. Fortunately, the linear form of our estimator in Equation (3)

Algorithm 1 The Metagraph-Based Posterior Density Estimation Algorithm

1: **Inputs:** subject imaging data X; model order k; number of sample points n; regularization constants c and b.

2: **Outputs:** Model weights $W = \{w_i\}_{i=1}^{k}$

3: **for** $i = 1$ to n **do** // Sample condition configuration space

4: Draw condition configuration $\mathbf{s} \sim p(\chi)$

5: $f_i := p(\chi = \mathbf{s} \,|\, X)$ // Via Equation 2

6: **end for**

7: Let $\mathcal{L}$ be the graph Laplacian of the Hamming hypercube over $|\mathbf{C}|$ conditions (not explicitly represented)

8: **for** $j = 1$ to k **do** // Construct GLM system

9: $\Lambda_{jj} := j^{\text{th}}$ smallest eigenvalue of $\mathcal{L}$

10: **for** $i = 1$ to n **do**

11: $\Phi_{ij} := i^{\text{th}}$ entry of jth eigenvector of $\mathcal{L}$ // Via formulas by Yackley et al., (2009) or Kondor and Lafferty (2002)

12: **end for**

13: **end for**

14: **return** $W := (\Phi^T \Phi + c\Lambda^b)\Phi^T f$ // Regularized least squares solution

15: // Now $p(\chi = \mathbf{s} \,|\, X) \approx \sum_{i=1}^{k} w_i \phi_{is}$ for all $s \in C$

makes this a tractable operation, so we can use the meta-graph estimator again. Further, if we can observe condition data (e.g., gender, age, etc.), then we can seek $p(N \,|\, X, \chi)$ and avoid the outer marginalization in (6) altogether.

Equation (6) gives us much more sophisticated estimation framework than does the first framework we illustrated in Section 2.1. By explicitly modeling condition sets, we can represent and account for the variability in the data due to conditions. Further, this framework supports reasoning about the effects of individual conditions or condition sets, allowing us to identify networks that depend on sets of conditions and to efficiently partition data among networks.

Conclusion

Confounding factors will always pose a practical challenge to science in general, but they are particularly difficult in neuroscience, given the extreme complexity of the system under study. We have argued that traditional controls, while powerful and correct, are constraining and difficult to work with in practice. Ignoring such variables leads to inappropriate averaging of different subpopulations, while controlling them by partitioning the data leads to an exponential decrease in the amount of available data.

In this chapter, we have argued that a different course is available to us: to place the entire system, including confounding variables, into a Bayesian inferential framework. Here we can treat confounds as simply additional variables in a coupled statistical system. When they are unobserved/unobservable, Bayesian inference can be used to estimate not only their values, but their influence on other variables (such as network structures). This yields a seamless estimation framework for the joint system, allowing us to answer questions such as "What brain activity network drives the observable data?", "Which members of the sample population fall into each sub-group?", or "Which activity networks are associated with a given condition (such as a mental illness)?"

While this Bayesian framework is mathematically unified, well principled, and more data -efficient than the traditional, frequentist approach, it is not without its challenges. For one, the Bayesian approach requires us to carefully enumerate our model assumptions and describe the relationships among variables so that we can write down a plausible model. For complicated assumption sets, like those of Sections 3.1 or 4.1, even stating the model precisely can be hard. A larger issue, though, is that many well-posed Bayesian models lead to seemingly intractable inference problems, typically because of a combinatoric explosion of possible system configurations. That challenge has been the subject of intense study for decades in the computer science and statistics communities and powerful methods are available to address some combinatoric challenges. Such methods have already been used to solve some very challenging problems in the analysis of neuroscience data, such as the inference of brain activity networks from functional neuroimaging data.

In this chapter, we have put forward proposals to address new combinatoric problems that arise in the context of analysis of shared and condition-specific networks and the analysis of comorbid conditions. While preliminary results with these methods are quite promising, much work remains to be done to flesh them out and fully validate them. If successful, however, they will provide us a powerful new tool to investigate complex phenomena in neuroscience, at levels not possible today.

REFERENCES

American Psychiatric Association (2000). *Diagnostic and Statistical Manual of Mental Disorders DSM-IV-TR* (4th Edition). American Psychiatric Publishing.

Anderson, B. and T. Lane (2009). Fast Bayesian network structure search using Gaussian processes. Technical Report TR-CS-2009-04, University of New Mexico, Albuquerque.

Bauman, M. D., P. Lavenex, W. A. Mason, J. P. Capitanio, and D. G. Amaral (2004). The development of social behavior following neonatal amygdale lesions in rhesus monkeys. *Journal of Cognitive Neuroscience, 16,* 1388–1411.

Beinlich, I., H. J. Suermondt, R. Chavez, and G. Cooper (1989). The ALARM monitoring system: A case study with two probabilistic inference techniques for belief networks. In *Proceedings of the Second European Conference on Artificial Intelligence in Medicine.*

Bertrand, C., M. Ohmi, R. Suzuki, and H. Kado (2001). A probabilistic solution to the MEG inverse problem via MCMC methods: The reversible jump and parallel tempering algorithms. *IEEE Transactions on Biomedical Engineering 48*(5), 533–542.

Bishop, C. M. (2006). *Pattern Recognition and Machine Learning.* Springer.

Blei, D., T. Griffiths, M. Jordan, and J. Tenenbaum (2003). Hierarchical topic models and the nested Chinese restaurant process. In S. Thrun, L. Saul, and B. Schölkopf (Eds.), *Advances in Neural Information Processing Systems 16* (NIPS 2003), Cambridge, Mass.: MIT Press.

Blei, D., A. Ng, and M. Jordan (2003). Latent Dirichlet allocation. *Journal of Machine Learning Research, 3,* 993–1022.

Buckner, R. L., A. Snyder, A. Sanders, R. Marcus, and J. Morris (2000). Functional brain imaging of young, nondemented, and demented older adults. *Journal of Cognitive Neuroscience, 12*(2), 24–34.

Burge, J. (2007, May). Learning Bayesian Networks from Hierarchically Related Data with a Neuroimaging Application. Ph. D. thesis, University of New Mexico, Albuquerque.

Burge, J. and T. Lane (2005, August). Learning class-discriminative dynamic Bayesian networks. In S. Dzeroski (Ed.), *Proceedings of the Twenty-Second International Conference on Machine Learning* (ICML-2005), Bonn, Germany, 97–104.

Burge, J. and T. Lane (2006, September). Improving Bayesian network structure search with random variable aggregation hierarchies. In J. Fürnkranz, T. Scheffer, and M. Spiliopoulou (Eds.), *Proceedings of the Seventeenth European Conference on Machine Learning* (ECML-2006), Berlin: Springer, 66–77.

Burge, J., T. Lane, H. Link, S. Qiu, and V. P. Clark (2009, January). Bayesian classification of fMRI data: Evidence for altered neural networks in dementia. *Human Brain Mapping 30,* 1, 122–137.

Casella, G. and R. L. Berger (1990). *Statistical Inference.* Pacific Grove, Calif.:Brooks/Cole.

Charniak, E. (1991). Bayesian networks without tears. *AI Magazine 12,* 4, 50–63.

Chung, F. R. K. (1997). *Spectral Graph Theory,* Volume 92 of *CBMS Regional Conference Series in Mathematics.* American Mathematical Society.

Coifman, R. R. and M. Maggioni (2006, July). Diffusion wavelets. *Applied and Computational Harmonic Analysis 21,* 1, 53–94.

Cormen, T. H., C. E. Leiserson, and R. L. Rivest (1990). *Introduction to Algorithms.* Cambridge: MIT Press.

Corona, E., T. Lane, C. Storlie, and J. Neil (2008, June). Using Laplacian methods, RKHS smoothing splines and Bayesian estimation as a framework for regression on graph and graph related domains. Technical Report TR-CS-2008-06, University of New Mexico, Albuquerque.

Daunizeau, J., C. Grova, G. Marrelec, J. Mattout, S. Jbabdi, M. Plgrini-Issac, J. M. Lina, and H. Benali (2007, May). Symmetrical event-related EEG/fMRI information fusion in a variational Bayesian framework. *NeuroImage 36*, 1, 69–87.

Dempster, A. P., N. M. Laird, and D. B. Rubin (1977). Maximum likelihood from incomplete data via the EM algorithm. *Journal of the Royal Statistical Society Series B, 39*, 1–38.

Doucet, A., N. de Freitas, and N. Gordon (Eds.) (2001). *Sequential Monte Carlo Methods in Practice*. Berlin: Springer-Verlag.

Duda, R. O., P. E. Hart, and D. G. Stork (2001). *Pattern Classification* (Second ed.). John Wiley & Sons.

Friedman, N. (1998). The Bayesian structural EM algorithm. In G. F. Cooper and S. Moral (Eds.), *Proceedings of the Fourteenth Conference on Uncertainty in Artificial Intelligence (UAI-98)*, Madison, Wisc.: Morgan Kaufmann.

Friedman, N. and D. Koller (2003, January). Being Bayesian about network structure: A Bayesian approach to structure discovery in Bayesian networks. *Machine Learning 50*, 1–2, 95–125.

Friston, K. J., J. T. Ashburner, S. J. Kiebel, T. E. Nichols, and W. D. Penny (Eds.) (2006). *Statistical Parametric Mapping: The Analysis of Functional Brain Images*. Academic Press.

Friston, K. J., L. Harrison, and W. Penny (2003, August). Dynamic causal modelling. *NeuroImage 19*, 4, 1273–1302.

Fukunaga, K. (1990). *Statistical Pattern Recognition* (2nd Edition). San Diego, CA: Academic Press.

Geman, S. and D. Geman (1984). Stochastic relaxation, Gibbs distributions, and the Bayesian restoration of images. *IEEE Transactions on Pattern Analysis and Machine Intelligence, 6*, 721–741.

Gilks, W. R. (1995, December). *Markov Chain Monte Carlo in Practice*. Chapman & Hall/CRC.

Hastie, T., R. Tibshirani, and J. Friedman (2001). *The Elements of Statistical Learning: Data Mining, Inference, and Prediction*. Springer.

Heckerman, D. (1999). A tutorial on learning with Bayesian networks. In M. Jordan (Ed.), *Learning in Graphical Models*. Cambridge: MIT Press.

Jensen, F. V. (2001). *Bayesian Networks and Decision Graphs*. Springer Verlag.

Jordan, M. I. (Ed.) (1999). *Learning in Graphical Models*. Cambridge: MIT Press.

Jordan, M. I., Z. Ghahramani, T. S. Jaakkola, and L. K. Saul (1999). An introduction to variational methods for graphical models. In M. I. Jordan (Ed.), *Learning in Graphical Models*. Cambridge: MIT Press.

Kim, D. I., J. Burge, T. Lane, K. A. Kiehl, G. D. Pearlson, and V. D. Calhoun (2008). Hybrid ICA-Bayesian network approach reveals distinct effective connectivity differences in schizophrenia. *NeuroImage, 42*, 1560–1568. Appeared online Jun 17, 2008.

Kondor, R. I. and J. Lafferty (2002, July). Diffusion kernels on graphs and other discrete input spaces. In C. Sammut and A. G. Hoffmann (Eds.), *Proceedings of the*

Nineteenth International Conference on Machine Learning (ICML-2002), Sydney, Australia: Morgan Kaufmann.

Lane, T. and C. E. Brodley (2003). An empirical study of two approaches to sequence learning for anomaly detection. *Machine Learning 51*, 1, 73–107.

Mahadevan, S. (2005, July). Representation policy iteration. In Chickering (Ed.), *Proceedings of the Twenty-First Conference on Uncertainty in Artificial Intelligence (UAI-2005)*, Edinburgh, Scotland.

Mitchell, T. M. (1997). *Machine learning.* New York: McGraw-Hill.

Mohar, B. (1991). The Laplacian spectrum of graphs. In Y. Alavi, G. Chartrand, O. Oellermann, and A. Schwenk (Eds.), *Graph Theory, Combinatorics and Applications,* Vol. 2. New York: Wiley, 871–898.

Moon, T. K. (1996, November). The expectation-maximization algorithm. *IEEE Signal Processing Magazine, 13*, 6, 47–59.

Murphy, K. (2002). *Dynamic Bayesian Networks: Representation, Inference and Learning.* Ph. D. thesis, University of California, Berkeley.

Murray, L. and A. Storkey (2008). Continuous time particle filtering for fMRI. In J. C. Platt, D. Koller, Y. Singer, and S. Roweis (Eds.), *Advances in Neural Information Processing Systems, 20*, pp. 1049–1056. Cambridge: MIT Press.

Neapolitan, R. E. (2003). *Learning Bayesian Networks.* Prentice Hall.

Pearl, J. (1988). *Probabilistic Reasoning in Intelligent Systems: Networks of Plausible Inference.* Morgan Kaufmann.

Pearl, J. (2000). *Causality: Models, Reasoning, and Inference.* New York: Cambridge University Press.

Penny,W., S. Kiebela, and K. Friston (2003, July). Variational Bayesian inference for fMRI time series. *Neuroimage, 19*, 3, 727–741.

Rabiner, L. and B. H. Juang (1993). *Fundamentals of Speech Recognition.* Englewood Cliffs, N.J: Prentice Hall.

Rabiner, L. R. (1989, February). A tutorial on hidden Markov models and selected applications in speech recognition. *Proceedings of the IEEE, 77*, 2, 257–286.

Ramo, S., J. R. Whinnery, and T. Van Duzer (1994). *Fields and Waves in Communication Electronics* (3rd Edition). New York: John Wiley & Sons.

Roy, S., T. Lane, C. Allen, A. Aragon, and M. Werner-Washburne (2006, December). A hidden-state Markov model for cell population deconvolution. *Journal of Computational Biology, 13*, 10, 1749–1774.

Roy, S., T. Lane, and M. Werner-Washburne (2009, June). Learning structurally consistent undirected probabilistic graphical models. In *Proceedings of the Twenty-Sixth International Conference on Machine Learning (ICML-2009)*, Montreal, Canada.

Roy, S., T. Lane, M. Werner-Washburne, and D. Martinez (2009, January). Inference of functional networks of condition-specific response: A case study of quiescence in yeast. In *Proc. 2009 Pacific Symposium on Biocomputing (PSB 2009)*, Hawaii.

Russell, S. J. and P. Norvig (2002, December). *Artificial Intelligence: A Modern Approach.* (2nd Edition). Prentice Hall.

Sander, D., J. Grafman, and T. Zalla (2003). The human amygdala: An evolved system for relevance detection. *Rev. Neuroscience, 14,* 303–316.

Sarvas, J. (1987). Basic mathematical and electromagnetic concepts of the biomagnetic inverse problem. *Phys Med Biol, 32,* 1, 11–22.

Schmidt, D. M., J. S. George, and C. C. Wood (1999). Bayesian inference applied to the electromagnetic inverse problem. *Human Brain Mapping, 7,* 195–212.

Smola, A. and R. Kondor (2003, August). Kernels and regularization on graphs. In M. Warmuth and B. Schölkopf (Eds.), *Proc. Sixteenth Annual Conference on Learning Theory,* Washington D.C.: Springer.

Smyth, P., D. Heckerman, and M. Jordan (1997). Probabilistic independence networks for hidden Markov models. *Neural Computation, 9,* 2, 227–269.

Somersalo, E., A. Voutilainen, and J. P. Kaipio (2003). Non-stationary magnetoencephalography by Bayesian filtering of dipole models. *Inverse Problems, 19,* 5, 1047–1063.

Stephan, K. E., W. D. Penny, J. Daunizeau, R. J. Moran, and K. J. Friston (2009, March). Bayesian model selection for group studies. *NeuroImage, 46,* 1004–1017.

Woolrich, M. W. and T. E. Behrens (2006). Variational Bayes inference of spatial mixture models for segmentation. *IEEE Transactions on Medical Imaging, 25,* 10, 1380–1391.

Woolrich, M. W., T. E. J. Behrens, and S. M. Smitha (2004). Constrained linear basis sets for HRF modelling using variational Bayes. *NeuroImage, 21,* 1748–1761.

Yackley, B., E. Corona, and T. Lane (2009). Bayesian network score approximation using a metagraph kernel. In D. Koller, D. Schuurmans, Y. Bengio, and L. Bottou (Eds.), *Advances in Neural Information Processing Systems 21 (NIPS 2008),* 1833–1840.

Zhou, D. and B. Schölkopf. (2004, July). A regularization framework for learning from graph data. In *Statistical Relational Learning and its Connections to Other Fields (SRL 2004),* Alberta, Canada.

Index

Brain activity networks, inferring the
structure of (*cont'd*)
clustering inference, 342–44
comorbidity condition, 349–60
Dynamic Causal Model (DCM), 347–49
estimation of $p\left(\chi_i \mid X_i\right)$, 352–54
in exponentially state spaces, 354–59
general linear model (GLM), 357–59
healthy state *vs* illness state, 339–42
hierarchical model, 347–49
latent variable model, 344–47
posterior probability distribution of
specific conditions, 355–59
Brain injuries, severe
anterior forebrain mesocircuit,
role of, 291
behavioral responsiveness, fluctuations
in, 283
cellular functions, 283
of central thalamus, 282–83
cognitive and motor impairment, 280–81
consciousness disorders, 282–83
cyclical variation in behavioral state, 280
deep brain stimulation (DBS)
study of, 287–91
degree of impaired cognitive
function, 280
disorders of consciousness and
fluctuations of behavioral
responsiveness, 279–83
locked-in state (LIS), 281
minimally conscious state (MCS), 281
neocortical neuronal cell death, 281–82
possible common "circuit-level"
mechanisms, 283–91
progressively severe disability, 282
regional changes, 286
responses to pharmacological and
electrophysiological interventions, 286
thalamocortical projections, 285
Broomhead/King (B/K)
eigenfunction, 307
Brownian motion affecting hair cells in
the auditory system, 52

C
Central pattern generators (CPGs), 105
Chaos
in neuronal network, 140
in nonlinear systems, 146

Chapman-Kolmogorov equations, 7, 18
Chronic depression, 355
"Circuit-level" mechanisms, common,
283–91
Cleaning of a signal, 142
Closed loop network configuration, 106
Cochlear neurons, firing of, 55
Cognitive state process, 5–6
Color discrimination, 219
Colpitts oscillators, 171, 177, 179–80
Coma Recovery Scale Revised (CRS-R),
288, 290
Common spatial patterns (CSP), 216
Competitive games
choice behaviors of rhesus monkeys,
259–63
cortical activity during matching
pennies task, 263–71
reinforcement learning in, 259–63
stochastic behavior, 257–59
Complicated cognitive processes, 339
Condition, notion of, 351
Conditional intensity function, 6
Conditional Lyapunov exponent (CLE),
146, 148–49
Condition-specific networks, 359–60
Confounding factors, 338, 349, 351
Confounding variables, 338
Continuous-valued reaction time
process, 10
Cortical neurons, activity during
competitive games, 263–71
Craniotomy, 96
Cross-validation technique, 358

D
Decision making models, 220–21, 256
Nash equilibrium, 258
of zero-sum games, 259–60
Deep brain stimulation (DBS) study,
of brain injuries, 287–91
Dementia, 345–46
Depression, 341, 349, 351, 355–56
Diagnosis, 349
Dirichlet prior distribution, 349
Discrete linear systems theory, 107
Discrete-time recursive estimation
algorithms, 7–8
Dorsal anterior cingulate cortex (ACCd),
263–71